Cancer Patients and Their Families

D1558322

Cancer Patients and Their Families:

Readings on Disease Course, Coping, and Psychological Interventions

Edited by Richard M. Suinn and Gary R. VandenBos

AMERICAN PSYCHOLOGICAL ASSOCIATION · WASHINGTON, DC

Published by
American Psychological Association
750 First Street, NE
Washington, DC 20002

Copies may be ordered from
APA Order Department
P.O. Box 92984
Washington, DC 20090-2984

In the U.K., Europe, Africa, and the Middle East, copies may be
ordered from
American Psychological Association
3 Henrietta Street
Covent Garden, London
WC2E 8LU England

Typeset in Times Roman by EPS Group Inc., Easton, MD

Printer: Port City Press, Inc., Baltimore, MD
Cover Designer: Naylor Design, Upper Marlboro, MD
Technical/production editor: Jennifer Powers

Library of Congress Cataloging-in-Publication Data
Cancer patients and their families / edited by Richard M. Suinn and
    Gary R. VandenBos.
        p.   cm.
    Includes bibliographical references.
    ISBN 1-55798-641-x (alk. paper)
    1. Cancer—Psychological aspects.   I. Suinn, Richard M.
    II. VandenBos, Gary R.

    RC262.C2914   1999
    362.1'96994—dc21

                                                                99-047782

British Library Cataloguing-in-Publication Data
A CIP record is available from the British Library.

Printed in the United States of America
First Edition

CONTENTS

CONTRIBUTORS

Melissa Alderfer
Barbara L. Andersen
Mary E. Avellone
Jamila Bookwala
Thomas G. Burish
Michael P. Carey
Charles S. Carver
Noel Chavez
Dimitri Christakis
Kimberley C. Clark
Sheldon Cohen
Mary Jo Coiro
Bruce E. Compas
Henry P. David
Christine Dunkel-Schetter
JoAnne E. Epping-Jordan
Roberta L. Falke
Lawrence G. Feinstein
Marian L. Fitzgibbon
Cynthia A. Forsthoff
Ronald Glaser
Kathryn E. Grant
Suzanne D. Harris
Susan M. Heidrich
Vicki S. Helgeson
David C. Howell

Sharon Hudson
Anne E. Kazak
Alfred S. Ketcham
Janice K. Kiecolt-Glaser
Judith E. Knapp
Beth Leedham
Vanessa L. Malcarne
Melvin M. Mark
Thomas J. Meyer
Beth E. Meyerowitz
Gina Mireault
Frederick L. Moffat, Jr.
Anne Moyer
Victoria Noriega
Christina Pozo
Jean Richardson
David S. Robinson
Michael F. Scheier
Richard Schulz
Melinda R. Stolley
Sharon Sugerman
Shelley E. Taylor
Sandra E. Ward
Gail M. Williamson
Nancy L. Worsham

PREFACE

In the United States, a technologically advanced country, cancer patients expect to receive comprehensive care, assuming that they are fortunate to have access to high quality care. However, changes in the organization and financing of U.S. health care can greatly complicate cancer treatment and care—often with the psychological aspects neglected. As a consequence, new scientific advances in cancer care do not always reach people who need them.

Understandably, this concern about adequate and quality care is greatest among patients and their families. Cancer, as an illness, is difficult and complex to manage, is devastating and greatly feared, and is emotionally and financially draining.

A 1999 Institute of Medicine (IOM) report estimates that in 1999, 3% of the U.S. population (some 8 million) will need some form of cancer care. Of this segment, 1.2 million will be newly diagnosed with cancer and will begin treatment. Some, diagnosed in previous years, will continue treatment; others, who have been successfully treated and no longer show evidence of cancer, will still require follow-up; and over 500,000 will die from the disease. In addition, many others in the general population will require some form of cancer screening.

The IOM has determined that many Americans with cancer find a wide gap between optimal care and the care they actually receive. Quality of care is inconsistent across health care systems, health care providers, and insurance companies. For instance, various effectively proven cancer control and treatment strategies, such as regular screening for cervical cancer and mammography in women over 50, are underused. Radical or modified mastectomies are still used for breast cancer instead of less invasive procedures that are equally effective. In addition, physicians often fail to recognize the immediate or long-term psychological effects of cancer and its treatment on patients and their families.

For patients with advanced cancer, health care providers sometimes fail to elicit, understand, and heed patient preferences. Each individual's experience with cancer is unique, depending on the type of cancer, its progression, the patient's socioeconomic status, insurance coverage, geographic location, and cultural beliefs and attitudes. Optimum cancer care involves taking into account all these factors and the psychosocial consequences, not just the biological aspects of the patient's care.

During my tenure as APA president, one initiative I took on and continue to work on is raising public awareness of the major role psychology can play in cancer prevention, research, and treatment. Although I have not treated cancer patients myself, I have seen firsthand the devastating impact of cancer. It became a reality as cancer took hold of greater and greater numbers of people I knew personally: a close family friend, a sister-in-law, a professional colleague, a student—people of all ages and backgrounds. I could see the catastrophe cancer brings when it invades a life and realized how many lives it currently invades and the psychological trauma it leaves. I believe it is important to try to offer solace and hope. But it is of utmost importance to share what psychologists are demonstrating through their research and practice: There are proven ways to enhance quality of life for cancer patients, to reduce their pain and emotional distress, and to help their families.

For at least a decade, research has confirmed the value of psychosocial interventions for controlling asthma, reducing hypertension, helping arthritis patients, and alleviating the disruptions to normal life from chronic disease. Turning to the more serious disorders of cancer, psychologists have demonstrated the effectiveness of psychoeducational group sessions for easing distress and emotional turmoil after diagnosis, strengthening the immune system, controlling pain, improving communications between patients and oncologists, raising patients' self-esteem and optimism, resolving the many problems of daily adjustment, and strengthening family and other support systems.

Research has documented the cost-effectiveness of adjunctive psychological treatment for medical patients. For instance, when psychological interventions are provided prior to surgery, patients spend fewer days in the hospital. One such study estimated savings per patient of more than $12,000. Yet psychosocial interventions are not offered routinely as a component in the overall care of seriously ill cancer patients. Cancer takes away from physicians one of their greatest assets: the ability to communicate confidence, to provide reassurance, and to convey unambiguous answers. Herein lies a crucial role for psychosocial interventions.

Cancer patients have limited access to psychosocial treatment because the public does not know to ask for it. Few are aware of what psychologists can do, and few psychologists are specifically trained in cancer care. When psychologists have expertise in psycho-oncology, their work generally goes unrecognized and unpublicized in our field. As psychologists we have identified ourselves well as mental health professionals, but not clearly enough as primary healthcare professionals. The medical community and the public need to understand the mind–body connection and the benefits of psychosocial interventions. Making this case is one of my major goals, and it should be the concern of all psychologists. Each psychologist should find several ways to educate the public. Psychologists could speak in public forums, inform the news media, include the topic in classroom materials, write articles, brief hospital groups, duplicate and distribute informational brochures (as the APA's Division 29 is doing), and identify and motivate prominent nonpsychologists to make the case. During my presidential year, I initiated a miniconvention on cancer at the APA convention in Boston. The miniconvention sessions focused on state-of-the-art reviews of what psychologists are doing to prevent and treat cancer and on helping individuals and their families cope with the disease.

Equally important as public awareness is the need for more psychologists to develop competence in psycho-oncology. We need training opportunities for psychologists. I urge regional and state psychological organizations and university-based psychology programs to design workshops to train psychologists in this specialty area. The APA Office of Continuing Education hopes to produce an independent study program based on this book, enabling individual psychologists as well as group practices to use the information for self-guided instruction in psycho-oncology. The American Cancer Society (ACS) and the National Cancer Institute (NCI) have contributed tremendously in promoting awareness of the importance of psychosocial interventions in cancer care. The ACS has recently undertaken a study of 100,000 cancer survivors and families and has supported assessments of quality of life among patients in culturally diverse populations.

The NCI has made basic and applied behavioral research a top priority by creating the Division of Cancer Control and Population Sciences in 1998. Psychologists can find research funding within many of the division's branches. Although the NCI funds the bulk of behavioral research on cancer, the U.S. Department of Defense, the ACS, and other National Institutes of Health departments also fund basic and applied behavioral research on cancer. Psychologists should take advantage of these opportunities.

To support training programs in psycho-oncology, we need tested training modules and patient workbooks on cancer treatment and care. Psychosocial programs for cancer patients should be able to assist focused groups on a solution-based approach to emotional issues, teach communication skills, support networking skills, and develop pain management techniques. For example, the APA's Practice Directorate, in collaboration with Blue Cross and Blue Shield of Massachusetts and the Linda Pollin Institute of the Harvard Medical School, has developed a group treatment manual and a psychoeducational workbook for women with primary breast cancer.

The APA is gradually publishing more on psychological aspects of cancer and the care of individuals with cancer. The June 1999 *APA Monitor* was a special issue on Psychology and Cancer. APA Books recently published *Helping Cancer Patients Cope: A Problem-Solving Approach* (1999). This volume, as well as an annotated bibliography on cancer and its consequences and psychological interventions, is now being released. The PsycINFO abstract database has new citations to relevant work on a monthly basis.

An Overview of the Readings

All but one of the chapters contained in this collection of readings were selected from articles appearing in APA published journals in recent years. The intent of this reprint reader is to highlight contributions by psychologists on psychological aspects of cancer. Selection of representative articles was determined, in part, by topic coverage. The five topic areas are (a) conceptualization, (b) coping and adjusting, (c) interventions and outcomes, (d) family dynamics, and (e) disease course.

Chapter 1, by Andersen, Kiecolt-Glaser, and Glaser, introduces a biobehavioral model of adjustment to cancer. Many studies document the deterioration in quality of life of cancer patients. "Quality of life" is a multidimensional construct that includes functional ability (activity), psychological functioning (e.g., mental health), social adjustment, and disease-related and treatment-related symptoms. Adults with long-term stressors experience not only high rates of adjustment difficulties (e.g., syndromal depression) but also important biological effects (e.g., persistent downregulation of elements of the immune system) and adverse health outcomes (e.g., higher rates of respiratory infections). Considering these and other data, Andersen et al. developed a biobehavioral model of adjustment to the stresses of cancer, identifying mechanisms by which psychological and behavioral responses may influence biological processes. They outline health outcomes on the basis of the model and propose strategies for testing the model through experiments using psychological interventions.

In the second section, we bring together four contributions on coping and adjusting to cancer. Such information is valuable in cancer rehabilitation and in developing a further understanding of the determinants of coping and adjustment.

Dunkel-Schetter, Feinstein, Taylor, and Falke investigate the determinants of coping behavior. In their research, they found coping behavior was not related to type of cancer, time since diagnosis, whether a person was currently in treatment, or the specific cancer-related problem (e.g., pain, fear of the future). However, perceptions of the stressfulness of cancer were related to significantly more coping through social support and also through cognitive and behavioral escape–avoidance strategies. More and more, the literature supports the contention that social support is a major help for stress reduction.

Helgeson and Cohen review the effects of three main types of supportive social interactions on psychological adjustment to cancer. Descriptive studies suggest that emotional support is most desired by patients, and correlational studies indicate that it does have the strongest associations with better adjustment. Peer discussion groups aimed at providing emotional support do not appear to be very helpful. Educational groups aimed at providing informational support appear to be only slightly more effective. Parenthetically, other research suggests that centering discussions around emotions can be of value if the emphasis is on problem solving and how to develop appropriate coping skills.

Heidrich, Forsthoff, and Ward look at the role of the self and adjustment. In a cross-sectional study of cancer patients, the authors examine how discrepancies between actual and ideal self-concepts influence adjustment and mediate the effects of disease-related health problems on psychological well-being. For cancer surgery such as mastectomy, or where prostate treatment involves impotence, self-image issues can become dominant psychological concerns.

Carver et al. discuss how the personality dimension of optimism–pessimism affects individuals' behavioral and psychological outcomes in the midst of adversity. The authors study the coping responses and distress levels of a sample of breast cancer patients at various points in their treatment and care. They discuss the role of various coping reactions in the process of adjustment and the mechanisms by which dispositional optimism versus pessimism appear to operate.

The third section of the book turns to interventions and outcomes. Although U.S. cancer incidence and death rates for all racial and ethnic groups have declined, millions of Americans continue to be diagnosed each year and must cope with the disease and with treatment. Accumulating data suggest that psychological interventions are important for reducing emotional distress, enhancing coping, and improving adjustment.

Andersen reviews experimental and quasi-experimental studies of psychological interventions and discusses treatment components and mechanisms, future research directions, and challenges to scientific advance. She notes that the research literature on psychological therapies for cancer patients has had a relatively brief history, but descriptive data documenting the psychologic–behavioral outcomes of cancer have grown rapidly. She discusses the impediments that have resulted in relatively few psychologists having a primary focus on cancer. The lack of attention to and funding of psychological intervention research by federal agencies have constricted the magnitude of clinical psychology's contribution to addressing the cancer problem. Psychological interventions can have a maximum impact on cancer patients, but not until psychologists are successful in advocating for their importance to policymakers and funding agencies.

Meyer and Mark assess the results of treatment-control studies of psychosocial interventions with adult cancer patients using meta-analysis. The focus of their study was on the effects of nonpharmacological interventions intended to improve the quality of life of adults who had been diagnosed with one of the neoplastic diseases. They argue that the cumulative evidence is sufficiently strong with respect to the efficacy of psychosocial interventions on emotional and functional adjustment and on treatment-related and disease-related symptoms. Research is needed to investigate direct comparisons of different treatments, the effects of psychosocial interventions on medical outcomes and survival, the mechanisms whereby psychosocial interventions have effects, ways of increasing the impact of interventions and of decreasing their cost, and ways of improving the acceptability of psychosocial interventions for both medical personnel and patients and ensuring easy accessibility.

Behavioral and psychosocial studies on cancer have focused largely on non-Hispanic Whites, despite the fact that cancer outcomes vary by ethnicity. The U.S. minority population is particularly vulnerable to cancer. The incidence and mortality rates for certain cancers are higher for minorities than for Whites. African Americans are about 30% more likely to die of cancer than Whites; cervical cancer is more than two times higher among Vietnamese women, with Hispanic women being next highest. Meyerowitz, Richardson, Hudson, and Leedham review behavioral and psychosocial studies that consider the relations between ethnicity and cancer-related behaviors, survival, and quality of life. They propose a mediational framework that links ethnicity and cancer outcomes through socioeconomic status, knowledge and attitudes, and access to medical care.

Cancer patients receiving chemotherapy routinely experience a wide range of distressing side effects, including nausea, vomiting, and dysphoria. These symptoms often compromise patients' quality of life and may lead to the decision to postpone or even reject potentially life-saving treatments. Carey and Burish discuss the hypotheses that have been offered to explain the development of such symptoms. They then review the research evidence for the efficacy of five treatments for such symptoms: hypnosis, progressive muscle relaxation training with guided imagery, systematic desensitization, attentional diversion or redirection, and biofeedback. They discuss the implications of this treatment research, paying particular attention to factors associated with treatment outcome, mechanisms of treatment effectiveness, and clinical application-related issues.

The last article on interventions and outcomes is a meta-analytic review of the literature comparing the psychosocial sequelae of newer breast-conserving treatments with mastectomy. Effective breast-conserving surgical techniques for early-stage disease were developed to improve breast cancer patients' quality of life. The psychosocial literature comparing these newer treatments with mastectomy is ambiguous and shows an unexpected lack of substantial benefits. Using meta-analysis, Moyer attempts to clarify the inconsistencies in the findings of 40 studies.

In Section IV we turn our attention to family dynamics. A diagnosis of cancer and its subsequent treatment are sources of considerable psychological stress for patients and their families. In turn, a strong social support system can contribute greatly to the well-being of a cancer patient. Understanding the family dynamics and possible developmental aspects of distress among family members can help in developing ways of preventing breakdown in the family structure.

Research points out that an important first step in studying stressors such as cancer is to document levels of psychological distress and identify individual differences among family members so as to set the stage for subsequent research on the processes that may contribute to distress.

Compas et al. examine markers of psychological distress in cancer patients, spouses, and their children. They assess anxiety/depression and stress response symptoms in adult cancer patients and their family unit to identify family members at risk for psychological maladjustment. They highlight implications for understanding the impact of cancer on the family.

Kazak, Christakis, Alderfer, and Coiro investigate adjustment in 10- to 15-year-old long-term survivors of childhood cancer and their parents at two points 1 year apart. They assess behavioral concerns, parental distress, anxiety, hopelessness, social support, and family functioning; they also consider gender and the presence of learning problems in their investigations. They found that levels of adjustment were near normative levels. However, gender differences were found, with male adolescents reporting low levels of anxiety and hopelessness. Survivors with learning difficulties appeared to be particularly vulnerable with respect to long-term adjustment.

The Fitzgibbon et al. article views family attitudes as the gatekeeper of daily habit patterns, such as food preferences. Some research suggests that there may be a relationship between dietary habits and the etiology of cancer of the colon, stomach, pancreas, and breast. Although controversy exists as to the precise role of diet in cancer prevention, prudence in one's dietary intake is a sensible approach to reducing one's risk to cancer. Fitzgibbon et al. explore changes in dietary behavior, nutrition knowledge, and parental support among inner-city, low-income, Hispanic American families. The authors found that parental support was related to changes in diet, nutrition knowledge, and attendance for both mothers and children. Additional research is needed to document behavioral changes after ethnic-specific interventions and the maintenance of those changes over time.

Finally, the last set of readings focuses on disease course. Disease course, progression, and ultimate survival are generally known to be dependent on initial disease severity, but it is widely debated whether secondary psychological factors also affect cancer progression. Overcoming cancer through mind-over-body techniques has been popularized in the media and in self-help books, but research is lacking in this line of inquiry. The available empirical evidence on the relationship between psychological factors and disease progression in cancer patients is mixed, and generalizations from this research are complicated because of differences in research design and variables being measured across studies.

Some researchers believe that emerging models of psychological stress, emotions, and disease can guide investigations on the relationship between psychological factors and cancer progression. Epping-Jordan, Compas, and Howell examine psychological symptoms, avoidance, and intrusive thoughts in cancer patients as predictors of cancer progression over a period of 1 year. These cancer patients differed in their diagnoses and initial disease-severity ratings. The researchers' longitudinal findings reveal that, after controlling for initial disease parameters and age, avoidance predicted disease status 1 year later, but neither psychological symptoms nor intrusive thoughts and emotions affected disease outcomes.

Schulz et al. examine the link between certain psychosocial factors and cancer mortality. The authors examine the independent effects on mortality of pessimism, optimism, and depression. They found that a pessimistic life orientation is an important risk factor for mortality, but only among younger patients. Replicating this finding using conceptually related constructs such as depression or optimism did not result in significant associations for either younger or older patients. The research findings lead the authors to believe that negative expectations about the future may contribute to cancer mortality in unique ways. They conclude that attempts to link psychosocial factors to cancer mortality should focus on specific psychological constructs instead of diffuse, global measures that cover many psychological phenomena. They think that the role of psychological processes in cancer mortality may vary dramatically depending on age.

The final chapter, by Henry David, is an interesting case study that illustrates how some of the ideas discussed in the previous chapters apply to an actual cancer case. Based on his understanding of the dynamics of psycho-oncology, David, a social psychologist, documents his personal experience as a victim of a rare and aggressive skin cancer. He discusses the psychological impact the cancer had on him; analyzes the psychological mechanisms he relied on for coping, adaptation, and assertive participation in his treatment; and reflects on how his successful confrontation with cancer led to his emotional growth. In documenting his illness, treatment, and recovery, he hopes his story will help others to "alleviate the terrifying sense of helplessness that can accompany diagnosis with a deadly disease."

This selection of readings is intended to introduce the reader to the psychosocial research on psychology and cancer. We hope it will motivate some psychologists to develop expertise in psycho-oncology, a vital area in health care where psychology can make significant contributions—an area with considerable potential for clinical work, research, and funding support. At the minimum, it will serve as a major resource for many who would become better informed about this crucial area of health care.

Richard M. Suinn, PhD
1999 APA President

Part I

Biobehavioral Model

Chapter 1
A BIOBEHAVIORAL MODEL OF CANCER STRESS AND DISEASE COURSE

Barbara L. Andersen, Janice K. Kiecolt-Glaser, and Ronald Glaser

Cancer is a major health problem, accounting for 23% of all deaths in the United States. Although death rates from heart diseases, stroke, and other conditions have been decreasing, deaths due to cancer have risen 20% in the past 30 years (American Cancer Society [ACS], 1993). This "big picture" holds for the major sites of disease, including lung, breast, and prostate cancer, for which death rates have shown large increases. The number-one killer, lung cancer, has shown huge increases in age-adjusted death rates in the past 30 years—an increase of 121% for men and 415% for women. The second most common site of cancer for men, prostate, has shown a 12% increase in the death rate. For women, breast cancer accounts for 32% of all new cases. During this decade alone, more than 1.5 million women (1 in 9) will be diagnosed and 30% of these women will die from the disease. Other sobering statistics indicate that since 1980 there has been a 24% increase in breast cancer incidence; despite major clinical studies (including trials of dramatic treatments, e.g., bone marrow transplantation), breast cancer mortality rates have been stable for the past 20 years. In sum, increasing numbers of individuals are being diagnosed, undergo difficult therapies, and somehow cope with 5-year relative survival rates of 53% for White Americans and 38% for Black Americans (ACS, 1993).

Although there are notable exceptions (e.g., Bard & Sutherland, 1952; Fox, 1976), research programs conducted by psychologists on the behavioral and psychological aspects of cancer did not begin in earnest until the late 1970s. Yet considerable advances have been made in describing the difficulties cancer patients face and examining the processes of adjustment (see discussions in Andersen, 1989; *Cancer*, 1991, Vol. 67, No. 3 Supplement). Much of the psychological research in cancer rehabilitation has been aimed toward preventing or reducing the psychological and behavioral burdens and improving quality of life. Although there are differing definitions, the term *quality of life* is a multidimensional construct that includes functional ability (activity), psychological functioning (e.g., mental health), social adjustment, and disease- and treatment-related symptoms. Thus, psychologists who study oncology focus on behavioral outcomes, as has been advocated (e.g., Kaplan, 1990).

A Biobehavioral Model

Several recent review articles, both qualitative (Kiecolt-Glaser & Glaser, 1988b; O'Leary, 1990; Weiss, 1992) and quantitative (Herbert & Cohen, 1993a, 1993b),

Reprinted from *American Psychologist, 49*(5), 389–404 (1994). Copyright © 1994 by the American Psychological Association. Used with permission of the author.

Robert M. Kaplan served as action editor for this article.

We thank John T. Cacioppo and the reviewers for helpful comments.

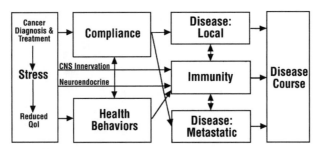

Figure 1. A biobehavioral model of the psychological (stress and quality of life), behavioral (compliance and health behaviors), and biologic pathways from cancer stressors to disease course. CNS = central nervous system.

have concluded that psychological distress and stressors (i.e., negative life events, both acute and chronic) are reliably associated with changes, that is, downregulation, in immunity.[1] Considering these and other data, we offer a biobehavioral model, shown in Figure 1, of adjustment to the stresses of cancer and propose mechanisms by which psychological and behavioral responses may influence biological processes and, perhaps, health outcomes. For simplicity, many paths move in one causal direction. We discuss, in turn, each component and pathway in the model.

The Cancer Stressor and Psychological Pathways

A cancer diagnosis and cancer treatments are objective, negative events. Although negative events do not always produce stress and an altered quality of life, data from many studies document severe emotional distress accompanying these cancer-related events. Several years ago, we studied gynecologic cancer patients within days of their diagnosis and prior to treatment (Andersen, Anderson, & deProsse, 1989a). Using the Profile of Mood States (POMS; McNair, Lorr, & Droppleman, 1981), we found that the scores for women with cancer were significantly greater than scores from matched women who were awaiting treatment for benign gynecologic diagnoses, which in turn were higher than the stresses of everyday life reported by a matched group of healthy women. These data underscore the acute stress of a life-threatening diagnosis. However, it is also clear that lengthy cancer treatments and the disruptions in major life areas that subsequently occur can produce chronic stress. For example, in a study of 60 male survivors of Hodgkin's disease, long after treatment had ended, men reported lower motivation for interpersonal intimacy, increased avoidant thinking about the illness (which is a characteristic of posttraumatic stress), illness-related concerns, and difficulty in returning to predisease employment status (Cella & Tross, 1986). Also, the majority of the patients (57%) reported low levels of physical stamina (Yellen, Cella, & Bonomi, 1993). Other permanent sequelae from cancer treatments, such as sexual problems or sterility (e.g., Kaplan, 1992), which have ramifications for intimate relationships and social support, are well documented

---

[1] Stress-associated changes in immune function occur as a result of the physiological changes that take place (i.e., alterations in levels of hormone and neuropeptides). These changes ultimately affect different aspects of immune function.

Table 1—*5-Year Survival Rates in Percentage for Selected Cancer Sites*

Site	Extent of disease at diagnosis		
	Localized	Regional	Distant
Esophagus	22	7	1
Lung	47	14	1
Female breast	94	74	19
Cervix	90	53	13
Ovary	89	36	17
Prostate	93	83	29

Note. Adapted from Boring, Squires, Tong, and Montgomery (1994).

(see Andersen, 1986, for a review). Unemployment, underemployment, job discrimination, and difficulty in obtaining health insurance can be problems for a substantial minority (e.g., 40% of bone marrow transplant survivors reported difficulty in obtaining insurance; Winegard, Curbow, Baker, & Piantadosi, 1991). Thus, many chronic stressors (e.g., continued emotional distress, disrupted life tasks, social and interpersonal turmoil, and fatigue and low energy) can occur with cancer.

We have considered the qualities of stressors that not only cause distress and a lowered quality of life, but that are also powerful enough to produce biological changes. Some of the effects may covary with the extent of the disease (which usually necessitates more radical treatment).[2] Considering psychological factors, Herbert and Cohen's (1993b) recent meta-analysis of the stress and immunity literature provides clarification. Their comparison of objective stressful events, such as bereavement, divorce, or caregiver stress, with self-reports of stress, such as reports of hassles, life events, or perceived stress, revealed that greater immune alteration (e.g., lower natural killer [NK] cell activity) occurred with objective events. Furthermore, analyses of stressor duration showed that long-term naturalistic stressors (e.g., be-

---

[2]The extent of disease or staging refers to the assignment of cancers to an appropriate category or stage according to their apparent local, regional, and distant anatomic extent. Stage groups are provided for cancers of similar anatomic sites, and prognosis is closely related to stage. Staging is a convenient means of communication, allowing easy identification of cancers of similar extent and prognostic importance. Staging also provides a logical means of selecting treatment options. There are several systems for cancer staging. The simplest one divides cancers into three categories. *Localized* indicates that the cancer is confined to the organ of origin (e.g., the cervix, the ovary, the breast, the prostate). *Regional* connotes that a spread beyond the organ of origin has occurred (e.g., to lymph nodes from the breast, to the seminal vesicles from the prostate), but not to distant sites. Regional spread may have occurred by direct growth to adjacent organs or tissues (e.g., from the ovary to the Fallopian tubes), by metastasis to regional lymph nodes, or by spread to both regional tissues and lymph nodes. *Distant spread* means that there is metastatic disease to locations distant from the organ of origin (e.g., from the ovaries to the lungs, from the prostate to the bone, from the larynx to the brain). Another staging system uses Roman numerals, and that system generally uses Stage I and II for localized diagnoses, Stage III for regional, and Stage IV for distant (metastatic) disease. As indicated, survival is closely related to stage of disease at diagnosis. As a rule of thumb, survival rates drop by approximately 50% when moving from one successive stage to another. Obvious exceptions are the more deadly forms of cancer, such as lung or pancreatic, which have dismal survival rates even when the disease is localized. The most common type of survival estimates are those for five years from diagnosis—that is, the percentage of individuals diagnosed with the specific site or stage of disease who will be alive five years following diagnosis and treatment. For illustration, Table 1 provides survival rates for common tumors.

reavement) may have a more substantial impact on NK cell function than do short-term stressors. Also, when events have interpersonal components, they too are related to greater immune alteration than are nonsocial events. The specific immune alterations that were sensitive to these stressor characteristics were NK cell activity, the helper:suppressor ratio, and the percentage of suppressor/cytotoxic T cells. Considering the objective, acutely stressful events of diagnosis and treatment and the chronic and interpersonally disruptive aspects of cancer recovery and survivorship described above, it would appear that cancer as a stressor includes the attributes that have documented linkages to immunity. Lowered NK cell activity may represent one of the more reliable markers of this process.

Behavioral Pathways

Health Behaviors

Evidence suggests that there are health behavior sequelae for individuals experiencing psychological stress from cancer (the arrow from stress to health behaviors in Figure 1). Distressed individuals often have appetite disturbances that are manifested by eating less often or eating meals of lower nutritional value. For example, in a survey of 800 cancer patients being cared for at home, 38% reported regular problems with a loss of appetite, which they reported as unrelated to other problems they were having, such as nausea or vomiting (Wellisch, Wolcott, Pasnau, Fawzy, & Landsverk, 1989). Individuals who are depressed, anxious, or both are also more likely to self-medicate with alcohol and other drugs; alcohol abuse can potentiate distress (Grunberg & Baum, 1985). Distressed individuals often report sleep disturbances, such as early morning awakening, sleep onset insomnia, or middle-night insomnia (Lacks & Morin, 1992). In a study of long-term survivors of Hodgkin's disease, 27% of the sample reported continuing sleep problems (Cella & Tross, 1986). Cigarette smoking and caffeine use, which often increase during periods of stress, can intensify the physiologic effects of psychosocial stress, such as increasing catecholamine release (Dews, 1984; Lane & Williams, 1985). In sum, poor health behaviors may potentiate the effects of stress, and their co-occurrence for the cancer patient may add psychological and biological burdens.

Cancer stressors may influence the initiation or frequency of positive health behaviors. Exercise is one important example, as reliable associations have been found between mental health and physical activity, and exercise can be an important primary or adjunctive therapy for mood disorders, including anxiety- and depression-related problems (Dubbert, 1992; LaPorte, Montoye, & Caspersen, 1985). To the extent that cancer patients engage in sufficient, regular exercise to secure these benefits, the psychologic effects of stressors may be lowered. In fact, positive mood effects as well as increased functional capacity have been found for breast cancer patients receiving chemotherapy and participating in a program of aerobic interval training (MacVicar, Winningham, & Nickel, 1989). Even so, exercise initiation and maintenance is difficult to achieve, even among young and healthy persons (Sallis et al., 1986), and so it may be more difficult for cancer patients, who as a group are older, symptomatic from the disease or treatments, and distressed. Also, the high frequency of other problems, particularly fatigue (Pickard-Holley, 1991; Rhodes,

Watson, & Hanson, 1988), may make it difficult to mobilize oneself to engage in positive health behaviors.

The contribution of stress to the alteration of health behaviors is made more complex by the direct effect that cancer treatments may have on some behaviors. For example, sensory changes may occur with radiation therapy (Smith, Blumsach, & Bilek, 1985) or chemotherapy (Bernstein, 1986), but they may occur at other times as well (Andrykowski & Otis, 1990). In turn, changes in eating patterns are well documented, with disruption and weight loss associated with learned taste aversions and changes in taste or smell acuity, as well as anorexia. Frequent clinical abnormalities that affect nutritional habits include elevated thresholds for sweet and salty tastes and lowered thresholds for bitter taste. The pathophysiology of weight loss, in particular, is not entirely understood but may be explained in part by the direct and interactive effects of energy balance and altered carbohydrate or protein metabolism (DeWys, 1982, 1985) from learning processes (Bernstein, 1986) as well as disease processes.

In the study of stress-immunity relationships, health behaviors as noted here are not always assessed, even though they may account for variance in immune function. We usually do not find that group differences in health behaviors between stressed and nonstressed samples are reliably related to immunological data in noncancer samples, including medical students (e.g., Kiecolt-Glaser, Garner, Speicher, Penn, & Glaser, 1984), divorced adults (e.g., Kiecolt-Glaser, Fisher, et al., 1987), and Alzheimer's disease caregivers (e.g., Kiecolt-Glaser, Glaser, Dyer, et al., 1987); this may be due in part to stringent health-screening criteria to control or rule out such factors at intake. In cancer studies, the omission of health–behavior variables has been unfortunate at times, as health–behavior mechanisms or compliance have been offered post hoc for some of the most notable findings (e.g., Spiegel, Bloom, Kraemer, & Gottheil, 1989).

Accumulating evidence exists for the direct effect of health behaviors on immunity (see arrow from health behaviors to immunity in Figure 1). The covariation of immunity and objective measures of sleep (Irwin, Smith, & Gillin, 1992), alcohol intake (MacGregor, 1986), smoking (Holt, 1987), and drug use (Friedman, Klein, & Specter, 1991) has been found. Moreover, problematic health behaviors can interact to further affect immunity. For example, substance abuse has direct effects on immunity (Jaffe, 1980), as well as indirect effects through alterations in nutrition (Chandra & Newberne, 1977). Poor nutrition is associated with a variety of immunological impairments, including cell-mediated immunity, phagocyte function, and mucosal immunity (Chandra & Newberne, 1977). In contrast, there is growing evidence that physical activity may also have positive immunological and endocrinological consequences, even among individuals with chronic diseases. For example, LaPerriere et al. (1990) showed a relationship between more positive immune responses and exercise and fitness in HIV-infected men. Thus, we posit that health behaviors are one plausible mechanism by which stress influences immune parameters.

Compliance

A second important behavioral pathway is (non)compliance. Data suggest that psychological or behavioral effects of cancer treatments can be so disruptive that patients become discouraged and fail to complete, or even refuse, treatment (see the arrow from stress to compliance in Figure 1). Noncompliance is a general health problem that crosses disease, treatment, and individual patient characteristics (e.g., Haynes, Taylor, & Sackett, 1979). It has, however, received relatively little research attention in cancer studies despite the potential of dramatic, negative consequences. Among the broader implications is the invalidation of clinical trials (Haynes & Dantes, 1987), and, for the individual patient, treatment noncompliance can result in a lowered chance of survival. Data from Bonadonna and Valagussa (1981) clearly demonstrated this latter effect, with differential survival rates for women receiving more than 85%, 65%–84%, or less than 65% of the recommended dosages of cyclophosphamide, methotrextate, and 5–fluorouracil (CMF) therapy for breast cancer. This was not a study of noncompliance per se, as the reasons for dosage reduction included toxicity (32%), refusal of treatment (8%), age (i.e., more than 60 years old; 10%), and other reasons (33%; e.g., desire to simplify drug administration). However, it illustrates the impact on survival that therapy alterations can have. Also, some reasons for therapy alterations may be correlated with the psychological and behavioral aspects of noncompliance (e.g., treatment toxicity related to emotional distress), whereas others may not be (e.g., physician preference, ease of administration, patient age). Within the context of cancer therapy, compliance will have many representations, and it is likely that there are different correlates for different behaviors. Predictors of compliance with appointments for chemotherapy regimens have included variables within the quality of life domain, including difficulty in coping with symptoms, symptom interference with normal activities, or depression (Richardson, Marks, & Levine, 1988), as well as non-quality of life variables, such as length of treatment regimen (Berger, Braverman, Sohn, & Morrow, 1988). Similarly, predictors of chemotherapy drug levels have included treatment environment (lower compliance in community vs. university clinics; Lebovits et al., 1990), income level (Lebovits et al., 1990), and complexity of the regimen (Richardson et al., 1987). Review of the noncancer literature affirms the generality of these findings and underscores quality of life factors, such as increased disability, as well as characteristics of the disease (i.e., frequency of symptoms) and regimen (i.e., duration and complexity of treatment), as correlates of noncompliance (DiMatteo & DiNicola, 1982). In contrast, global personality factors have not proved to be illuminating (Kaplan & Simon, 1990); instead, social factors might be important (Dunbar-Jacob, Dwyer, & Dunning, 1991).

The model also notes that poor compliance can affect local control (arrow from Compliance to Disease: Local in Figure 1) as well as distant control of the disease (arrow from Compliance to Disease: Metastatic in Figure 1). The selection of the route(s) would depend on characteristics of an individual's noncompliance for the particular treatment regimen. Noncompliance leading to failure of local control includes the following examples. Irregular daily attendance to radiotherapy would allow more time for regeneration of cancer cells at the tumor site, reversing the balance that is in favor of normal tissue cell repair in a course of fractionated radiotherapy. Or, premature termination of the course (e.g., quitting therapy after 4 weeks of a 6-week course) would increase risk for local failure (i.e., disease-involved tissue at the primary site might not receive an adequate dosage to affect the biologic status of the tumor). Noncompliance leading to failure of metastatic control could include the following examples. Not ingesting systemic chemotherapy may lead to a more rapid spread of micrometastases, because therapeutic drug levels would not be achieved at the cellular level. Or, a patient may comply with initial therapy but fail to return for follow-up and thus lengthen the time of detection and treatment of recurrent disease; in many tumors, such as those caused by ovarian cancer, success at retreatment is directly related to tumor volume.

Figure 1 also has a double-headed arrow between compliance and health behaviors, suggesting that the factors may interact; even synergy is possible. That is, those cancer patients who are compliant may expect better health outcomes and because of this may find it easier to comply with diet, exercise, sleep, and so forth, or to engage in other behaviors indicative of "good health." Conversely, those individuals who are noncompliant with therapy may have poor linkages to the health care system, and they might not receive information on, for example, diet, that others might receive during treatment or follow-up. The interaction of behavioral phenomena such as these and the effect of the personality factors that may govern them (e.g., conscientiousness; see relevant discussion in Friedman et al., 1993, or Andersen, in press) may account in part for the positive main effect for compliance in randomized clinical trials of drug versus placebo for coronary heart disease. That is, better disease outcomes are found for placebo-compliant versus placebo-noncompliant patients, along with the expected finding of better outcomes for compliant versus noncompliant patients who receive active drugs (Coronary Drug Project Research Group, 1980; Epstein, 1984).

Biological Pathways

A variety of data suggest that stress sets into motion important biological effects, including those influencing the autonomic, endocrine, and immune systems. As illustrated in Figure 1, stress may be routed to the immune system by the central nervous system (CNS) by activation of the sympathetic nervous system (adrenergic nerves terminating in the lymphoid organs; Felten & Felten, 1991; Felten et al., 1987) or through neuroendocrine-immune pathways (i.e., the release of hormones). In the latter case, a variety of hormones released under stress have been implicated in immune modulation. Examples include the catecholamines epinephrine and norepinephrine, which are secreted by the adrenal medulla; cortisol, which is secreted by the adrenal cortex; and growth hormone prolactin and endogenous opioid peptides, produced by the pituitary, the adrenal medulla, the brain, or the immune system itself (see Baum, Grunberg, & Singer, 1982; Bonneau, Sheridan, Feng, & Glaser, in press; Cohen & Williamson, 1991; Morley, Benton, & Solomon, 1991; Rabin, Cohen, Ganguli, Lysle, & Cunnick, 1989; Sabharwal et al., 1992).

Regardless of the impact of stress, the immune system may be one of the more important biological determinants in the control of certain malignant diseases. There is considerable evidence for both the classical and natural immune responses in host resistance against progression and metastatic spread of tumors. In fact, the evidence for some components of the immune system, for example, NK cells, is more compelling in controlling metastases than for surveillance (Herberman, 1991). The presence of cancer can induce antitumor immune responses involving T cells, antibody-producing B cells, or both. Also, tumor-bearing individuals may have general alterations in their immune system, with depression of a variety of immunological activities, such as decreased cellular immune reactivity (as demonstrated in vivo by delayed cutaneous hypersensitivity and in vitro by lymphoproliferative responses to mitogen or alloantigens), decreased macrophage responsiveness (Cianciolo & Snyderman, 1983), and decreased NK cell activity. These impairments have been most consistent in patients with advanced, metastatic disease, but some studies have shown abnormalities among individuals with localized disease (Stein, Adler, & BenEfran, 1976). In addition to the alterations in cellular immunity noted above, cancer may affect the relative proportions and absolute numbers of T and B cells, as many cancer patients, including some with localized disease, have decreased percentages of T-cell subpopulations (e.g., Kikuchi, Kita, & Oomori, 1988). For our model, there are at least two important questions regarding stress–immune relationships: What is the evidence for either stress-mediated immune responses, and what is the evidence for stress-mediated health effects?

Evidence for a Stress—Quality of Life Mediated Immune Response

There are three lines of supporting data. First, time-limited (acute) stressors can produce immunologic changes in relatively healthy individuals. Data from our psychoneuroimmunology (PNI) laboratory studies with healthy medical students taking academic examinations have provided strong and reliable demonstrations of this effect. They have shown, for example, that during the stressful exam period, significant declines in NK cell activity and decreases in T-cell killing of Epstein-Barr virus (EBV)-infected target cells have occurred, along with dramatic decreases in gamma interferon production by lymphocytes stimulated with concanavalin A (Con A; e.g., Glaser et al., 1987; Glaser, Rice, Speicher, Stout, & Kiecolt-Glaser, 1986).

Although the emotional distress of medical students taking exams and the distress of cancer patients have not been directly compared, convergent data support the acute emotional crisis with a life-threatening diagnosis and the correlated immune responses. For example, Ironson et al. (1990) prospectively assessed men taking the HIV-1 antibody test and found differential immune responses among men who tested seropositive and those who tested seronegative. As would be expected, men who tested seropositive reported significant acute anxiety responses and traumatic stress, with significant negative correlations between self-reported anxiety and NK activity ($-.69$).

Returning to cancer, we showed that for women with gynecologic cancer who had been assessed with the POMS, emotional distress within days of diagnosis and prior to their treatment was significantly greater than that for two relevant comparison groups (Andersen, Anderson, & deProsse, 1989a). A follow-up study (Andersen & Turnquist, 1985) on the covariation of affective distress and immunity was conducted with newly diagnosed but as yet untreated cervical and endometrial patients. On the first visit to the tertiary care hospital for their diagnostic workup, women's emotional distress was assessed with the POMS, and a morning blood sample was drawn. A subgroup of the women had a repeat blood sample drawn approximately 10 days later, on the day before surgery. First, differences between disease sites were examined; no emotional distress or immune variable or white blood cell (WBC) count differed significantly. However, because differential immune effects for sites are unknown, within-site analyses were conducted. Using a hierarchical multiple regression model, total mood disturbance on the POMS significantly predicted WBC counts at the initial and presurgery assessments beyond that predicted by the relevant disease risk, stage, and immune-moderating factors. Additional analyses with the POMS Depression subscale revealed similar significant relationships at both the initial and the presurgery assessments. These effects were replicated for the endometrial sample; the POMS was significantly related to WBC counts at the initial assessment, and depression and confusion were related to WBC counts at presurgery. These data were encouraging as they were the first tests of covariation of emotional distress and one general measure of immune status in cancer patients prior to their treatment. Also, the subscales that the prospective longitudinal study had indicated as relevant for women with cancer (Depression and Confusion; Andersen, Anderson, & deProsse, 1989b) were also relevant for the prediction of WBC counts.

More recent data replicated and extended these findings (Roberts, Andersen, & Lubaroff, 1994). Subjects were women with cervical (Stage I, $n = 27$; Stage II, $n = 10$) or endometrial (Stage I, $n = 17$; Stage II, $n = 4$) cancer assessed on two occasions (separated by approximately one week) following their diagnosis and prior to treatment. Distress measures included self-reported distress (POMS) and interviewer-rated distress and disturbance of affect (a modified version of a Schedule for Affective Disorders and Schizophrenia—SADS; Endicott & Spitzer, 1978—interview) to address inconsistencies in previous research (e.g., Levy, Herberman, Maluish, Schlein, & Lippman, 1985). Twenty age-matched healthy women were included to validate emotional distress indicators. Descriptive analyses indicated that, as expected, cancer subjects exhibited greater psychological distress across all measures. A multivariate analysis of variance (MANOVA) for the quantitative immune measures revealed significant differences between WBC and NK, with follow-ups indicating increased WBC counts and decreased numbers of large unclassified (NK) cells between the cancer group and healthy group. Regression analyses focused on the prediction of large unclassified (NK) cell counts. As before, relevant variables correlating with outcome (i.e., cell counts at Time 1, age, stage, and a functional performance rating) were entered as prior steps. Thirty-two percent of the variance was predicted, with the final step of the POMS and interviewer-rated distress ratings accounting for an additional, significant 17% of the variance in predicting large unclassified cell counts at the second assessment. In sum, data from healthy, HIV-infected, and cancer subjects indicate that the occurrence and magnitude of stress accompanying time-limited stressors or acutely stressful periods is correlated with at least certain aspects of immune downregulation.

Second, chronic stressors are associated with continuing downregulation of immunoresponsiveness rather than adaptation. This effect is evident in longitudinal studies for a range of lengthy or permanent stressors, including environmental stressors, such as living next to a damaged nuclear reactor (McKinnon, Weisse, Reynolds, Bowles, & Baum, 1989), or PNI laboratory studies of close relationship failures (e.g., divorce, separation, or marital distress; Kiecolt-Glaser, Fisher, et al., 1987) and caregiving for a family member with progressive dementia (Kiecolt-Glaser, Dura, Speicher, Trask, & Glaser, 1991). In the latter example, quality of life factors (the caregivers' social support) moderated immune functioning. Again, direct comparisons between chronic stressors of this sort and cancer have not been made, but we have noted the many commonalities between these chronic stressors and the cancer experience.

One implication of the chronic stressor data reported thus far is that the immune changes associated with the stressor do not habituate. For example, recent PNI data from the Alzheimer caregiver study showed lower NK cell cytotoxicity in caregivers than in controls when NK cells were stimulated by interferon gamma; similar results were obtained with the generation of lymphokine-activated killer (LAK) cells by interleukin-2. Moreover, even after the chronic stresses of caregiving had ended, bereaved caregivers did not differ from continuing caregivers; both groups had significantly lower NK-augmented cytotoxicity than did the controls (Esterling, Kiecolt-Glaser, Bodnar, & Glaser, in press), suggesting nonhabituating stress effects for bereaved persons. The latter data parallel Baum's (1990) data on the longer-term downregulation in immune function among residents who continue to live next to the Three Mile Island nuclear reactor. The physiological effect of long-term secretion of stress-relevant hormones (e.g., catecholamine) has been noted, with the result that neuroendocrine receptor number and availability is altered (Baum, 1990; Sapolsky, Krey, & McEwen, 1986). Assuming a continuously interactive system, such changes could in turn result in a new, lower baseline.

Convergent evidence from several laboratories suggests that a psychological factor—social support—may interact with chronic stressors to produce differences in sympathetic nervous system (SNS) reactivity, neuropeptide release, and immune function. Our data indicate that family caregivers of relatives with Alzheimer's disease who are high in social support display different patterns of age-related heart rate reactivity and blood pressure than do caregivers who are low in social support (Uchino, Kiecolt-Glaser, & Cacioppo, 1992). Our earlier data from the same sample had shown that caregivers had poorer immune function than did controls and that low social support was associated with greater declines in immune function over the course of a year (Kiecolt-Glaser, Cacioppo, Malarkey, & Glaser, 1992). Similarly, Irwin, Brown, et al. (1992) found higher levels of neuropeptide Y (NPY) in Alzheimer's disease caregivers than in controls; levels of NPY, a sympathetic neurotransmitter released during emotional stress, were inversely correlated with NK cell activity. Related data come from a study of social support among wives of cancer patients. Baron, Cutrona, Hicklin, Russel, and Lubaroff (1990) have shown greater immunocompetence on two of three measures (NK cytotoxicity and phenohemagglutin, PHA, but not Con-A) among those wives reporting higher levels of social support.

Chronic stress has also been implicated as a factor in enhanced cardiovascular reactivity as well as in higher levels of urinary catecholamine in two studies from Baum's laboratory (Fleming, Baum, Davidson, Rectanus, & McArdle, 1987; McKinnon et al., 1989). Because individuals with high cardiovascular reactivity appear to show magnified endocrine and cellular immune responses to experimental psychological stressors (Kiecolt-Glaser et al., 1991; Sgoutas-Emch et al., in press), enhanced SNS reactivity could have important physiological consequences.

In addition to these biological mechanisms, which could serve to maintain downregulation of certain aspects of immune function, behavioral adaptations made in the lengthy coping process could produce related effects on immunity. Some coping behaviors may be adaptive but others may not be, or it may be difficult (or impossible, in some cases) to resume prestressor adjustment levels. For example, the behavioral data from the longitudinal study of Alzheimer's disease caregivers indicates that former caregivers who now are bereaved show similarly high rates of syndromal depression, depressive symptoms, and lower social support as do the continuing caregivers, with both of these groups having significantly poorer immune function than age-matched noncaregivers (Esterling et al., in press). Although early surveys suggested that well-being increased once caregiving ended (George & Gwyther, 1984), our longitudinal data indicate no reconstitution of social networks, but rather the continuation of intrusive and avoidant thoughts about the experience for as long as two years after the disabled relative's death (Bodnar & Kiecolt-Glaser, in press). Similarly, Baum and his colleagues (Fleming et al., 1987) found that when chronic stress was associated with avoidant or intrusive thinking about the stressor, enhanced cardiovascular reactivity was one possible consequence. These findings are consistent with other data on environmental stressors that suggest that long-term stressors may erode social support (Lepore, Evans, & Schneider, 1991) and have continuing, negative, cognitive effects. Taken together, however, they provide suggestive evidence for several pathways through which behavioral mechanisms could promote continued immune downregulation in concert with long-term stressors.

Third, studies with cancer patients provide data linking quality of life components and immunity. In an early study by Levy et al. (1985), 75 women with Stage I or II breast cancer were assessed following surgery (lumpectomy or mastectomy with node dissection) and before initiation of other therapy. Women who were rated as better adjusted to their illness but who reported higher fatigue (as assessed with the POMS) had lower NK cell levels. Another study (Levy et al., 1990) reported on different psychosocial variables at three months after treatment (lumpectomy or mastectomy with or without adjuvant therapy) for 66 women with Stage I or II disease. In addition to estrogen receptor status (an important prognostic indicator) predicting NK cell lysis, social support added significantly to the model in predicting higher NK cell activity. These data are somewhat inconsistent but are generally in line with data from healthy individuals with positive indicators of quality of life (e.g., social adjustment) predicting higher NK cell levels and negative–distress indicators (e.g., emotional distress) predicting lower NK cell levels.

Finally, relevant animal studies have come from the laboratory of Liebeskind and colleagues (Ben-Eliyahu, Yirmirya, Liebeskind, Taylor, & Gale, 1991) that suggest a link between pain-induced immune suppression of NK cell activity and the development of syngenetic mammary tumors. In this model, tumor development and metastatic spread has been shown to be significantly controlled by NK cells. Using Fisher rats that were exposed to an acute stressor (pain from surgery), a substantial decrease in NK cell lysis in vitro was found using the tumor cells as target cells. When in vivo studies were performed using animals undergoing the surgery stressor, there was a decrease in NK cell cytotoxicity concomitant with an increase in tumor metastases. Although the applicability of animal tumor data to cancer processes in humans is complex and best achieved with narrow, hypothesis-driven comparisons (Moulder, Dutreix, Rockwell, & Sieman, 1988), these animal data support stress-induced modulation of certain aspects of the immune system (i.e., NK cells) known to be important for surveillance and tumor control.

Evidence for Stress or Decrements in Quality of Life Having Health Consequences

Two lines of data suggest negative health consequences. Some investigators have tested the direct role of stress, whereas others have tested an indirect route through immune indicators. First, there is solid evidence for the link between acute stress and illness, specifically, infectious illness in young, healthy individuals. Cohen, Tyrrell, and Smith (1991) inoculated 357 volunteers with either a cold virus or a placebo. They found that rates of both respiratory infection and clinical colds increased in a does–response manner with increases in psychological stress using five different strains of "cold viruses," providing a controlled demonstration of increased infection associated with increased stress. Consistent with Cohen's data, we found that stress influenced medical students' responses to a hepatitis B vaccination. Students received each of three injections of the vaccine on the last day of a three-day examination period to study the effects of academic stress on the students' ability to generate an immune response to a primary antigen (Glaser et al., 1992). A quarter of the students seroconverted (produced an antibody response to the vaccine) after the first injection; early seroconverters were significantly less stressed and less anxious than those students who did not seroconvert until the second injection. In addition, students who reported greater social support demonstrated a stronger immune response to the vaccine at the time of the third inoculation, as measured by antibody titers to the virus and a virus-specific T-cell response to a purified viral polypeptide. Thus, these data suggest that the immune response to a vaccine (and, by extension, to other primary antigens) can be modulated by a mild stressor—even in young, healthy adults who have a long history of exposure to (and mastery of) this very stressor. Moreover, these data provide a window on the body's response to other pathogens, such as viruses or bacteria. The more stressed and more anxious students seroconverted later; these same individuals might also be slower to develop an antibody response to other pathogens and, in turn, be at risk for more severe illness.

Data are accumulating for the health effects from chronic stressors. Data from our PNI laboratories (Kiecolt-Glaser et al., 1991) have shown that "at risk" Alzheimer caregivers (i.e., caregivers with consistent immune downregulation across functional assays) had more and longer-lasting upper respiratory tract infections than did the remainder of the sample. Baum (1990), using physician's data, found that numbers of both physical complaints and prescriptions written for Three Mile Island-area residents were greater than those for control subjects for two years after the accident. Moreover, although physician-measured blood pressure had been comparable for Three Mile Island residents and controls in the year preceding the nuclear reactor accident, Three Mile Island-area residents showed greater elevations on both systolic and diastolic blood pressure than did controls in the year following the accident.

The few data from diagnosed cancer groups are most relevant. All of the health outcomes that have been studied have been disease endpoints. However, infections and infectious illnesses, for example, would seem relevant, as infectious pathogens are a major cause of morbidity and mortality for cancer patients (e.g., Innagaki, Rodriguez, & Bodey, 1974; Ketchel & Rodriguez, 1987). Although it is not an endpoint, the extent of disease at initial diagnosis (i.e., number of positive nodes) is important prognostically. Levy et al. (1985) found self-reports of fatigue (POMS) obtained shortly following initial treatment to be a predictor of nodal status in women with breast cancer, but there was no effect for fatigue if NK cell levels were first entered into the regression equation. We also examined disease progression to the lymph nodes in women with gynecologic cancer (Roberts et al., 1994). Unlike Levy et al.'s study, which confounded collection of distress and immunity data with knowledge of nodal status, here nodal status was learned afterward, approximately 16 days from the initial assessment (Time 1) and 5 days from the presurgery (Time 2) immune assessment. After the clinical stage and the two assessments of NK cell lysis, interviewer-rated disturbance of affect (i.e., blunted, inappropriate, and depressed affect) contributed significantly (14% of the variance) to the prediction of the number of positive nodes.

Psychological studies predicting cancer endpoints, however, have the most relevance for the model.[3] Levy, Herberman, Lippman, D'Angelo, and Lee (1991) examined variables predicting disease-free intervals (DFIs) and recurrence in 90 women with initial Stage I or II breast cancer with data gathered at postsurgery and at 3- and 15-month follow-ups. DFI was predicted by number of positive nodes ($-.27$) and distress (POMS; $-.41$) at 15 months, with neither NK cell lysis at postsurgery nor 15 months later as significant predictors. In contrast, POMS scores did not predict recurrence; instead, recurrence was predicted by NK cell activity at postsurgery ($-.35$) and 15 months later (.75). Finally, Levy, Lee, Bagley, and Lippman (1988) examined time to death following recurrence for 36 women with breast cancer. Along with the medically relevant variables of DFIs, physician-rated prognosis, and number of metastatic sites, positive affect (Joy) reported at recurrence predicted a longer survival time.

Summary

Data from healthy samples suggest that stress variables are predictive of immune downregulation, and accumulating data with cancer groups support the same general conclusion. Because the phenomena appear to be reliable, investigators are beginning to examine the clinical relevance of the effect. That is, are these immune changes related to health consequences? Here the data are sparse, but the most controlled analysis, the study by Cohen et al. (1991), shows a direct, replicable relationship between stress and infections and colds. Many researchers question whether the latter findings are relevant to persons with cancer or to those with other chronic illnesses, such as HIV infection or AIDS. The most frequent argument waged against psychological and behavioral effects (even if large) significantly affecting biologic processes is because of the presumed downregulating effects of the disease or the treatments. That is, both our data and those of Levy and colleagues come from correlational designs that tested the contribution of psychological factors, and the directional hypotheses for all variables—psychological–behavioral and disease–treatment effects—are in the same direction, downregulation.

In this context we offer one observation and one suggestion for continued study.

---

[3]In clinical cancer research, a major research design decision is the selection of the important endpoint, or criterion, to be predicted. Survival time (time alive since diagnosis and treatment) is one of the most common, but often is not the most helpful because of the variable course of most cancers. Endpoints fall into four broad categories. Response to therapy includes, for example, judgments of complete response, partial response, stable disease, and failure or progression of disease. Time intervals associated with control of disease include disease-free interval following initial therapy, survival, disease-free survival, interval of local control, or time before development of metastatic disease. Toxicity-related endpoints also are considered, such as degrees of therapy modification because of toxicity, highest grade of toxicity encountered, occurrence and grade of late effects, and time to appearance of late effects. Finally, there is increasing interest in establishing quality of life endpoints in cancer.

First, the directional effects of cancer on the immune system remain to be documented; however, there are sufficient data to state that cancer effects are not unidirectional (i.e., downward), within or across sites. For example, T-cell levels may be slightly decreased, whereas T-cell function appears to be intact in early stage ovarian cancer (Mandell, Fisher, Bostick, & Young, 1979). In contrast, cervical cancer patients often have an increase in B cells and gamma interferon levels, with a decrease in T-cell function (Sharma, Gupta, & Kadian, 1979). Variability on other immune measures, such as delayed hypersensitivity to antigens and contact allergens, can occur across cervical, endometrial, and ovarian cancers (Khoo, MacKay, & Daunter, 1979; Nalick, DiSaia, Rea, & Morrow, 1974). The model we and other psychologists test, however, is in line with the immune theory that posits an influential role of NK cells in host resistance against metastasis (Gorelik & Herberman, 1986). The latter theory rests on the association between depressed immune activity and increased metastases in animal models.

We have proposed a biobehavioral model of variables and pathways believed to lead to immune and health effects. Regarding the health effects, we have discussed disease progression and related variables (e.g., DFI) as endpoints; however, the model may be relevant to other health outcomes, such as a higher incidence of infections and infectious (viral) illnesses (infections are a major obstacle in health care management of cancer patients and also are a major cause of death; Bodey, 1986). Further correlational studies of diagnosed cancer patients would need to be performed to document the reliability of the stress–immunity–cancer link. However, a stronger test would be, of course, to experimentally manipulate a variable in the model. Despite the numerous difficulties entailed, a randomized intervention trial offers a powerful test. A psychological–behavioral intervention is powerful because the prediction for the intervention would be for immune enhancement, more positive health outcomes, or both, in contrast to the prediction for a no-treatment control of downward regulation, poorer health outcomes, or both.

We have reviewed the effects of psychological interventions on moderating immunity in noncancer populations (Kiecolt-Glaser & Glaser, 1992). There we noted that researchers have used diverse strategies to modulate immune function, including relaxation, hypnosis, exercise, self-disclosure, and cognitive–behavioral interventions, and these interventions have generally produced positive changes. For example, our PNI laboratory tested the immune effects of a relaxation training and social contact intervention (Kiecolt-Glaser et al., 1985) with a cancer-relevant sample, elderly adults (mean age of 74 years) living in independent living facilities. Subjects were randomized to (a) relaxation training, (b) social contact, or (c) no contact. Subjects in the two intervention conditions were seen individually three times a week for a month (12 sessions). Blood samples and self-report data were obtained at pretreatment, posttreatment, and one-month follow-up. Analysis of the psychological data indicated that the relaxation intervention had quality of life effects, as indicated by significant reductions on the Hopkins Symptom Checklist (Derogatis, Lipman, Rickels, Uhlenhuth, & Covi, 1974), a measure of affective distress. Also, all subjects (including controls) reported a significant increase in self-rated quality of sleep, a positive health behavior. Analyses of the immune data indicated that the relaxation intervention produced significant increases (approximately 30%) in NK cell activity (see Figure 1 in Kiecolt-Glaser et al., 1985), with the highest percentage lysis of target cells occurring immediately after treatment. It is because of promising data such as these (see Kiecolt-Glaser & Glaser, 1992, for a review) that we conclude with a brief discussion of the role psychological interventions may play in answering stress and immunity questions in cancer.

Testing the Model

Research Design: A Role for Experimental Trials of Psychological and Behavioral Interventions

We have previously reviewed the evidence for psychological and behavioral interventions with cancer patients (see Andersen, 1992, for a discussion). Several controlled trials have demonstrated that such efforts can reduce distress, hasten resumption of routine activities, and improve social outcomes for groups at high risk for quality of life morbidity, such as patients with disseminated or recurrent disease, as well as patients at lower risk, such as those with localized disease and time-limited cancer therapy. We have suggested here that appropriately designed psychosocial interventions can reduce stress and enhance quality of life as well as improve behavioral responses, such as health behaviors and compliance. This research progress in behavioral oncology—the prospect of randomly assigning individuals to conditions that will result in differential psychological and behavioral outcomes—provides one of the necessary conditions for an experimental test of the model.

Therapy components for psychological interventions have included an emotionally supportive context to address fears and anxieties about the disease (e.g., Cain, Kohorn, Quinlan, Latimer, & Schwartz, 1986; Capone, Good, Westie, & Jacobson, 1980; Forester, Kornfeld, & Fleiss, 1985; Maguire, Brooke, Tait, Thomas, & Sellwood, 1983), information about the disease and treatment (e.g., Cain et al., 1986; Fawzy et al., 1990; Houts, Whitney, Mortel, & Batholomew, 1986; Jacobs, Ross, Walker, & Stockdale, 1983; Maguire et al., 1983), behavioral coping strategies (e.g., role playing difficult discussions with family or the medical staff; Fawzy et al., 1990; Houts et al., 1986), cognitive coping strategies (Cain et al., 1986; Davis, 1986; Houts et al., 1986; Telch & Telch, 1986), relaxation training to lower "arousal" or enhance one's sense of control (Davis, 1986; Fawzy et al., 1990), and focused interventions for disease-specific problems (e.g., sexual functioning for gynecologic or breast cancer; Capone et al., 1980).

It is more difficult to enumerate the intervention components that can affect health behaviors. Despite their importance, health behaviors have not been included as outcomes in cancer studies, even though many psychosocial interventions include educational components designed for them. Of the very few studies focusing on compliance per se, the data suggest similar interventions, including information about the disease and treatment (Richardson et al., 1987; Robinson, 1990), enlistment of help of significant others (i.e., social support; Richardson et al., 1987), and practitioner counseling (i.e., prompts by a physician to be compliant; Robinson, 1990). For reference, the extensive literature on compliance with antihypertensive regimens (e.g., Dunbar-Jacob et al., 1991) suggests different techniques for different compliance targets. Specifically, mailed reminders and home visits by nursing personnel have been used to improve appointment keeping, whereas education, behavioral strategies (e.g., self-monitoring, contingency contracting), and enhanced social support have been used to improve medication compliance.

In considering an experimental trial to affect immunity or disease endpoints, a simple experimental design—treatment versus no treatment—would be the strategic next step. At present, there are insufficient data to choose among intervention components that would be expected to affect the immune system, but these and related findings would suggest an emphasis on relaxation, coping, social support, and disease-specific components (Andersen, 1992; Kiecolt-Glaser & Glaser, 1992). Such a design would not provide the basis for ruling out secondary hypotheses of therapist characteristics separate from treatment techniques, patient characteristics separate from psychological and behavioral difficulties, or specific therapeutic techniques as separate from nonspecific or placebo effects. What it can do, however, is establish cause–effect conclusions for the presence of intervention-producing enhanced psychological and behavioral outcomes, immune responses, and health effects. Once an effect is reliably demonstrated, it would then be relevant to study component questions. In the interim, investigators should document the content, the reliability of intervention delivery, and the involvement of the patients, for hypothesis generation in follow-up studies. Previous studies have omitted documentation and process measures (but see Gordon et al., 1980, for an example of number of individual therapy sessions; or Telch & Telch, 1986, for monitoring of homework assignments).

There already is suggestive evidence in support of the model, with data that indicate positive immune and health consequences for psychological interventions, and taken together they provide a basis for further scientific inquiry. One study included immune measures and disease endpoints, and two others reported disease endpoints. All of the studies used extensive psychological assessments, but none examined behavioral variables (i.e., health behaviors and compliance). For the first study, Fawzy et al. (1990) studied newly treated Stage I or II melanoma patients randomly assigned to either no intervention or a structured short-term (10 sessions) group support intervention. At posttreatment and the six-month follow-up, significant psychological and coping outcomes for the intervention subjects were evident, as well as increases in the percentage of large granular lymphocytes, the NK cell phenotype, an increase in NK cell numbers (as determined by markers), and other positive findings, such as interferon alpha-augmented NK activity. These data are relevant to the findings of Kiecolt-Glaser et al. (1985), who found intervention differences in NK activity. Importantly, the magnitude of the NK changes Fawzy et al. found was frequently greater than 25% for the intervention subjects. Finally, the correlation data of immune and affective change provides additional support for the model in that interferon-augmented NK cytotoxic activity increased with concomitant reductions in anxiety ($-.37$) and depression ($-.33$). We believe the NK cell data are particularly important, because it has been shown that there is a reduction in NK cell activity with tumor progression (Akimoto et al., 1986; Takasugi, Ramseyer, & Takasugi, 1977). It is also known that the ability of NK cells to respond to interleukin-2 (IL-2) or gamma interferon is different in cancer patients who are managed with different types of therapy.

Six-year follow-up data on disease endpoints are also available (Fawzy et al., 1993). Analyses of DFIs to death have indicated significant group differences, with 29% of controls and 9% of experimental subjects dying in the six-year interval. Analyses of DFIs to recurrence were in the same direction but only approached significance ($p = .09$). Follow-up analyses suggested that the former effects were primarily due to the men in the control group dying and, in particular, men with the highest Breslow depth rating (a disease-related prognostic indicator; higher values indicate poorer prognosis). Considering the latter factor, 9 of 10 experimental subjects in the highest Breslow category were alive, versus only 1 of 9 control patients.

In the same follow-up, other analyses examined baseline and six-month psychological and immune parameters by survivor group and gender. The majority of the effects reside within the male group, so it is useful to consider the surviving versus the deceased males. These comparisons indicate that from baseline to the six-month assessment, the surviving males reported significant decreases in affective distress, increases in active behavioral coping, and increases in CD16 NK cells and interferon alpha-augmented NK cell activity (i.e., immune up-regulation). In contrast, males who died showed no significant changes on any of these variables, that is, no quality of life improvement or immune enhancement. It also should be noted that the deceased males began the study reporting significantly lower overall levels of distress (i.e., 34 vs. 64 on the baseline Total Mood Disturbance of the POMS for the deceased vs. surviving males, respectively), but their immune responses were within the same range as those of the survivors.

Fawzy et al.'s (1990, 1993) investigation was the first intervention study to combine psychological, immune, and disease endpoint data. The initial outcome data indicated that early, brief psychological efforts produced immediate (posttreatment) effects as well as long term (six-month) changes. We have suggested that the maintenance of gains may be a crucial foothold for immune effects to emerge (Andersen, 1992); data from a relaxation intervention study suggest this as well. Gruber et al. (1993) studied 13 Stage I, node-negative breast cancer patients who received electromyograph (EMG) biofeedback-assisted relaxation training. Weekly immune assessments during the nine-week intervention indicated significant differences between the treatment and control groups in the expected direction: WBC values were stable for the intervention group but declined for the control, and Con-A and mixed lymphocyte response values were higher for the intervention group. NK cell values significantly increased from pre- to posttreatment. Considering immune data taken each of the nine study weeks, there was suggestive evidence that the immune effects became evident only after several weeks into the intervention.

Other data relevant to the model come from samples very different from these good prognosis patients. Specifically, women with recurrent breast cancer and lung cancer patients have been studied. Spiegel, Bloom, and colleagues (Spiegel, Bloom & Yalom, 1981; Spiegel & Bloom, 1983) randomly assigned women with metastatic breast disease to a no-treatment condition or to a group treatment condition that met weekly for at least one year. The intervention subjects were also randomly assigned to a no additional treatment condition or to a self-hypnosis condition for pain problems. The intervention group subjects reported significantly lower emotional distress (POMS) and fewer maladaptive coping responses than did the control subjects, with the magnitude of the difference increasing during the intervention year. Data also suggested that the hypnosis component provided an additive analgesic effect to other group treatment components. A 10-year follow-up was conducted, at which time only three women, all of whom were intervention participants, remained alive (Spiegel et al., 1989). A striking survival difference was found between the control subjects (18.9 months) and the intervention subjects (36.6 months) from study entry until death. Survival time differences between the groups began to emerge approximately 8 months after termination of the year-long intervention.

As might be expected, the publication of Spiegel et al.'s (1989) survival follow-up study unleased a torrent of interest in the role of psychological factors in cancer in both academic and popular circles (e.g., Moyers, 1993; ten Have-de Labije & Balner, 1991; Temoshok & Dreher, 1992). One critic of the findings, however, was LeShan (1991, 1992), who suggested that the survival effects might have been due to adverse effects on the control group (i.e., perceived rejection implied by being randomly selected out of the treatment group) rather than to positive effects on the intervention group. In fact, Fox's (1992) comparison of the study's survival data with national survival rate data has supported the implication of LeShan's concern: "The survival of the intervention group was somewhat worse than the survival of the national sample, while the survival of the control group was considerably worse (p. 83)." Despite this, Fox argued that it is unlikely that the control group died at a faster rate for "perceived rejection" reasons. He posited that this explanation is unlikely for several reasons, including the lack of national enthusiasm for group support interventions at the time of the study (late 1970s), no suggestion at all to the study participants that the study had any relevance to survival, and, more likely, that the differences reflect chance deviation of the entire study sample (consisting of only 84 women) from the population of women represented in national trends.

Finally, contradictory data come from Linn, Linn, and Harris (1982), who offered a death and dying intervention program to male cancer patients, 46% of whom had lung cancer. Despite favorable quality of life outcomes for the intervention subjects (e.g., lower stress [POMS], higher life satisfaction, lower alienation), there were no functional status or body system impairment differences between the control group and the intervention group. Survival analyses also revealed no significant differences. Aside from the many methodology differences between this and the Spiegel et al. (1989) study, two disease factors may account for the discrepancy in survival outcomes. First, there is a shorter survival window for metastatic lung cancer in contrast to metastatic breast cancer. (Five-year survival rates are 13% and 73%, respectively, for initial Stage III disease and 1% and 19%, respectively, for initial Stage IV disease; Boring et al., 1993.) Second, hormonal and immune factors may be more important in breast cancer than in lung cancer (see subsequent discussion below).

Methodology: Maximizing the Signal to Noise Ratio

It is an understatement to characterize this as "a most difficult area of research" (Fox, 1978, p. 117), and one that, like AIDS and HIV, is methodologically complex for behavioral immunology researchers (Kiecolt-Glaser & Glaser, 1988a). We cannot adequately address all of the methodology challenges that tests of the biobehavioral model pose; however, we reference here some of the more difficult ones at the interface of behavioral oncology and immunology and we refer the reader to other methodology discussions of variables predicting risk for psychosocial morbidity, and individual-differences variables that may covary with psychosocial outcomes or intervention effectiveness (Andersen, 1994, in press).

First, the term *cancer* refers to a heterogeneous group of diseases of multiple etiologies that vary in their tissue of origin, cell type, biologic behavior, anatomic site, and degree of differentiation (stage and degree of malignancy). Although we have used the generic term *cancer* in this article, it is likely that quality of life and stress and health behavior factors would interact with immune function only in selected cases. Many hypothesized cancer-causing mechanisms are associated with immunological downregulation. However, the likelihood of psychological or behavioral factors interacting with the immune system to influence disease progression would be expected to differ across sites. Cancers that are etiologically linked to hormonal stimuli (e.g., breast, ovarian, endometrial, and prostate) or to the immune system (e.g., leukemias, lymphomas) may be most susceptible to influence; Epstein-Barr virus (EBV)-associated tumors (i.e., EBV-associated B-cell lymphomas; Levine, Ablashi, Nonoyama, Pearson, & Glaser, 1987), viral (e.g., cervical; Goodkin, Antoni, Sevin, & Fox, 1993a, 1993b), and genetically linked forms (e.g., some types of breast and colon cancer) may be somewhere in the middle, and those cancers believed to be due to physical or chemical carcinogens (e.g., lung cancer linked to tobacco usage) may be the least susceptible to influence. Also, it is known that the risk of cancer increases with age, and as the immune system ages it becomes less efficient. It has been suggested that psychological and stress factors may be most relevant for middle-aged persons (age 35–65) rather than for very young or very old persons, because of the disproportionate influence of hereditary factors on young cancer patients and the influence of aging factors on older persons (Fox, 1978).

Thus, the proposed model may evidence the best fit for some sites (e.g, breast, ovary, prostate), and even for some forms within sites, as opposed to others. Application of the model to other chronic illnesses would require further refinement. Testing of the model might be additionally optimized when samples are as homogeneous as possible on other major dimensions, such as prognostic factors; such variables might be chosed for stratification or at least for documentation (e.g., the case with Breslow depth in the Fawzy et al., 1990, 1993, study). Selection of variables would be based on their unique importance to the disease site being studied. This is the same tactic taken in moderate-sized clinical trials of medical therapies in which the effect of the prognostic variables is anticipated to be greater than the effect of the new cancer treatment. For most sites it is more feasible to stratify on disease or prognostic variables than to attempt to control for cancer treatment. There are diverse treatment regimens now available, and choices among them are made on several bases, including, but not limited to, current data on the treatment regimens' relationship with prognostic variables; patient choice, if possible; physician preference, expertise, or specialty; and data from new trials (e.g., new uses of Taxol are occurring on a monthly basis). Because this is the scenario for most of the prevalent disease sites (e.g., breast, prostate, colon), careful selection of major prognostic indicators can result in de facto control of treatment, even when the available cancer therapies change during the course of the study. For example, the variables of nodal status, hormone receptor status, and menopausal status might be considered for a study of women with breast cancer (see Clark & McGuire, 1992, for a discussion). These variables would, in various combinations, determine most of the treatment pathways, influencing, for example, the occurrence and extent of surgery, the type of chemotherapy for premenopausal (adjuvant chemotherapy) versus postmenopausal women (adjuvant Tamoxifen), or the likelihood of extreme treatments, such as bone marrow transplant.

Second, the model posits immune effects from psychological and behavioral factors beyond any immune downregulation that may accrue either from malignant disease processes or from cancer treatment effects. Some researchers believe intervention trials of this sort are misguided at best, because the immunosuppressive effects of the disease or treatments would override any positive effects from a psychological intervention. In fact, attempting to address this concern with evidence, such as determining the magnitude of immunosuppressive effects from disease or cancer treatments, is surprisingly difficult because of the dearth of basic immunology data. Also, data that are available are not always confirmatory. For example, Ludwig et al. (1985) found unaltered immune function in patients with nondisseminated breast cancer (Stages I through III) at diagnosis, with the significant reductions (e.g., depressed PHA responsiveness) found only among women with metastatic (Stage IV) disease. Regarding cancer treatments—surgery, radiotherapy, chemotherapy, chemoradiation (chemotherapy that is radiosensitizing and given with radiation), and combination therapy—all have immunosuppressive effects, but much of the detail about the nature of the effects is unknown. It has been found that lymphocyte transformation is depressed during radiotherapy but may rebound within two months after therapy; there is also specificity due to site of treatment, as greater depression is found for pelvic–abdominal sites versus chest or head–neck sites (Slater, Ngo, & Lau, 1976). Considering chemotherapies, some will suppress lymphocyte proliferation, yet others are designed to enhance lymphocyte proliferation; but more typically, the immune-moderating effects of most chemotherapies are unknown. One of the more well-studied drugs (from an immune standpoint) is cyclophosphamide (CY). It consistently causes a sharp reduction in circulating peripheral blood lymphocytes and lymphoproliferative responses to mitogens, although the effect on antibody production is more variable (Ehrke, Mihich, Berd, & Mastrangelo, 1989). In contrast, CY can augment immunity to clinically relevant antigens; the leading hypothesis for how this occurs is that CY has selective toxicity for suppressor T cells or their precursors. Another drug, less well-studied from an immune standpoint, but one as widely used clinically, is adriamycin (ADM). The most prominent immunosuppressive effect of ADM is that it induces myelosuppression, which is likely due to the well-established antiproliferative effects of such anthracycline antibiotics. Although the immunopotentiation effects have not been studied as extensively, clinical studies with cancer patients have suggested that long-term ADM therapy does not appear to alter cell-mediated immunity, but data suggest that recovery is complete by one to three weeks after therapy (Kempf & Mitchell, 1984a, 1984b).

We acknowledge the complexity of these issues and suggest special care in the selection of stratification variables (see prior discussion) so that it might be possible to de facto equate groups on the heterogeneous treatment options that might be available for a single site of disease. Of course, full documentation of the nature of the regimens for subjects, including dosages and timing of delivery, is essential. In addition to following basic guidelines for behavioral immunology studies (Kiecolt-Glaser & Glaser, 1988a), investigators will need to consider strategies for controlling variation in blood draws for cancer patients; for example, scheduling blood draws before chemotherapy administration may maximize the likelihood of tapping recovered responses at the end of cycles rather than any acute dysregulation with drug administration per se. Multiple blood draws to monitor immunity after patients are off therapy will also be important. Unfortunately, contextual factors relevant to blood draws may also be important for chemotherapy patients. Data from Bovbjerg et al.

(1990) suggest that psychological factors may operate for conditioned immune suppression following cytotoxic chemotherapy much as they do for other chemotherapy side effects, such as anticipatory nausea and vomiting.

Third, skeptics often note a related concern—the magnitude of change from psychological and behavioral factors that would be needed to affect immunity (or cancer progression) is unknown. We agree that such data are unavailable. However, the absence of this data is not unique to the PNI field but characterizes much of the basic research in immunology and cancer. For example, there are no such data linking changes in immune responses and disease progression for many of the current biological response modifiers (e.g., lymphokine-activated killer cells or interferons) being tested as cancer therapies. Immunotherapies are tested on the basis of their mechanisms at the level of the cell, and their effect on clinical outcomes (i.e., disease progression) is unknown but is seen as the relevant question to determine through clinical trials. The inability to specify the magnitude of change is not unique to this paradigm test for a psychological therapy, as the same criticism could be leveled against the testing of any new chemotherapeutic or chemopreventive agent. To illustrate, the current testing of Tamoxifen for breast cancer prevention is based on relevant but indirect lines of support. There is experimental support that Tamoxifen affects both the initiation and promotion of tumors in animal studies, and it has lengthened disease-free survival and reduced the incidence of contralateral disease in women with breast cancer (Fisher, 1991; NSABP Protocol P-1). These data (and the fact that toxicity from Tomoxifen is low) were sufficiently encouraging to embark on a chemopreventive trial with 16,000 healthy women—even without two critical lines of evidence: (a) the precise mechanisms through which Tomoxifen achieves its effect are unknown and (b) there is only limited support for Tomoxifen's ability to increase survival rates in women with breast cancer (Fisher, 1991). Thus, it would seem unusual to hold tests of psychological therapies (which by their nature are nontoxic) to higher standards than the ones used for clinical trials of immunotherapies, new agents, or new uses of old agents.

Finally, a related methodologic concern is that the effects of stress on immune responses are small and are usually within normal ranges. We agree with this characterization, as it holds for the correlations with stress (Herbert & Cohen, 1993b), the psychological intervention studies (Kiecolt-Glaser & Glaser, 1992; Kiecolt-Glaser, Glaser, et al., 1985), and experimental studies of self-disclosure (Pennebaker, Kiecolt-Glaser, & Glaser, 1988) or relevant (personality) disclosure styles (Esterling, Antoni, Fletcher, Margulies, & Schneiderman, in press). But in all of these lines of research—research programs that use different paradigms, different subject populations, and documentation of psychological changes—the findings are consistent for the direction of the effect (i.e., immune downregulation with heightened distress) and for the effects to covary with experimental manipulation via psychological interventions or methods (e.g., ranging from brief self-disclosure for healthy individuals to eight-week interventions for cancer patients). Thus, although the immune effects are small, they are robust across samples and manipulations. Furthermore, these supportive findings include studies with cancer patients (Fawzy et al., 1990) and the same type of manipulations (Esterling et al., in press; Kiecolt-Glaser, Glaser, et al., 1985) that would be offered in psychological therapies.

Conclusion

Several studies have documented that quality of life benefits, such as reduced emotional distress, enhanced social adjustment, adaptive behavioral coping, symptom improvement (e.g., pain reduction or stabilization), and so forth, accrue from a psychosocial intervention offered to cancer patients. In contrast, health behaviors and compliance have rarely been intervention targets, although data suggest that such a broadened approach would be very effective. We view stress (quality of life), health behaviors, and compliance as the major factors in adjustment to the cancer stressor. Also, part of the biobehavioral model is the biological system, which may be one of the more important ones for moderating the effects of stress on disease processes, the immune system. The framework we have outlined addresses an important research need, as prior quality of life intervention studies have been in large part atheoretical. The proposed model endeavors to clarify the importance of psychological and behavioral factors for cancer patients and to clarify the routes by which such factors might have important health consequences.

References

Akimoto, M., Nakajima, Y., Tan, M., Ishii, H., Iwasaki, H., & Abe, R. (1986). Assessment of host immune response in breast cancer patients. *Cancer Detection and Prevention, 9,* 311–317.

American Cancer Society. (1994). *Cancer facts and figures—1993.* New York: Author.

Andersen, B. L. (Ed.). (1986). *Women with cancer: Psychological perspectives.* New York: Springer-Verlag.

Andersen, B. L. (1989). Health psychology's contribution to addressing the cancer problem: Update on accomplishments. *Health Psychology, 8,* 683–703.

Andersen, B. L. (1992). Psychological interventions for cancer patients to enhance the quality of life. *Journal of Consulting and Clinical Psychology, 60,* 552–568.

Andersen, B. L. (1994). Predicting sexual and psychological morbidity and improving quality of life for women with gynecologic cancer. *Cancer, 71,* 1678–1690.

Andersen, B. L. (in press). Surviving cancer. *Cancer.*

Andersen, B. L., Anderson, B., & deProsse, C. (1989a). Controlled prospective longitudinal study of women with cancer: I. Sexual functioning outcomes. *Journal of Consulting and Clinical Psychology, 57,* 683–691.

Andersen, B. L., Anderson, B., & deProsse, C. (1989b). Controlled prospective longitudinal study of women with cancer: II. Psychological outcomes. *Journal of Consulting and Clinical Psychology, 57,* 692–697.

Andersen, B. L., & Turnquist, D. C. (1985, May). *Emotions and immunity: Response to the diagnosis of cancer.* Paper presented at the meeting of the Midwestern Psychological Association, Chicago.

Andrykowski, M. A., & Otis, M. L. (1990). Development of learned food aversions in humans: Investigation in a "natural laboratory" of cancer chemotherapy. *Appetite, 14,* 145–158.

Bard, M., & Sutherland, A. M. (1952). Adaptation to radical mastectomy. *Cancer, 8,* 656–671.

Baron, R. S., Cutrona, C. E., Hicklin, D., Russel, D. W., & Lubaroff, D. M. (1990). Social support and immune function among spouses of cancer patients. *Journal of Personality and Social Psychology, 59,* 344–352.

Baum, A. (1990). Stress, intrusive imagery, and chronic distress. *Health Psychology, 9,* 653–675.

Baum, A., Grunberg, N., & Singer, J. (1982). The use of psychological and neuroendocrinological measurements in the study of stress. *Health Psychology, 1,* 217–236.

Ben-Eliyahu, S., Yirmirya, R., Liebeskind, J. C., Taylor, A. N., & Gale, R. P. (1991). Stress increases metastatic spread of a mammary tumor in rats: Evidence for mediation by the immune system. *Brain, Behavior, and Immunity, 5,* 193–205.

Berger, D., Braverman, A., Sohn, C. K., & Morrow, M. (1988). Patient compliance with aggressive multimodal therapy in locally advanced breast cancer. *Cancer, 61,* 1453–1456.

Berkman, L. F., & Syme, S. L. (1979). Social networks, host resistance, and mortality: A nine year follow-up study of Alameda County residents. *American Journal of Epidemiology, 109,* 186–204.

Bernstein, I. L. (1986). Etiology of anorexia in cancer. *Cancer, 58,* 1881–1886.

Bodey, G. P. (1986). Infection in cancer patients: A continuing association. *American Journal of Medicine, 61,* 11–26.

Bodnar, J. C., & Kiecolt-Glaser, J. K. (in press). Caregiver depression after bereavement: Chronic stress isn't over when it's over. *Psychology and Aging.*

Bonadonna, G., & Valagussa, P. (1981). Dose-response effect of adjuvant chemotherapy in breast cancer. *New England Journal of Medicine, 304,* 10–46.

Bonneau, F. H., Sheridan, J. F., Feng, N., & Glaser, R. (in press). Stress-induced modulation of the primary cellular immune response to herpes simplex virus infection is mediated by both adrenal-dependent and adrenal-independent mechanism. *Journal of Neuroimmunology.*

Boring, C. C., Squires, T. S., Tong, T., & Montgomery, S. (1994). Cancer statistics, 1994. *Ca-A Cancer Journal for Clinicians, 44*(1), 7–26.

Bovbjerg, D. H., Redd, W. H., Maier, L. A., Holland, J. C., Lesko, L. M., Niedzwiecki, D., Rubin, S. C., & Hakes, T. B. (1990). Anticipatory immune suppression and nausea in women receiving cyclic chemotherapy for ovarian cancer. *Journal of Consulting and Clinical Psychology, 58,* 153–157.

Cain, E. N., Kohorn, E. I., Quinlan, D. M., Latimer, K., & Schwartz, P. E. (1986). Psychosocial benefits of a cancer support group. *Cancer, 57,* 183–189.

Capone, M. A., Good, R. S., Westie, K. S., & Jacobson, A. F. (1980). Psychosocial rehabilitation of gynecologic oncology patients. *Archives of Physical Medicine and Rehabilitation, 61,* 128–132.

Cella, D. F., & Tross, S. (1986). Psychological adjustment to survival from Hodgkin's disease. *Journal of Consulting and Clinical Psychology, 54,* 616–622.

Chandra, R. K., & Newberne, P. M. (1977). *Nutrition, immunity, and infection: Mechanisms of interactions.* New York: Plenum.

Cianciolo, G. J., & Snyderman, R. (1983). Neoplasia and mononuclear phagocyte function. In R. B. Herberman & H. Friedman (Eds.), *The reticuloendothelial system: A comprehensive treatise: Vol. 5. Cancer* (pp. 193–216). New York: Plenum.

Clark, G. M., & McGuire, W. L. (1992). Defining the high-risk breast cancer patient. In I. C. Henderson (Ed.), *Adjuvant therapy of breast cancer* (pp. 161–187). Norwell, MA: Kluwer Academic.

Cohen, S., Tyrrell, D. A., & Smith, A. P. (1991). Psychological stress in humans and susceptibility to the common cold. *New England Journal of Medicine, 325,* 606–612.

Cohen, S., & Williamson, G. M. (1991). Stress and infectious disease in humans. *Psychological Bulletin, 109,* 5–24.

Coronary Drug Project Research Group. (1980). Influence of adherence to treatment and response of cholesterol on mortality in the Coronary Drug Project. *New England Journal of Medicine, 303,* 1038–1041.

Davis, H. (1986). Effects of biofeedback and cognitive therapy on stress in patients with breast cancer. *Psychological Reports, 59,* 967–974.

Derogatis, L. R., Lipman, R. S., Rickels, K., Uhlenhuth, E. H., & Covi, L. (1974). The Hopkins Symptom Checklist (HSCL): A measure of primary symptom dimensions. In P. Pichot (Ed.), *Psychological measurements in psychopharmacology: Modern problems in pharmacopsychiatry* (Vol. 7, pp. 79–110). Basel, Switzerland: Karger.

Dews, P. B. (Ed.). (1984). *Caffeine.* New York: Springer-Verlag.

DeWys, W. (1982). Pathophysiology of cancer cachexia: Current understanding and areas for future research. *Cancer Research, 42,* 721–726.

DeWys, W. (1985). Nutritional problems in cancer patients: Overview and perspective. In T. G. Burish, S. M. Levy, & B. E. Meyerowitz (Eds.), *Cancer, nutrition, and eating behavior: A biobehavioral perspective* (pp. 135–148). Hillsdale, NJ: Erlbaum.

DiMatteo, M. R., & DiNicola, D. D. (1982). *Achieving patient compliance.* Elmsford, NY: Pergamon Press.

Dubbert, P. M. (1992). Exercise in behavioral medicine. *Journal of Consulting and Clinical Psychology, 60,* 613–618.

Dunbar-Jacob, J., Dwyer, K., & Dunning, E. J. (1991). Compliance with antihypertensive regimen: A review of the research in the 1980's. *Annals of Behavioral Medicine, 13,* 31–39.

Ehrke, M. J., Mihich, E., Berd, D., & Mastrangelo, M. J. (1989). Effects of anticancer drugs on the immune system in humans. *Seminars in Oncology, 16,* 230–253.

Endicott, J., & Spitzer, R. L. (1978). A diagnostic interview: The Schedule for Affective Disorders and Schizophrenia. *Archives of General Psychiatry, 35,* 837–844.

Epstein, L. (1984). The direct effects of compliance upon outcome. *Health Psychology, 3,* 385–393.

Esterling, B. A., Antoni, M. H., Fletcher, M. A., Margulies, S., & Schneiderman, N. (in press). Emotional disclosure through writing or speaking modulates latent Epstein-Barr virus reactivity reactivation. *Journal of Consulting and Clinical Psychology.*

Esterling, B. A., Kiecolt-Glaser, J. K., Bodnar, J. C., & Glaser, R. (in press). Chronic caregiving stress in older adults is associated with a depression in the natural killer cell response to cytokines. *Health Psychology.*

Fawzy, F. I., Fawzy, N. W., Hyun, C. S., Gutherie, D., Fahey, J. L., & Morton, D. (1993). Malignant melanoma: Effects of an early structured psychiatric intervention, coping, and affective state on recurrence and survival six years later. *Archives of General Psychiatry, 50,* 681–689.

Fawzy, F. I., Kemeny, M. E., Fawzy, N. W., Elashoff, R., Morton, D., Cousins, N., & Fahey, J. L. (1990). A structured psychiatric intervention for cancer patients: I. Changes over time in immunological measures. *Archives of General Psychiatry, 47,* 729–735.

Felten, D. L., & Felten, S. Y. (1991). Innervation of lymphoid tissue. In R. Ader, D. L. Felten, & N. Cohen (Eds.), *Psychoneuroimmunology* (pp. 87–101). San Diego, CA: Academic Press.

Felten, D. L., Felten, S. Y., Bellinger, D. L., Carlson, S. L., Ackerman, K., Madden, K. S., Olschowki, J. A., & Livnat, S. (1987). Noradrenergic sympathetic neural interactions with the immune system: Structure and function. *Immunological Reviews, 100,* 225–260.

Fisher, B. (1991, December 20). *NSABP (National Surgical Adjuvant Breast Program) Protocol P-1: A clinical trial to determine the worth of Tamoxifen for preventing breast cancer.* (Available from National Cancer Institute)

Fleming, I., Baum, A., Davidson, L. M., Rectanus, E., & McArdle, S. (1987). Chronic stress as a factor in physiologic reactivity to challenge. *Health Psychology, 6,* 221–237.

Forester, B., Kornfeld, D. S., & Fleiss, J. L. (1985). Psychotherapy during radiotherapy: Effects on emotional and physical distress. *American Journal of Psychiatry, 142,* 22–27.

Fox, B. H. (1976). Psychosocial epideminology of cancer. In J. W. Cullen, B. H. Fox, & R. N. Isom (Eds.), *Cancer: The behavioral dimension* (pp. 11–22). New York: Raven Press.

Fox, B. H. (1978). Premorbid psychological factors as related to cancer incidence. *Journal of Behavioral Medicine, 1*, 45–133.

Fox, B. H. (1992). LeShan's hypothesis is provocative, but is it plausible? *Advances, The Journal of Mind-Body Health, 8*(2), 82–84.

Friedman, H., Klein, T., & Specter, S. (1991). Immunosuppression by marijuana and components. In R. Ader, D. L. Felten, & N. Cohen (Eds.), *Psychoneuroimmunology* (pp. 66–85). San Diego, CA: Academic Press.

Friedman, H. S., Tucker, J. S., Tomlinson-Keasey, C., Schwartz, J. E., Wingard, D. L., & Criqui, M. H. (1993). Does childhood personality predict longevity? *Journal of Personality and Social Psychology, 65*, 176–185.

George, L. K., & Gwyther, L. P. (1984, November). *The dynamics of caregiver burden: Changes in caregiver well-being over time.* Paper presented at the annual meetings of the Gerontological Society of America, San Antonio, TX.

Glaser, R., Kiecolt-Glaser, J. K., Bonneau, R., Malarkey, W., Kennedy, S., & Hughes, J. (1992). Stress-induced modulation of the immune response to recombinant hepatitis B vaccine. *Psychosomatic Medicine, 54*, 22–29.

Glaser, R., Rice, J., Sheridan, J., Fertel, R., Stout, J. C., Speicher, C. E., Pinsky, D., Kotur, M., Post, A., Beck, M., & Kiecolt-Glaser, J. K. (1987). Stress-related immune suppression: Health implications. *Brain, Behavior, and Immunity, 1*, 7–20.

Glaser, R., Rice, J., Speicher, C. E., Stout, J. C., & Kiecolt-Glaser, J. K. (1986). Stress depresses interferon production concomitant with a decrease in natural killer cell activity. *Behavioral Neuroscience, 100*, 675–678.

Goodkin, K., Antoni, M. H., Sevin, B., & Fox, B. H. (1993a). A partially testable, predictive model of psychosocial factors in the etiology of cervical cancer: I. Biological, psychological and social aspects. *Psycho-oncology, 2*, 79–98.

Goodkin, K., Antoni, M. H., Sevin, B., & Fox, B. H. (1993b). A partially testable, predictive model of psychosocial factors in the etiology of cervical cancer: II. Bioimmunological, psychoneuroimmunological and socioimmunological aspects, critique and prospective integration. *Psycho-oncology, 2*, 99–121.

Gordon, W. A., Freidenbergs, I., Diller, L., Hibberd, M., Wold, C., Levine, L., Lipkins, R., Ezrachi, O., & Lucido, O. (1980). Efficacy of psychosocial investigation with cancer patients. *Journal of Consulting and Clinical Psychology, 48*, 743–759.

Gorelik, E., & Herberman, R. B. (1986). Role of natural killer cells in the control of tumor growth and metastatic spread. In R. B. Herberman (Ed.), *Cancer immunology: Innovative approaches to therapy* (pp. 151–176). Dordrecht, The Netherlands: Martinus Nijhoff.

Gruber, B. L., Hersh, S. P., Hall, N. R., Waletzky, L. R., Kunz, J. F., Carpenter, J. K., Kverno, K. S., & Weiss, S. M. (1993). Immunological responses of breast cancer patients to behavioral interventions. *Biofeedback and Self-Regulation, 18*, 1–22.

Grunberg, N. E., & Baum, A. (1985). Biological commonalities of stress and substance abuse. In S. Shiffman & T. A. Wills (Eds.), *Coping and substance use* (pp. 25–62). San Diego, CA: Academic Press.

Haynes, R. B., & Dantes, R. (1987). Patient compliance and the conduct and interpretation of therapeutic trials. *Controlled Clinical Trials, 8*, 12–19.

Haynes, R. B., Taylor, R. B., & Sackett, D. L. (Eds.). (1979). *Compliance in health care.* Baltimore: Johns Hopkins University Press.

Herberman, R. B. (1991). Principles of tumor immunology. In A. I. Holleb, D. J. Fink, & G. P. Murphy (Eds.), *Textbook of clinical oncology* (pp. 69–79). Atlanta, GA: American Cancer Society.

Herbert, T. B., & Cohen, S. (1993a). Depression and immunity: A meta-analytic review. *Psychological Bulletin, 113*, 472–486.

Herbert, T. B., & Cohen, S. (1993b). Stress and immunity in humans: A meta-analytic review. *Psychosomatic Medicine, 55*, 364–379.

Holt, P. G. (1987). Immune and inflammatory function in cigarette smokers, *Thorax, 42,* 241–249.

Houts, P. S., Whitney, C. W., Mortel, R., & Bartholomew, M. J. (1986). Former cancer patients as counselors of newly diagnosed cancer patients. *Journal of the National Cancer Institute, 76,* 793–796.

Innagaki, J., Rodriguez, V., & Bodey, G. P. (1974). Causes of death in cancer patients. *Cancer, 33,* 568–573.

Ironson, G., LaPerriere, A., Antoni, M., O'Hearn, P., Schneiderman, N., Klimas, N., & Fletcher, M. A. (1990). Changes in immune and psychological measures as a function of anticipation and reaction to news of HIV-A antibody status. *Psychosomatic Medicine, 52,* 247–270.

Irwin, M., Brown, M., Patterson, T., Hauger, R., Mascovich, A., & Grant, I. (1992). Neuropeptide Y and natural killer activity: Findings in depression and Alzheimer caregiver stress. *FASEB J, 5,* 3100–3107.

Irwin, M., Smith, T. L., & Gillin, J. C. (1992). Electroencephalographic sleep and natural killer activity in depressed patients and control subjects. *Psychosomatic Medicine, 54,* 10–21.

Jacobs, C., Ross, R. D., Walker, I. M., & Stockdale, F. E. (1983). Behavior of cancer patients: A randomized study of the effects of education and peer support groups. *American Journal of Clinical Oncology, 6,* 347–353.

Jaffe, J. H. (1980). Drug addiction and drug abuse. In A. G. Gilman, L. S. Goodman, & A. Gilman (Eds.), *The pharmacological basis of therapeutics* (6th ed., pp. 150–175). New York: Macmillan.

Kaplan, R. M. (1990). Behavior as the central outcome in health care. *American Psychologist, 45,* 1211–1220.

Kaplan, R. M. (1992). Controversies in dietary intervention. *Annals of Behavioral Medicine, 14,* 99–100.

Kaplan, R. M., & Simon, H. J. (1990). Compliance in medical care: Reconsideration of self-predictions. *Annals of Behavioral Medicine, 12,* 66–71.

Kempf, R. A., & Mitchell, M. S. (1984a). Effects of chemotherapeutic agents on the immune response: I. *Cancer Investigation, 2,* 459–466.

Kempf, R. A., & Mitchell, M. S. (1984b). Effects of chemotherapeutic agents on the immune response: II. *Cancer Investigation, 3,* 23–33.

Ketchel, S. J., & Rodriguez, V. (1987). Acute infections in cancer patients. *Seminars in Oncology, 5,* 167–179.

Khoo, S. K., MacKay, E., & Daunter, B. (1979). Dinitrochlorobenzene reactivity of women with cancer of the ovary, cervix, and corpus uteri. *International Journal of Gynaecology and Obstetrics, 17,* 58–65.

Kiecolt-Glaser, J. K., Cacioppo, J. T., Malarkey, W. B., & Glaser, R. (1992). Acute psychological stressors and short-term immune changes: What, why, for whom, and to what extent? *Psychosomatic Medicine, 54,* 680–685.

Kiecolt-Glaser, J. K., Dura, J. R., Speicher, C. E., Trask, O. J., & Glaser, R. (1991). Spousal caregivers of dementia victims: Longitudinal changes in immunity and health. *Psychosomatic Medicine, 53,* 345–362.

Kiecolt-Glaser, J. K., Fisher, L., Ogrocki, P., Stout, J. C., Speicher, C. E., & Glaser, R. (1987). Marital quality, marital disruption, and immune function. *Psychosomatic Medicine, 49,* 13–34.

Kiecolt-Glaser, J. K., Garner, W., Speicher, C. E., Penn, G., & Glaser, R. (1984). Psychosocial modifiers of immunocompetence in medical students. *Psychosomatic Medicine, 46,* 7–14.

Kiecolt-Glaser, J. K., & Glaser, R. (1988a). Methodological issues in behavioral immunology research with humans. *Brain, Behavior, and Immunity, 2,* 67–78.

Kiecolt-Glaser, J. K., & Glaser, R. (1988b). Psychological influences on immunity: Implications for AIDS. *American Psychologist, 43,* 892–898.

Kiecolt-Glaser, J. K., & Glaser, R. (1992). Psychoneuroimmunology: Can psychological interventions modulate immunity? *Journal of Consulting and Clinical Psychology, 60,* 569–575.

Kiecolt-Glaser, J. K., Glaser, R., Dyer, C., Shuttleworth, E., Ogrocki, P., & Speicher, C. E. (1987). Chronic stress and immunity in family caregivers of Alzheimer's disease victims. *Psychosomatic Medicine, 49,* 523–535.

Kiecolt-Glaser, J. K., Glaser, R., Willinger, D., Stout, J., Messick, G., Sheppard, S., Ricker, D., Romisher, S. C., Briner, W., Bonnell, G., & Donnerberg, R. (1985). Psychosocial enhancement of immunocompetence in a geriatric population. *Health Psychology, 4,* 25–41.

Kikuchi, T., Kita, T., & Oomori, K. (1988). Interleukin-2 activity in peripheral blood mononuclear cells of patients with gynecologic malignancies. *Medical Oncology Tumor Pharmacotherapy, 5,* 85–90.

Lacks, P., & Morin, C. M. (1992). Recent advances in the assessment and treatment of insomnia. *Journal of Consulting and Clinical Psychology, 60,* 586–594.

Lane, J. D., & Williams, R. B. (1985). Caffeine affects cardiovascular responses to stress. *Psychophysiology, 22,* 648–655.

LaPerriere, A. R., Antoni, M. H., Schneiderman, N., Ironson, G., Klimas, N., Caralis, P., & Fletcher, M. A. (1990). Exercise intervention attenuates emotional distress and natural killer cell decrements following notification of positive serologic status for HIV-A. *Biofeedback and Self-Regulation, 15,* 229–242.

LaPorte, R. E., Montoye, H. J., & Caspersen, C. J. (1985). Assessment of physical activity in epidemiologic research: Problems and prospects. *Public Health Reports, 100,* 131–146.

Lebovits, A. H., Strain, J. J., Schleifer, S. J., Tanaka, J. S., Bhardwaj, S., & Messe, M. R. (1990). Patient noncompliance with self-administered chemotherapy. *Cancer, 65,* 17–22.

Lepore, S. J., Evans, G. W., & Schneider, M. L. (1991). Dynamic role of social support in the link between chronic stress and psychological distress. *Journal of Personality and Social Psychology, 61,* 899–909.

LeShan, L. (1991). A new question in studying psychosocial interventions and cancer. *Advances, The Journal of Mind–Body Health, 7,* 69–71.

LeShan, L. (1992). Whatever we do, we should do with as full consciousness as possible of the possible dangers to our patients. *Advances, The Journal of Mind-Body Health, 8,* 86–87.

Levine, P. H., Ablashi, D. V., Nonoyama, M., Pearson, G. R., & Glaser, R. (Eds.). (1987). *Epstein-Barr virus and human disease.* Clifton, NJ: Humana Press.

Levy, S. M., Herberman, R. B., Lee, J., Whiteside, T., Kirkwood, J., & McFeeley, S. (1990). Estrogen receptor concentration and social factors as predictors of natural killer cell activity in early-stage breast cancer patients. *Natural Immunity and Cell Growth Regulation, 9,* 313–324.

Levy, S. M., Herberman, R. B., Lippman, M., D'Angelo, T., & Lee, J. (1991, Summer). Immunological and psychosocial predictors of disease recurrence in patients with early stage breast cancer. *Behavioral Medicine,* 67–75.

Levy, S. M., Herberman, R. B., Maluish, A. M., Schlein, B., & Lippman, M. (1985). Prognostic risk assessment in primary breast cancer by behavioral and immunological parameters. *Health Psychology, 4,* 99–113.

Levy, S. M., Lee, J., Bagley, C., & Lippman, M. (1988). Survival hazards analysis in first recurrent breast cancer patients: Seven-year followup. *Psychosomatic Medicine, 50,* 520–528.

Linn, M. W., Linn, B. S., & Harris, R. (1982). Effects of counseling for late stage cancer patients. *Cancer, 49,* 1048–1055.

Ludwig, C. U., Hartmann, D., Landmann, R., Wesp, M., Rosenfelder, G., Stucki, D., Buser, M., & Obrecht, J. P. (1985). Unaltered immunocompetence in patients with nondisseminated breast cancer at the time of diagnosis. *Cancer, 55,* 1673–1678.

MacGregor, R. R. (1986). Alcohol and immune defense. *Journal of the American Medical Association, 256,* 1474–1479.

MacVicar, M., Winningham, M., & Nickel, J. (1989). Effects of aerobic interval training on cancer patients' functional capacity. *Nursing Research, 38,* 348–351.

Maguire, P., Brooke, M., Tait, A., Thomas, C., & Sellwood, R. (1983). The effect of counselling on physical disability and social recovery after mastectomy. *Clinical Oncology, 9,* 319–324.

Mandell, G. L., Fisher, R. I., Bostick, F., & Young, R. C. (1979). Ovarian cancer: A solid tumor with evidence of normal cellular immune function but abnormal B-cell function. *American Journal of Medicine, 66,* 621–627.

McKinnon, W., Weisse, C. S., Reynolds, C. P., Bowles, C. A., & Baum, A. (1989). Chronic stress, leukocyte subpopulations, and humoral response to latent viruses. *Health Psychology, 8,* 399–402.

McNair, D. M., Lorr, M., & Droppleman, L. F. (1981). *Profile of Mood States.* San Diego, CA: Educational and Testing Service.

Morley, J. E., Benton, D., & Solomon, G. F. (1991). The role of stress and opioids as regulators of the immune response. In J. A. McCubbin, P. G. Kaufmann, & C. B. Nemeroff (Eds.), *Stress, neuropeptides and systemic disease* (pp. 221–231). San Diego, CA: Academic Press.

Moulder, J. E., Dutreix, J., Rockwell, S., & Sieman, D. W. (1988). Applicability of animal tumor data to cancer therapy in humans. *International Journal of Radiation Oncology and Biological Physics, 14,* 913–927.

Moyers, W. (1993). *Healing and the mind.* New York: Bantam, Dell, & Doubleday.

Nalick, R. H., DiSaia, R. J., Rea, T. H., & Morrow, C. P. (1974). Immunocompetence and prognosis in patients with gynecologic cancer. *Gynecologic Oncology, 2,* 81–85.

O'Leary, A. (1990). Stress, emotion, and human immune function. *Psychological Bulletin, 108,* 363–382.

Pennebaker, J. W., Kiecolt-Glaser, J. K., & Glaser, R. (1988). Disclosure of traumas and immune function: Health implications for psychotherapy. *Journal of Consulting and Clinical Psychology, 56,* 239–245.

Pickard-Holley, S. (1991). Fatigue in cancer patients. *Cancer Nursing, 14,* 13–19.

Rabin, B. S., Cohen, S., Ganguli, R., Lysle, D. T., & Cunnick, J. E. (1989). Bidirectional interaction between the central nervous system and the immune system. *Critical Reviews in Immunology, 9,* 279–312.

Richardson, J. L., Marks, G., Anderson Johnson, C., Graham, J. W., Chan, K. K., Selser, J. N., Kishbaugh, C., Barranday, Y., & Levine, A. M. (1987). Path model of multidimensional compliance with cancer therapy. *Health Psychology, 6,* 183–207.

Richardson, J. L., Marks, G., & Levine, A. (1988). The influence of symptoms of disease and side effects of treatment on compliance with cancer therapy. *Journal of Clinical Oncology, 6,* 1746–1752.

Rhodes, V., Watson, P., & Hanson, B. (1988). Patients' descriptions of the influence of tiredness and weakness on self-care abilities. *Cancer Nursing, 11,* 188–194.

Roberts, D., Andersen, B. L., & Lubaroff, A. (1994). *Stress and immunity at cancer diagnosis.* Manuscript in preparation.

Robinson, J. K. (1990). Behavior modification obtained by sun protection education coupled with removal of a skin cancer. *Archives of Dermatology, 126,* 477–481.

Sabharwal, P. J., Glaser, R., Lafuse, W., Liu, Q., Arkins, S., Koojiman, R., Lutz, L., Kelley, K. W., & Malarkey, W. B. (1992). Prolactic synthesis and secretion by human peripheral blood mononuclear cells: An autocrine growth factor for lymphoproliferation. *Proceedings of the National Academy of Science, 89,* 7713–7716.

Sallis, J. F., Haskell, W. L., Fortmann, S. P., Vranizan, K. M., Taylor, C. B., & Solomon, D. S. (1986). Lifetime history of relapse from exercise. *Addictive Behaviors, 15,* 573–579.

Sapolsky, R. M., Krey, L. C., & McEwen, B. S. (1986). The neuroendocrinology of stress and aging: The glucocorticoid cascade hypothesis. *Endocrine Review, 7,* 284–301.

Sgoutas-Emch, S. A., Cacioppo, J. T., Uchino, B., Malarkey, W., Pearl, D., Kiecolt-Glaser, J. K., & Glaser R. (in press). The effects of an acute psychological stressor on cardiovascular, endocrine, and cellular immune responses: A prospective study of individuals high and low in heart rate reactivity. *Psychophysiology.*

Sharma, D., Gupta, R. M., & Kadian, V. (1979). Clinical and immunological study of patients with cancer of the cervix. *Indiana Journal of Medical Research, 70,* 793–801.

Slater, J. M., Ngo, E., & Lau, B. H. S. (1976). Effect of therapeutic irradiation on the immune responses. *Journal of Radiology, 126,* 313–320.

Smith, J. C., Blumsach, J. T., & Bilek, F. S. (1985). Radiation-induced taste aversions in rats and humans. In T. G. Burish, S. M. Levy, & B. E. Meyerowitz (Eds.), *Cancer, nutrition, and eating behavior: A biobehavioral perspective* (pp. 77–101). Hillsdale, NJ: Erlbaum.

Spiegel, D., Bloom, H. C., Kraemer, J. R., & Gottheil, E. (1989, October 14). Effect of psychosocial treatment on survival of patients with metastatic breast cancer. *The Lancet,* 888–901.

Spiegel, D., & Bloom, J. R. (1983). Group therapy and hypnosis reduce metastatic breast carcinoma pain. *Psychosomatic Medicine, 45,* 333–339.

Spiegel, D., Bloom, J. R., & Yalom, I. (1981). Group support for patients with metastatic cancer: A randomized outcome study. *Archives of General Psychiatry, 38,* 527–533.

Stein, J. A., Adler, A., & BenEfran, S. (1976). Immunocompetence, immunosuppression and human breast cancer: I. An analysis of their relationship by known parameters of cell-mediated immunity in well-defined clinical stages of disease. *Cancer, 38,* 1171–1187.

Takasugi, M., Ramseyer, A., & Takasugi, J. (1977). Decline of natural non-selective cell mediated cytotoxicity in patients with tumor progression. *Cancer Research, 37,* 413–418.

Telch, C. F., & Telch, M. J. (1986). Group coping skills instruction and supportive group therapy for cancer patients: A comparison of strategies. *Journal of Consulting and Clinical Psychology, 54,* 802–808.

Temoshok, L., & Dreher, H. (1992). *Type C and cancer.* New York: Random House.

ten Have-de Labije, J., & Balner, H. (1991). *Coping with cancer and beyond: Cancer treatment and mental health.* Lisse, The Netherlands: Swets & Zeitlinger.

Uchino, B. N., Kiecolt-Glaser, J. K., & Cacioppo, J. T. (1992). Age and social support: Effects on cardiovascular functioning in caregivers of relatives with Alzheimer's disease. *Journal of Personality and Social Psychology, 63,* 839–846.

Weiss, C. S. (1992). Depression and immunocompetence: A review of the literature. *Psychological Bulletin, 111,* 475–489.

Wellisch, D. K., Wolcott, D. L., Pasnau, R. O., Fawzy, F. I., & Landsverk, J. (1989). An evaluation of the psychosocial problems of the homebound cancer patient: Relationship of patient adjustment to family problems. *Journal of Psychosocial Research, 7,* 55–76.

Winegard, J. R., Curbow, B., Baker, F., & Piantadosi, S. (1991). Health, functional status, and employment of adult survivors of bone marrow transplantation. *Annals of Internal Medicine, 114,* 113–118.

Yellen, S. B., Cella, D. F., & Bonomi, A. (1993). Quality of life in people with Hodgkin's disease. *Oncology, 7*(8), 41–45.

Part II

Coping and Adjusting

Chapter 2
PATTERNS OF COPING WITH CANCER

Christine Dunkel-Schetter, Lawrence G. Feinstein, Shelley E. Taylor, and
Roberta L. Falke

For many years, there has been interest in how people cope with cancer. Important descriptive studies were completed in the 1950s (e.g., Bard & Sutherland, 1955; Quint, 1965; Shands, Finesinger, Cobb, & Abrams, 1951) emphasizing unconscious defenses such as denial and maladaptive coping patterns (see Meyerowitz, Heinrich, & Schag, 1983, for a review). Weisman (1979) and Weisman and Worden (1976–1977) later conducted systematic research on coping with cancer using a variety of assessment methods and revealed relationships between patterns of coping and emotional distress. Weisman (1979) defined coping as "what one does about a perceived problem in order to bring about relief, reward, quiescence, or equilibrium" (p. 27). Lazarus and Folkman (1984) defined coping similarly—as cognitive and behavioral efforts to manage demands appraised as taxing or exceeding resources.

Coping efforts may be distinguished from their effects on the stressful situation, on emotional well-being, and on subsequent health and adjustment. Such efforts have been shown to be a function of both person and situation factors (Fleishman, 1984; Folkman, Lazarus, Gruen, & DeLongis, 1986; Holahan & Moos, 1987; Parkes, 1986). However, little is known about what predisposes individuals with cancer to cope in specific ways. Why does one cancer patient construe his or her situation in a positive light, whereas another does not? What predisposes a person to use avoidant coping strategies, such as fantasizing or social withdrawal, in response to cancer? Which individuals are most likely to respond by seeking and using available support? Such information would be valuable in cancer rehabilitation and in developing a further understanding of the determinants of coping in general.

The goal of this research was to examine factors identified in the stress and coping literature that might predispose a person to cope with cancer in various ways. Past research has indicated that an individual will cope differently as a function of the particular stressful situation involved (Folkman & Lazarus, 1980; McCrae, 1984; Pearlin & Schooler, 1978). Cancer includes a wide range of situations with which to cope—such as painful or frightening symptoms, ambiguity about the prognosis, and changes in social relationships. An adaptive strategy for coping with physical discomfort might be problem focused (e.g., seeking the advice of one's physician or taking medication), whereas the best strategies for dealing with ambiguity about the future might be emotion regulating (e.g., distraction or avoidance).

Situational factors—site of cancer, stage of the disease, time since diagnosis,

Reprinted from *Health Psychology, 11*(2), 79–87. (1992). Copyright © 1992 by the American Psychological Association. Used with permission of the author.

This research was supported by National Cancer Institute Grant US-PHS CA 36409 to Shelley E. Taylor, by National Institute of Mental Health (NIMH) Research Scientist Development Award MH 00311 to Shelley E. Taylor, and by NIMH Institutional Training Grant MH15750 to Christine Dunkel-Schetter and Shelley E. Taylor.

We are grateful to Anne Rocheleau and D. Garrett Gafford for assistance.

and whether the person is currently in treatment—are additional possible influences on coping behavior in cancer patients. People with more acute and severe medical conditions are likely to apply more of the many different coping strategies than those with less acute and less severe disease states. However, stress and coping theories emphasize subjective appraisals of the stressful situation (Hobfoll, 1989; Lazarus & Folkman, 1984; McGrath, 1970). Given the demonstrated importance of stress appraisals (Folkman, Lazarus, Dunkel-Schetter, DeLongis, & Gruen, 1986; Folkman, Lazarus, Gruen, & DeLongis, 1986), the cancer patient's perception of the degree of current stress should influence how he or she is coping at least as much as medical condition. Thus, both were expected to be significant determinants of coping.

Another set of variables that has been found to predispose individuals to cope in particular ways is sociodemographic characteristics. Higher socioeconomic status (SES) has been linked fairly consistently to particular methods of coping, although not with cancer samples (Billings & Moos, 1981; Holahan & Moos, 1987; Menaghan, 1983; Pearlin & Schooler, 1978). For example, Billings and Moos (1981) found that better educated respondents relied more on problem-focused coping and less on avoidance coping for dealing with daily problems. To what extent does this finding extend to coping with cancer? We also examined age, sex, religion, and religiosity for relationships to coping. Links between these variables and coping might offer practical implications as to which cancer patients should receive which coping interventions.

Socioenvironmental factors, such as the presence of a social network, have also been found to be related to coping (Billings & Moos, 1981; Dunkel-Schetter, Folkman, & Lazarus, 1987). For example, Cronkite and Moos (1984) found that women without family support were more likely to engage in avoidance coping. In our study, we considered whether structural aspects of the cancer patient's social network—such as marital status, number of children, and whether the person lived alone—were associated with coping. Based on past research, we expected that the absence of social relationships would be associated with more avoidance coping.

A final aim was to examine relationships between patterns of coping and emotional distress. We expected that highly distressed cancer patients would cope differently than less distressed cancer patients based on two pertinent earlier investigations (Felton, Revenson, & Hinrichsen, 1984; Weisman & Worden, 1976–1977). In both studies, positive reinterpretation was associated with less distress, and escape–avoidance was associated with more distress. However, one of the studies (Weisman & Worden, 1976–1977) found that attempts to forget the cancer were associated with high distress, whereas the other study (Felton et al., 1984) found that similar attempts, labeled *threat minimization*, were unrelated to distress. There were many differences in the samples, designs, and measures of these investigations, which may account for the discrepancy. Also, neither study controlled for severity of disease or for interindividual differences in stress appraisals in testing for relationships between distress and coping. The present study afforded opportunities (a) to clarify the relationship between coping with cancer by distraction and level of emotional distress and (b) to replicate the relationships between coping through positive reinterpretation or avoidance and emotional distress.

A major roadblock in studying coping in general and in studying cancer specifically has been the lack of consensus on the particular dimensions of coping behavior and on how to measure these dimensions (Moos & Billings, 1982; Singer, 1984; Taylor, 1984). Thus, a preliminary step to testing for correlates of coping was to identify reliable patterns or dimensions of coping with cancer. An ongoing study of cancer patients afforded an excellent opportunity to delineate patterns of coping with cancer and to investigate their correlates within the tradition of stress and coping research. In keeping with this approach, an adapted version of the most commonly used self-report coping instrument, the Ways of Coping Inventory (WOC), was used (Folkman & Lazarus, 1980; Lazarus & Folkman, 1984). In addition to gathering information on correlates of coping, we also present descriptive information on coping styles (Carver, Scheier, & Weintraub, 1989) and on flexibility of coping (Pearlin & Schooler, 1978).

Method

Procedure

The present research was conducted as part of an investigation on self-help groups and cancer (Taylor, Falke, Mazel, & Hilsberg, 1988; Taylor, Falke, Shoptaw, & Lichtman, 1986) in which a large sample of cancer patients was obtained—heterogeneous with respect to type and severity of cancer and to other characteristics such as age and SES. Cancer patients were recruited from two referral sources. Fifteen Los Angeles area oncologists whose names were obtained through the University of Southern California Cancer Center were contacted and asked to provide names and addresses of patients in their practices. In addition, leaders of 21 Southern California cancer support groups were contacted and asked to supply mailing lists of members' names and addresses. Prospective participants were mailed a letter from the research team and a letter from the physician or support group leader. These letters introduced the investigators in the study, indicated that a questionnaire would arrive within a few days, and assured respondents of the confidentiality of their answers. A return postcard permitted individuals to decline to participate. A 31-page questionnaire was later mailed to anyone who had not returned the postcard declining to participate. If the prospective respondent did not return the questionnaire within 2 weeks, a reminder postcard was sent followed by a replacement questionnaire shortly afterward. To preserve patients' confidentiality, the names obtained from physicians and self-help groups were given to a typist—blind to the topic of the study and to the sources of the names—for the purpose of typing envelopes. The researchers did not have access to the names.

One thousand sixty-eight potentially eligible individuals were contacted. Of these, 178 indicated that they were not interested (6% refusal rate), and 223 did not return the questionnaire. The research team subsequently randomly sampled nonrespondents and determined that a large percentage had died before the mailing or were ineligible to participate in the study (e.g., children or hematology patients inadvertently included on oncologists' lists). After the estimated number of ineligible participants determined by the telephone survey was subtracted, the response rate was estimated to be 80%.

Subjects

The sample consisted of 668 cancer patients. Seventy-eight percent were women, and 22% were men. They ranged in age from 21 to 88 years, with a median age of 58 years. The sample varied considerably in education and income, although 93% were White. Many sites and all stages of cancer were represented in the sample. The most common primary site of cancer was the breast (42%). Thirteen percent of the sample had gastrointestinal cancers, 11% had circulatory or lymph cancers, 9% had female reproductive cancers, 8% had respiratory cancer, 6% had musculoskeletal cancer, 5% had head and neck cancers, and 6% had other cancers (which included smaller percentages of male reproductive cancer, skin cancer, and eye cancer). Time since diagnosis ranged from newly diagnosed to first diagnosed several years ago. Seventy-two percent of the subjects had been diagnosed with initial cancers in the previous 5 years, more than 50% had been diagnosed in the previous 3 years, and about 25% had been diagnosed in the previous 18 months.

Of the 668 subjects who completed the questionnaire, 35 indicated that they had no current cancer-related stress and were not engaging in any coping. An additional 30 respondents failed to answer three or more items on the coping inventory. Consequently, the present results are based on a subsample of 603 individuals with complete coping data.

Materials

The 31-page questionnaire included sociodemographic and personal background items and items on the patient's medical condition, health care providers, social networks and support, psychotherapeutic experiences (particularly experiences with self-help groups), and stress and adjustment. Only a subset of these items was relevant to the hypotheses and questions of the present article. In addition, the questionnaire included the WOC (Lazarus & Folkman, 1984), adapted by our research team for cancer patients, and the bipolar version of the Profile of Mood States (POMS-BI; Lorr & McNair, 1982). The 72 adjectives on the POMS-BI are each rated regarding mood at present and can be scored into six bipolar subscales (e.g., Composed–Anxious, Agreeable–Hostile, Elated–Depressed). For these analyses, the subscales were combined into one index of emotional state, with high scores corresponding to more positive emotional states and low scores corresponding to more negative emotional states. The Cronbach alpha coefficient for the overall index in this study was .92.

WOC–Cancer Version (WOC–CA)

The WOC–CA was adapted in several ways to suit the present research purposes. Because it was devised for repeated assessments, the original WOC asks subjects to select a stressful episode. When single assessments are made, as in this study, the procedure would provide an isolated and possibly unrepresentative instance of the individual's coping responses. Asking about how people coped with cancer "in general," however, seemed too nonspecific. Therefore, we delineated a small set of specific cancer-related stressors based on results from past studies (Dunkel-Schetter,

1982; Revenson & Felton, 1985): (a) fear and uncertainty about the future due to cancer; (b) limitations in physical ability, appearance, or life style due to cancer; (c) acute pain, symptoms, or discomfort from illness or treatment; and (d) problems with family or friends related to cancer. These problems were listed, and respondents were asked to pick whichever one had been most stressful for them or to designate one of their own. Subjects were also asked to indicate how stressful the problem had been for them in the past 6 months on a scale ranging from *not stressful* (1) to *extremely stressful* (5).

The 51 items making up the eight factors in the revised WOC (Folkman, Lazarus, Dunkel-Schetter et al., 1986) were next evaluated for their applicability to cancer. Six items were dropped because they appeared inappropriate for cancer patients. In addition, 4 of the 67 items on the earlier version of the WOC that did not load on Folkman, Lazarus, Dunkel-Schetter et al.'s (1986) eight factors were included in our instrument because they appeared to be relevant to cancer. Three of these concerned the future (i.e., waiting or preparing for it), and 1 concerned comparison of one's own situation to hypothetical outcomes. A few of the 49 items taken from the WOC were also reworded slightly to be clearer or briefer. In addition, 4 items were added to represent various coping behaviors commonly observed in cancer patients (Dunkel-Schetter, 1982) but not already captured. The preface to the coping items read as follows:

> When we experience stress in our lives, we usually try to manage it by trying out different ways of "coping." Sometimes our attempts are successful in helping us solve a problem or feel better, and other times they are not. The next set of items is on the ways of coping you may have used in trying to manage the most stressful part of your cancer. Please read each item below and indicate *how often you tried this* in the past six months in attempting to cope with the specific problem circled above.

The response options were *does not apply/never* (0), *rarely* (1), *sometimes* (2), *often* (3), and *very often* (4). A final open-ended item asked whether subjects applied any other particular coping techniques or strategies besides those mentioned.

Other Variables

Other variables used for these analyses were:

1. Sociodemographic variables—sex, age, employment status, education, income, religion, and religiosity (one item on reported strength of spiritual belief).
2. Medical background—site of cancer, time elapsed since initial diagnosis, whether cancer was currently in remission, whether currently receiving medical treatment (chemotherapy, radiation, or recovering from surgery), and extent of functional limitations on activity.
3. Appraisal of cancer—frequency of worries about cancer in general and, from the WOC–CA, (a) what problem associated with cancer has been most stressful and (b) how stressful it was.
4. Social network—marital status, children, and living alone or with others.
5. Psychotherapeutic experiences—whether the respondent had ever attended a cancer self-help group and how frequently, evaluation of the group ex-

perience, and whether the individual had ever had psychotherapy for any
reason other than cancer.

Results

Stressful Aspects of Cancer

The most frequent problem associated with cancer in this sample was fear or uncertainty about the future, endorsed by 41% of the sample. Limitations in physical
ability were the most stressful for 24%, pain was most stressful for 12%, and problems in social relationships were most stressful for 3%. Another 9% had experienced
more than one of the problems listed, and 5% wrote in their own stressor. The
remaining 6% of the sample had not had any stress from cancer in the prior 6 months.
The mean stressfulness rating of cancer problems was 3.04 or *somewhat stressful*
(SD = 1.49).

Patterns of Coping and Their Prevalence

Factor analysis was conducted on data obtained from all subjects who specified at
least one problem with which they were coping (*N* = 603). Oblique rotation was
selected in order to permit correlation among factors (Folkman, Lazarus, Dunkel-
Schetter et al., 1986). Based on a review of coping research, we specified four
through eight factors to obtain a manageable number of coping dimensions. A five-
factor solution appeared to be most coherent and most consistent with earlier research. Table 1 lists the items for each of the five factors, their factor loadings, and
the alpha coefficients for each factor.[1]

   We labeled the factors *Seek and Use Social Support, Focus on the Positive,
Distancing, Cognitive Escape–Avoidance*, and *Behavioral Escape–Avoidance*. The
interfactor correlation coefficients were all positive, ranging from .07 to .47. Seek
and Use Social Support and Positive Focus were the most highly correlated factors,
and Seek and Use Social Support and Distancing were the least correlated factors.
Factor scores were computed based on the factor loadings in Table 1. These scores
reflect both the number of strategies used (i.e., items endorsed) of a particular type
as well as the intensity of their use.[2]

   A second method of scoring coping—proportional scores—was used for descriptive purposes (Vitaliano, Russo, Carr, Maiuro, & Becker, 1985). We computed
the proportion of each subject's total coping efforts of each of the five types. Subjects

---

   [1]The factor analysis procedures were repeated on subsets of the sample to determine whether factor
pattern results would vary as a function of several variables including recency of diagnosis, stage of
cancer, which cancer-related problem subjects coped with, and self-help group participation or nonpar-
ticipation. The factors produced in these analyses were very similar to the ones reported for the sample
as a whole, generally varying only in the order in which items loaded on the five factors.

   [2]Separate scoring of intensity of coping efforts and number of behaviors of each type resulted in
very highly correlated indices and similar patterns of results. That is, in this study, the effort exerted to
cope in a particular way was highly associated with the number of behaviors of that type a person
reported.

Table 1—*Coping Factors Derived from WOC–CA*

Scale	Item number	Item description	Factor loading
Seek and Use Social Support[a]	4	Talked to someone to find out more	.80
	34	Talked to someone about how feeling	.80
	22	Talked to someone who could do something	.72
	20	Let my feelings out somehow	.68
	16	Tried to get professional help	.58
	49	Tried to find out as much as I could	.53
	13	Looked for sympathy or understanding	.52
	31	Asked a friend or relative for advice	.52
	6	Tried not to close off options	.42
	19	Made a plan of action and followed it	.40
	1	Concentrated on the next step	.39
Cognitive Escape– Avoidance[b]	7	Hoped a miracle would happen	.60
	44	Prayed	.59
	45	Prepared for the worst	.56
	42	Wished the situation would go away or be over	.54
	43	Had fantasies/wishes about how it might turn out	.49
	46	Went over in my mind what I would say or do	.42
	8	Went along with fate	.31
	51	Depended mostly on others to handle things	.31
	12	Slept more than usual	.25
Distancing[c]	40	Tried to keep my feelings from interfering	.69
	30	Didn't let it get to me; refused to think about it	.65
	33	Made light of it; refused to get too serious	.59
	9	Went on as if it were not happening	.58
	10	Tried to keep my feelings to myself	.58
	11	Looked for silver lining, looked on bright side	.51
	50	Treated the illness as a challenge	.48
	37	Knew what had to be done, so increased efforts	.46
	15	Tried to forget the whole thing	.46
	32	Kept others from knowing how bad things were	.46
	48	Reminded myself how much worse things could be	.43
	52	Lived one day at a time/took one step at a time	.25
Focus on the Positive[d]	26	Found new faith	.77
	27	Rediscovered what is important in life	.71
	17	Changed or grew as a person in a good way	.70
	41	Changed something about myself	.62
	21	Came out of the experience better than before	.57
	28	Changed something so things will turn out	.57
	14	Was inspired to be creative	.39
	47	Thought of how a person I admire would act	.35
Behavioral Escape– Avoidance[e]	29	Avoided being with people	.62
	23	Tried to make myself feel better by eating, drinking, smoking, or drug use	.57
	24	Took a big chance and did something risky	.55
	35	Took it out on other people	.45

Table 1—(*Continued*)

Scale	Item number	Item description	Factor loading
	39	Came up with different solutions	.43
	18	Waited to see what would happen before acting	.34
	5	Criticized or lectured myself	.33
	3	Did something just to do something	.26
	25	Tried not to act too hastily	.26
Dropped due to low loadings	2	The only thing to do was wait	
	36	Drew on past experiences from similar situations	
	38	Refused to believe it would happen	

[a]Alpha = .86, mean item–total correlation = .55.
[b]Alpha = .78, mean item–total correlation = .46.
[c]Alpha = .80, mean item–total correlation = .45.
[d]Alpha = .85, mean item–total correlation = .57.
[e]Alpha = .74, mean item–total correlation = .41.

tended to use distancing techniques most frequently (on average, 26% of subjects' total coping effort). Seeking support, positive focus, and cognitive escape–avoidance were used about equally often; approximately 20% of coping effort was of each type (21%, 21%, and 20%, respectively). Behavioral escape–avoidance was used least (11%).

Subjects' primary coping methods were also examined as derived from the proportional coping scores. A primary coping method was operationalized as any method that was used at least 5% more often than all others. By this criterion, more than half the sample (55%) had no primary coping method. Of the remainder, 42% used distancing as their primary method of coping, 22% used positive focus, 19% used social support, and 17% used cognitive escape–avoidance. No one in the sample used behavioral escape–avoidance as a primary method of coping.

We examined further whether subjects were flexible in their use of coping methods (Pearlin & Schooler, 1978). Subjects were asked to indicate how many of the five coping methods make up at least 15% of their total coping effort. The median number of coping methods used was four. About 13% of the sample used all five methods of coping, 54% used four of the five, 27% used three, 4% used two, and 1% used only one. In short, the majority of the sample was highly flexible in methods of coping used.

Relationship of Coping Indices to Other Variables

All variables (i.e., sociodemographics, medical, appraisals, social network, psychotherapeutic factors) were first tested for bivariate relationships to the five coping factors with analyses of variance and Pearson project–moment correlations. Next, multiple-regression equations were constructed to examine the unique contributions of certain variables to each of the five patterns of coping while controlling for other variables. Significant bivariate results that were not redundant with the results of regression analyses are noted in the Discussion section.[3]

---

[3]Full results of bivariate tests are not presented here due to space limitations but can be obtained from Christine Dunkel-Schetter.

Variables were selected for regression analyses by theoretical criteria and were based on bivariate correlations so as to maximize power and to avoid multicollinearity. The 12 variables selected as possible predictors of coping in regressions are grouped into four conceptual groups:

1. Personal/environmental variables—sex, age, education, religiosity, whether the person had ever attended a support group, and whether the person lived alone as a proxy for availability of social support.
2. Appraisal-of-cancer variables—whether the problem selected as most stressful in recent months was "fear and uncertainty about the future" or was "physical" in nature (combining physical limitations and pain) and the perceived stressfulness of this problem.
3. Medical-condition variables—type of cancer (recoded as breast vs. other sites), recency of diagnosis, and whether the person was currently in treatment.
4. Emotional distress—POMS–BI.

Correlation coefficients computed among all 12 variables used as predictors in regression analyses showed only three of the intercorrelations higher than .20 and none higher than .50.

Each of the five coping patterns was regressed on the 12 variables, which were entered as a set simultaneously using listwise deletion of cases with missing values. Standardized betas, adjusted R squares, overall Fs, and ps appear in Table 2.[4] Four of the five equations are highly significant, accounting for 24% to 29% of the variance in coping. The exception was coping through distancing oneself from the cancer-related problem, which was not well predicted by these variables, although the overall equation is significant at the .05 level. Significant regression coefficients are discussed.

Of the personal/environmental factors entered into the equations, younger age was associated with more support seeking, more focusing on the positive, and more behavioral escape–avoidance. Less education (i.e., less than a high school diploma) was related to more distancing and more cognitive escape–avoidance. Religiosity was associated with more cognitive escape–avoidance and more focusing on the positive. Participation in mutual support groups was related to more support use and more focusing on the positive but also with somewhat greater behavioral and cognitive escape–avoidance. Living alone was associated with more coping through support seeking and more behavioral escape–avoidance. Sex of subject was unrelated to coping.

Of the stress appraisal variables, the specific problem with which subjects were coping did not relate significantly to patterns of coping. In contrast, perceived stressfulness of the current problem was associated with significantly greater coping through support, and significantly greater use of both forms of escape–avoidance. Of the medical condition variables, respondents with breast cancer were slightly more inclined to seek support than those with cancer in other sites, but there were no further effects of type of cancer on coping. Time since diagnosis was also associated only with one pattern of coping; the greater the time that had elapsed since the first

---

[4]The standard error terms for all betas ranged from .40 to .60.

Table 2—*Results of Regression Analyses on Predictors of Coping*

Predictor of coping	WOC–CA scale				
	Seek and use social support	Focus on the positive	Distancing	Cognitive escape– avoidance	Behavioral escape– avoidance
Personal/environmental					
1. Sex[a]	−.07	−.06	.09	.01	−.04
2. Age	−.14**	−.18***	.02	−.01	−.19***
3. Education[b]	−.01	.01	−.13**	−.19***	−.02
4. Religiosity	.04	.35***	.09	.32***	−.01
5. Live alone[c]	.17***	.08	.02	.03	.20***
6. Support groups[c]	.19***	.19***	.03	.10*	.12**
Appraisal of cancer					
7. Problem	.01	.00	.00	−.05	.06
8. Degree of stress	.40***	.05	−.02	.29***	.24***
Medical condition					
9. Breast cancer[c]	.11*	.03	.01	−.02	.00
10. Time since diagnosis	−.01	−.05	.01	−.02	.12**
11. In treatment[c]	.07	−.01	.04	.06	−.07
Emotional distress					
12. POMS–BI[d]	.20***	.22***	.13*	−.11*	−.25***
Adjusted R^2	.24	.25	.02	.29	.24
F	10.98***	11.65***	1.78*	13.97***	10.95***

[a]1 = male.
[b]Recoded 1 = high school or less, 2 = some college or more.
[c]0 = no, 1 = yes.
[d]High scores = positive affect, low scores = negative affect.
*$p < .05$.
**$p < .01$.
***$p < .001$.

cancer diagnosis, the more frequently people coped with cancer-related problems by behavioral escape–avoidance. Whether a person was currently in treatment was not significantly related to coping in regression analyses with other variables controlled.

Finally, emotional state was associated significantly with all five patterns of coping in regression results. Less emotional distress was significantly associated with more coping through social support, focusing on the positive, and distancing. More distress was associated with using more of both types of escape–avoidance.

Discussion

Patterns of Coping With Cancer

Five patterns of coping with cancer were identified: seeking or using social support, focusing on the positive, distancing, cognitive escape–avoidance, and behavioral escape–avoidance.[5] These are the first coping patterns to be identified with a large and heterogeneous sample of cancer patients, and they are similar to those identified earlier with smaller samples of cancer patients (Felton et al., 1984; Ray, Lindop, & Gibson, 1982; Weisman & Worden, 1976–1977) and large samples of community residents experiencing a variety of life stresses (Aldwin & Revenson, 1987; Folkman, Lazarus, Dunkel-Schetter et al., 1986). It appears that they may be representative of universal dimensions of coping and are not specific to cancer, except as noted later.

There was little evidence of coping styles in these cancer patients. Most subjects in the study coped in multiple ways with the stressful aspects of cancer. Even the subjects who used only one or two of the five patterns of coping did not report any single pattern of coping much more frequently than the others. People who have had cancer appear to use a large repertoire of behaviors to cope flexibly with any one threat from the disease, rather than rigidly adhering to a particular coping style (Folkman & Lazarus, 1980; Folkman, Lazarus, Gruen, & DeLongis, 1986).

Distancing was the most common form of coping in this study. However, coping by distancing was predicted relatively poorly by the variables in our model—especially compared to the other four coping patterns, which were predicted quite well. Although distancing was negatively associated with education, it was unrelated to every other variable tested in both multivariate and bivariate tests. It appears that most individuals with cancer cognitively and behaviorally distance themselves from the disease and its adverse effects most of the time, perhaps due to the ambiguity of the outcome of most cancers and the uncontrollability of the disease (Felton & Revenson, 1984). That distancing was the most common primary method of coping is also consistent with this conclusion. Distancing was not associated with time since diagnosis, however, which suggests that it is not disproportionately prevalent in people with newly diagnosed cancers.

The remaining four patterns of coping were used in different degrees depending on the characteristics of the person with cancer and her or his currently appraised situation. For example, social support and focusing on the positive were the two most highly correlated patterns of coping in this study, yet each had meaningfully different correlates. Focusing on the positive was most common among individuals who were very religious and who were younger. Differences among religious groups in this coping factor were also highly significant; Catholics were most likely to focus on the positive followed by Protestants, who used this coping method more than Jews, and those with no religious preference coped this way least often. In bivariate tests, focusing on the positive was also associated with being employed. Focusing on the positive, however, was not associated with degree of appraised stress. Overall, coping with cancer by focusing on the positive seems to originate more from personal characteristics (e.g., age or religion) of individuals than from situational factors (e.g., disease state or degree of stress). In fact, in bivariate tests, coping by focusing on

[5]Some of the factors were not themselves unidimensional. For example, the three items loading lowest on the Seek and Use Social Support factor were problem-solving behaviors, which is consistent with the existence of a higher order problem-focused coping factor (Dunkel-Schetter et al., 1987). However, this is to be expected in that, although only five factors were interpretable and internally consistent, more than five eigenvalues were greater than 1. Examination of the written responses to the open-ended item on "other ways subjects coped" revealed only behaviors easily coded as one of the five core factors and did not reveal any additional dimensions not tapped by our item pool.

the positive was most characteristic of individuals not in treatment and those currently in remission. In contrast, use of social support was strongly related to greater
perceived stress from cancer and was associated in bivariate tests with more functional limitations, more frequent worry about cancer, and higher levels of education.

Two distinguishable escape–avoidance coping patterns were detected in this
study. These patterns have not been differentiated in studies of coping in community
samples (Aldwin & Revenson, 1987; Folkman, Lazarus, Dunkel-Schetter et al.,
1986), but they are similar to two factors reported in the study by Felton et al. (1984)
on coping with chronic illness—suggesting that they may be manifested primarily
in response to illness. In this study, the Cognitive Escape–Avoidance factor included
several items on fantasizing or wishful thinking together with hints of fatalism, res-
ignation, and preparing for a poor outcome. The Behavioral Escape–Avoidance factor involved behavioral signs of avoidance likely to be maladaptive, such as social
withdrawal, drug use, and impulsivity. A self-blame item also loaded on this factor,
consistent with earlier research (Dunkel-Schetter et al., 1987).

Cognitive escape–avoidance was associated with less education and greater religiosity in regression analyses. Bivariate correlations also showed significant relationships of use of cognitive escape–avoidance to lower income, unemployment, and
greater likelihood of a Christian religious preference (i.e., Catholics and Protestants).
Analyses further indicated that cognitive escape–avoidance coping was more common in those individuals with recurrent disease, those currently in treatment, and
those with more functional limitations. Because both methods of escape–avoidance
coping were associated with degree of perceived stress, they appear to be situation-
ally influenced patterns of coping. However, cognitive escape–avoidance seems to
occur more in response to currently problematic medical conditions, whereas behavioral escape–avoidance seems to occur more in response to past cancer treatment
and any residual problems from it.

Behavioral Escape–Avoidance was the only coping factor associated with time
since diagnosis; the more time elapsed since diagnosis, the more frequently people
coped with cancer-related problems in this way. People who coped with cancer by
behavioral escape–avoidance were also more likely to live alone, but living alone
was associated with coping more through social support as well. Similar results were
obtained for marital status and parental status in bivariate tests: People without partners and without children were more likely to cope by behavioral escape–avoidance
and support seeking. Yet, avoidance of others was the highest loading item on the
Behavioral Escape–Avoidance factor, which is puzzling. Why should people without
social ties engage in both avoidance of others and support seeking? Individuals using
this form of coping were also less recently diagnosed and, as a result, may vacillate
between avoiding and seeking out others in connection with the cancer. This aspect
of our results may be worth follow-up given that social networks can play an important role in shaping coping responses (Dunkel-Schetter et al., 1987; Holahan &
Moos, 1987; Umberson, 1987).

Predictors of Coping Behavior

The level of appraised stress from cancer was related to three of the five patterns of
coping, as expected, whereas the specific cancer-related problem with which subjects

were coping was not predictive of the ways people coped, contrary to predictions. Similarly, medical factors (i.e., type of cancer, time since diagnosis, and whether the cancer was currently being treated) were not strongly associated with coping when other factors were controlled. These results are highly consistent with past stress and coping research in which appraisal processes are a central mediator of coping behavior (Folkman, Lazarus, Gruen, & DeLongis, 1986; Vitaliano, DeWolfe, Maiuro, Russo, & Katon, 1990). One implication is that research on psychosocial adjustment to cancer might focus less on biomedical and disease characteristics often presumed to be determinants of coping and more on subjective appraisals of stress from cancer and their effects. Biomedical factors cannot be ignored—particularly in sampling, in which homogeneity is advised if small samples are studied. Nonetheless, medical factors seem to influence coping only as they are filtered through the person's cognitive appraisal system.

Of the personal characteristics studied, age, education, and religiosity proved to be especially important in explaining how people coped. For example, more-religious people in the sample were more likely to use methods of coping involving cognitively reframing the stressful situation. Our results, together with recent evidence suggesting "religious coping" is protective in the face of stress (Park, L. H. Cohen, & Herb, 1990), offer interesting hypotheses about differences among religious groups in coping and adjustment to cancer. In general, cancer patients may be predisposed by virtue of premorbid factors such as life stage, SES, or personal beliefs to cope in particular ways with their illness (Holahan & Moos, 1987).

Our results raise the question of the amenability of coping behavior to change—which is an important assumption underlying much of coping research. Are some patterns of coping, specifically use of social support, more modifiable than others in cancer patients or in general? Although positive attitude is often promoted as a method of coping with cancer in media sources, self-help groups, and trade books (Simonton, Matthews-Simonton, & Creighton, 1978), a positive approach may not be feasible as a means of coping for everyone (Viney & Westbrook, 1982). Our results suggest that older and less religious cancer patients may find it difficult to adopt a positive stance. Popular sources advocating a positive attitude may be misleading and even harmful if a cancer patient is not able to adopt this perspective toward the disease. On the other hand, use of social support was not as strongly related to as many specific characteristics of individuals—suggesting that this coping method may be available to a wider range of cancer patients. The prevalence of support interventions for cancer patients may reflect the assumption of health care providers that it is easier to encourage use of support than it is to alter patients' well-established views of the world.

Rehabilitation efforts for cancer patients might take some of these findings into account in targeting interventions. Age was inversely related to three methods of coping with cancer and in bivariate tests was positively associated with coping by distancing. Older age may reduce perceptions of cancer as a threat and perceptions of the number of coping options one has. A greater understanding of the impact of cancer on older individuals compared to younger individuals seems valuable from the standpoint of psychosocial intervention and given the disproportionate occurrence of cancer among older people.

There was no evidence in this study for sex differences in coping with cancer, and there were very few effects of having breast versus other types of cancer. There were consistent effects of support group attendance, however, and attenders were more likely to be female. Support group attenders (those who attended a group at least once) applied more coping efforts of all types, except distancing, to manage their cancers compared to those who had never met with a group. Attenders were particularly likely to report seeking support and focusing on the positive, as were individuals who had previously been in therapy for any reason. Whether these coping methods predispose individuals to get psychological assistance or whether such assistance enhances the use of particular coping methods is not clear, but both appear to be probable occurrences. If self-help groups are disproportionately composed of individuals using problem-focused coping, individuals who cope in other ways, such as by distancing, may be difficult to assist by this means. The absence of sex differences in coping might be explained by selection bias in sampling such that avoidant men were less represented in the study. However, this selection bias would apply to avoidant women as well. It is also possible that differences between men and women in coping are less striking than differences between cancer patients in other factors such as age, religiosity, or perceived stress.

This study replicated earlier evidence that escape–avoidance coping is associated with more emotional distress and that positive reinterpretations (termed here *focusing on the positive*) are associated with less emotional distress (Felton et al., 1984; Weisman & Worden, 1976–1977). In addition, our analyses controlled for individual stress appraisals and whether the person was in treatment (which to some extent reflects severity of disease, albeit imperfectly). Distancing was associated with slightly less emotional distress in this study, whereas the earlier research found either no relationship or a positive one. Further post hoc analyses revealed that frequency of coping by distancing was related to emotional distress in a curvilinear manner (see also Meyerowitz, 1983). Distancing was most frequent at moderate levels of distress and least frequent under conditions of very low or very high distress. This finding may account for conflicting past results and can be understood if distress is viewed as a determinant of coping. Stressful conditions causing slight distress may not warrant the use of distancing as a means of coping, and those conditions causing extreme distress may make it impossible to distract oneself. At moderate levels of distress, which most of our cancer sample was experiencing, distancing was most common. We suspect that, under these circumstances, coping by distancing is more feasible and more adaptive.

Limitations of the present study include those common in coping research—for instance, lack of certainty as to whether self-reports of coping behavior reflect accurately how a person behaves. Observational studies and informant reports are needed to validate coping inventories (F. Cohen, 1987; Tennen & Herzberger, 1985). Concerns about confounded variables such as mood, personality, and social desirability can be partially addressed by the multivariate analyses, which controlled many factors. However, further studies of coping behavior are much needed to address some of the remaining questions in this domain of research. Finally, inferences about causality are difficult in cross-sectional designs such as this one. Although some alternatives could be ruled out in this study (i.e., effects of coping on age), others (e.g., third-variable causation) remain plausible and must be untangled in longitudinal or experimental designs.

Conclusion

Five patterns of coping were delineated and labeled *seeking and using social support, focusing on the positive, distancing, cognitive escape–avoidance, and behavioral escape–avoidance*. These conform well to how individuals cope with other major life stresses and were related in meaningful ways to factors hypothesized to be determinants of coping. Cognitive appraisals of stress from cancer were associated with three of the five coping patterns. However, medical factors such as site of cancer and time since diagnosis were not related to coping patterns after appraisals of stress were controlled. Type of cancer threat also was not associated significantly with coping. There was evidence for links between some aspects of social networks and coping. Finally, emotional distress was associated with focusing on the positive and escape–avoidance coping, and results on the relationship of distress to distancing clarify equivocalities in prior studies.

The coping literature was once described as a "three-car garage filled to the rafters with junk" and badly in need of rigorous housecleaning (Taylor, 1984, p. 2313). This article provides information on five patterns of coping with cancer within an established theoretical tradition, a practical method of assessing these patterns, and indications of the factors associated with the patterns. Such information has implications for the provision of psychosocial assistance to cancer patients as well as for further basic research on coping.

References

Aldwin, C. A., & Revenson, T. A. (1987). Does coping help? A reexamination of the relation between coping and mental health. *Journal of Personality and Social Psychology, 53,* 337–348.

Bard, M., & Sutherland, A. M. (1955). Psychological impact of cancer and its treatment: Adaptation to radical mastectomy. *Cancer, 8,* 656–672.

Billings, A. G., & Moos, R. H. (1981). The role of coping responses and social resources in attenuating the stress of life events. *Journal of Behavioral Medicine, 4,* 157–189.

Carver, C. S., Scheier, M. F., & Weintraub, J. K. (1989). Assessing coping strategies: A theoretically based approach. *Journal of Personality and Social Psychology, 56,* 267–283.

Cohen, F. (1987). Measurement of coping. In S. V. Kasl & C. L. Cooper (Eds.), *Stress and health: Issues in research methodology* (pp. 283–305). New York: Wiley.

Cronkite, R. C., & Moos, R. H. (1984). The role of predisposing and moderating factors in the stress–illness relationship. *Journal of Health and Social Behavior, 25,* 372–393.

Dunkel-Schetter, C. (1982). *Social support and coping with cancer.* Unpublished doctoral dissertation, Northwestern University, Evanston, IL.

Dunkel-Schetter, C., Folkman, S., & Lazarus, R. (1987). Correlates of social support receipt. *Journal of Personality and Social Psychology, 53,* 71–80.

Felton, B. J., & Revenson, T. A. (1984). Coping with chronic illness: A study of illness controllability and the influence of coping strategies on psychological adjustment. *Journal of Consulting and Clinical Psychology, 52,* 343–353.

Felton, B. J., Revenson, T. A., & Hinrichsen, G. A. (1984). Coping and adjustment in chronically ill adults. *Social Science and Medicine, 18,* 889–898.

Fleishman, J. A. (1984). Personality characteristics and coping patterns. *Journal of Health and Social Behavior, 25,* 229–244.

Folkman, S., & Lazarus, R. S. (1980). An analysis of coping in a middle-aged community sample. *Journal of Health and Social Behavior, 21,* 219–239.

Folkman, S., Lazarus, R. S., Dunkel-Schetter, C., DeLongis, A., & Gruen, R. (1986). Dynamics of a stressful encounter: Cognitive appraisal, coping, and encounter outcomes. *Journal of Personality and Social Psychology, 50,* 992–1003.

Folkman, S., Lazarus, R. S., Gruen, R. J., & DeLongis, A. (1986). Appraisal, coping, health status, and psychological symptoms. *Journal of Personality and Social Psychology, 50,* 571–579.

Hobfoll, S. E. (1989). Conservation of resources: A new attempt at conceptualizing stress. *American Psychologist, 44,* 513–524.

Holahan, C. J., & Moos, R. H. (1987). Personal and contextual determinants of coping strategies. *Journal of Personality and Social Psychology, 52,* 946–955.

Lazarus, R. S., & Folkman, S. (1984). *Stress, appraisal, and coping.* New York: Springer.

Lorr, M., & McNair, D. (1982). *Profile of Mood States: Bi-polar form (POMS–BI).* San Diego: Educational and Industrial Testing Service.

McCrae, R. R. (1984). Situational determinants of coping responses: Loss, threat, and challenge. *Journal of Personality and Social Psychology, 46,* 919–928.

McGrath, J. E. (1970). A conceptual formulation for research on stress. In J. E. McGrath (Ed.), *Social and psychological factors in stress* (pp. 10–21). New York: Holt, Rinehart & Winston.

Menaghan, E. (1983). Individual coping efforts: Moderators of the relationship between life stress and mental health outcomes. In H. B. Kaplan (Ed.), *Psychosocial stress: Trends in theory and research* (pp. 157–191). New York: Academic.

Meyerowitz, B. E. (1983). Postmastectomy coping strategies and quality of life. *Health Psychology, 2,* 117–132.

Meyerowitz, B. E., Heinrich, R. L., & Schag, C. C. (1983). A competency-based approach to cancer. In T. G. Burish & L. A. Bradley (Eds.), *Coping with chronic disease* (pp. 137–158). New York: Academic.

Moos, R. H., & Billings, A. G. (1982). Conceptualizing and measuring coping resources and processes. In L. Goldberger & S. Breznitz (Eds.), *Handbook of stress: Theoretical and clinical aspects* (pp. 212–230). New York: Free Press.

Park, C., Cohen, L. H., & Herb, L. (1990). Intrinsic religiousness and religious coping as life stress moderators for Catholics versus Protestants. *Journal of Personality and Social Psychology, 59,* 562–574.

Parkes, K. R. (1986). Coping in stressful episodes: The role of individual differences, environmental factors, and situational characteristics. *Journal of Personality and Social Psychology, 51,* 1277–1292.

Pearlin, L. I., & Schooler, C. (1978). The structure of coping. *Journal of Health and Social Behavior, 19,* 2–21.

Quint, J. C. (1965). Institutionalized practices of information control. *Psychiatry, 28,* 119–132.

Ray, C., Lindop, J., & Gibson, S. (1982). The concept of coping. *Psychological Medicine, 12,* 385–395.

Revenson, T. A., & Felton, B. J. (1985, November). *Perceived stress in chronic illness: A comparative analysis of four diseases.* Paper presented at the meeting of the Gerontological Society of America, New Orleans.

Shands, H. Z., Finesinger, J. E., Cobb, S., & Abrams, R. D. (1951). Psychological mechanisms in patients with cancer. *Cancer, 4,* 1159–1170.

Simonton, O. C., Matthews-Simonton, S., & Creighton, J. (1978). *Getting well again.* New York: Tarcher.

Singer, J. E. (1984). Some issues in the study of coping. *Cancer, 53*(Suppl. 10), 2303–2313.

Taylor, S. E. (1984). Some issues in the study of coping: A response. *Cancer, 53*(Suppl. 10), 2313–2315.

Taylor, S. E., Falke, R. L., Mazel, R. M., & Hilsberg, B. L. (1988). Sources of satisfaction and dissatisfaction among members of cancer support groups. In B. H. Gottlieb (Ed.), *Marshaling social support: Formats, processes, and effects* (pp. 187–208). Beverly Hills, CA: Sage.

Taylor, S. E., Falke, R. L., Shoptaw, S. J., & Lichtman, R. R. (1986). Social support, support groups and the cancer patient. *Journal of Consulting and Clinical Psychology, 54,* 608–615.

Tennen, H., & Herzberger, S. (1985). Ways of Coping scale. In D. J. Keyser & R. C. Sweetland (Eds.), *Test critiques* (Vol. 3, pp. 686–697). Kansas City, MO: Test Corporation of America.

Umberson, D. (1987). Family status and health behaviors: Social control as a dimension of social integration. *Journal of Health and Social Behavior, 28,* 306–319.

Viney, L. L., & Westbrook, M. T. (1982). Coping with chronic illness: The mediating role of biographic and illness-related factors. *Journal of Psychosomatic Research, 26,* 595–605.

Vitaliano, P. P., DeWolfe, D. J., Maiuro, R. D., Russo, J., & Katon, W. (1990). Appraised changeability of a stressor as a modifier of the relationship between coping and depression: A test of the hypothesis of fit. *Journal of Personality and Social Psychology, 59,* 582–592.

Vitaliano, P. P., Russo, J., Carr, J. E., Maiuro, R. D., & Becker, J. (1985). The Ways of Coping checklist: Revision and psychometric properties. *Multivariate Behavioral Research, 20,* 3–26.

Weisman, A. (1979). *Coping with cancer.* New York: McGraw-Hill.

Weisman, A., & Worden, J. W. (1976–1977). The existential plight in cancer: Significance of the first 100 days. *International Journal of Psychiatry in Medicine, 7*(1), 1–15.

Chapter 3
SOCIAL SUPPORT AND ADJUSTMENT TO CANCER:
Reconciling Descriptive, Correlational, and Intervention Research

Vicki S. Helgeson and Sheldon Cohen

Increasing cure rates and remissions have led to a 5-year survival rate, averaged across all sites of cancer, of more than 50% (American Cancer Society, 1992; National Cancer Institute, 1984). To date, 4 million people are living with cancer (American Cancer Society, 1992). Thus, health care professionals are faced with a new challenge: helping people live with cancer or live with having had cancer (Scott & Eisendrath, 1986). An important determinant of cancer patients' ability to live with their illness is their social environment.

There are at least two reasons that the social environment is a particularly important domain in the study of cancer. First, aspects of the social environment have been shown to promote well-being and to protect persons from the deleterious effects of stressful life events, of which cancer is one (Cohen & Wills, 1985). Both the structural aspects of social networks (e.g., size) and the functional aspects of social supports (e.g., emotional support) have been related to cancer morbidity and mortality (see Glanz & Lerman, 1992, for a review; Reynolds & Kaplan, 1990). Second, cancer is a stressful event that influences interpersonal relationships (e.g., Peters-Golden, 1982). Because cancer is a potentially fatal illness and often is characterized by a stigma, cancer patients' network members may withdraw or react inappropriately. Cancer also may affect relationships indirectly by restricting patients' social activities, which will affect their access to interpersonal resources (Bloom & Kessler, 1994; Bloom & Spiegel, 1984). Thus, people diagnosed with cancer may have difficulties obtaining social resources just when they are most needed (Dakof & Taylor, 1990; Dunkel-Schetter, 1984; Wortman & Conway, 1985).

The experience of cancer depends on a host of variables, including patient demographics (age, sex, socioeconomic status), site of malignancy (e.g., breast, pelvic), stage of disease, and type of treatment (e.g., surgery, chemotherapy, radiation). Despite this diversity in experience, we believe that persons diagnosed with cancer confront a number of common psychosocial issues and, as a consequence, have similar needs that can be met by people in their social environment.

A diagnosis of cancer challenges basic assumptions about the self and the world (Janoff-Bulman & Frieze, 1983), and successful adjustment involves restoration of these assumptions (Taylor, 1983). Specifically, a diagnosis of cancer may lead to a sense of personal inadequacy, diminished feelings of control, increased feelings of vulnerability, and a sense of confusion (Lesko, Ostroff, & Smith, 1991; Rowland,

Reprinted from *Health Psychology, 15*(2), 135–148. (1996). Copyright © 1996 by the American Psychological Association. Used with permission of the author.

Preparation of this article was supported by a grant from the National Cancer Institute (CA61303) and a Research Scientist Development Award from the National Institute of Mental Health (MH00721).

1989). People in the social environment can behave in ways that influence these reactions to illness.

There are three main types of supportive social interactions: emotional, informational, and instrumental (House, 1981; House & Kahn, 1985; Kahn & Antonucci, 1980; Thoits, 1985). In theory, each kind of support can influence one or more of the illness reactions described above. *Emotional support* involves the verbal and nonverbal communication of caring and concern. It includes listening, "being there," empathizing, reassuring, and comforting. Emotional support can help to restore self-esteem or reduce feelings of personal inadequacy by communicating to the patient that he or she is valued and loved. It also can permit the expression of feelings that may reduce distress. Emotional support can lead to greater attention to and improvement of interpersonal relationships, thus providing some purpose or meaning for the disease experience. *Informational support* involves the provision of information used to guide or advise. Information may enhance perceptions of control by providing patients with ways of managing their illness and coping with symptoms. Learning how to manage the illness also may enhance patients' optimism about the future and thus reduce feelings of future vulnerability. Informational support also can help to ameliorate the sense of confusion that arises from being diagnosed with cancer by helping the patient understand the cause, course, and treatment of the illness. *Instrumental support* involves the provision of material goods, for example, transportation, money, or assistance with household chores. This kind of support may offset the loss of control that patients feel during cancer treatment by providing tangible resources that they can use to exert control over their experience. Provision of instrumental support, however, also may increase feelings of dependence and undermine self-efficacy in patients (Wortman & Dunkel-Schetter, 1987).

Our goal in this article is to determine the conditions under which the social environment beneficially influences adjustment to cancer. We review studies that examine the effect of the social environment on psychological adjustment, and we include the very small literature on the role of the social environment in the progression of disease. Psychological adjustment refers to adaptation to disease without continued elevations of psychological distress (e.g., anxiety, depression) and loss of role function (i.e., social, sexual, vocational). Disease progression refers to severity of symptoms and longevity.

We first examine descriptive and correlational evidence on social interactions and adjustment to cancer to determine which interactions are associated with the greatest benefits. Then, we describe intervention research in which aspects of the social environment were manipulated to determine which interactions lead to the greatest benefits. Because the conclusions reached by these literatures are contradictory, we then discuss ways of reconciling the discrepancies and offer suggestions for future research.

Descriptive and Correlational Research on Adjustment to Cancer

The nonexperimental research on social support and cancer has addressed two issues. First, descriptive data have been collected on the kinds of support patients desire from each of their network members. Second, correlational research has been conducted on the kinds of support related to cancer adjustment.

Helpful and Unhelpful Support

In three separate studies, researchers asked patients to describe the interactions they found helpful or unhelpful during the illness experience. Each study showed that patients identify emotional support as the most helpful kind of support, regardless of which network member is involved, and informational support as helpful from health care professionals but unhelpful from family and friends.

Dunkel-Schetter (1984) interviewed 79 breast and colorectal cancer patients between 7 and 20 months following diagnosis. Respondents were asked to describe the most helpful and unhelpful behaviors and the sources of such behaviors. Behaviors were coded into four categories: emotional (love, concern, understanding, reassurance, encouragement), instrumental (aid, assistance), informational (advice, problem-solving information), and appraisal (approval). Emotional support was identified most often as helpful, and instrumental support was identified least often as helpful.

When the source of support was considered, emotional and instrumental support were perceived to be helpful from any source, whereas informational support was perceived to be helpful only if the source was a health care professional. A lack of information from a physician was problematic, whereas too much information from family and friends was problematic; the converse (complaints of too much information from a physician and lack of information from family and friends) did not apply.

A similar set of findings emerged from Neuling and Winefield's (1988) longitudinal study of 58 women recovering from breast surgery. They interviewed women three times: in the hospital after surgery, 1 month after surgery, and 3 months after surgery. At each time of assessment, patients rated the frequency with which family, friends, and surgeons provided each of the following kinds of support: emotional (listening, encouragement, talking, understanding, love), informational (advice, telling what to expect, answering questions), instrumental (helping with chores, providing transportation, providing child care), and reassurance. The findings suggest that (a) needs for emotional support, especially from family, are particularly high; (b) emotional support is the kind of support most received but is also perceived to be the least adequate; and (c) patients desire informational support but only from physicians.

Dakof and Taylor (1990) replicated the findings on emotional and informational support. They asked 55 cancer patients (with a variety of cancer sites) who were within 6 years of diagnosis or recurrence to identify the most helpful and unhelpful support behaviors. Behaviors were coded into one of three categories: Emotional support included physical presence, concern, empathy, affection, and understanding; informational support included information, optimism about prognosis, and being a positive role model; instrumental support (tangible support) included practical assistance and medical care. Among the kinds of support, emotional support was perceived to be the most helpful if present and the most harmful if absent when the source was a spouse, family member, or friend. When the source was a physician, informational support was the most helpful if present, and both informational and emotional support were harmful when absent. Instrumental support was identified as more helpful among poor-prognosis patients.

A fourth study examined support needs among 64 patients (with a variety of cancer sites, but 59% had breast cancer) who were an average of 18 months from diagnosis (Rose, 1990). Patients rated the extent to which they needed emotional, instrumental, and informational support from three sources: family, friends, and health care professionals. Some aspects of emotional support were desired equally from the three sources, whereas other aspects were desired more from different sources. For example, one kind of emotional support—opportunity for ventilation —was desired more from family and friends than from health care professionals. Patients desired instrumental support from family more than from friends or health care professionals but informational support from health care professionals more than from family or friends. Finally, patients indicated a desire for one type of informational support—modeling—from friends, especially when the friend had cancer.

Another approach to determining perceptions of helpful and unhelpful behaviors involved a comparison of attitudes toward cancer among 100 healthy lay people and 100 women with breast cancer who had been diagnosed between 3 weeks and 21 years prior to the interview (Peters-Golden, 1982). This work identified several misconceptions lay people had about cancer patients' needs and desires. Whereas the majority of potential support providers said that they would try to cheer up a cancer patient, the majority of cancer patients said that "unrelenting optimism" disturbed them. Another misconception of healthy people was that it is harmful for cancer patients to discuss their illness. In addition, healthy people believed patients' major concerns were cosmetic (i.e., losing a breast), whereas patients' major concerns centered on recurrence and death. One expectation of lay people borne out by patients is that others avoid those with cancer.

Other studies have identified similar unhelpful behaviors. Prominent unhelpful behaviors noted by cancer patients include minimizing the problem, forced cheerfulness, being told not to worry, medical care being delivered in the absence of emotional support, and insensitive comments of friends (Dakof & Taylor, 1990; Dunkel-Schetter, 1984). Dakof and Taylor (1990) found that a particularly hurtful behavior was others' avoidance of the patient. This behavior characterized friends rather than spouse and family.

The most frequently reported unhelpful behaviors could be construed as the failure to provide emotional support. Avoiding the patient, minimizing the patient's problems, and forced cheerfulness all keep the patient from discussing the illness. The availability of someone with whom the patient can discuss illness-related concerns is central to the concept of emotional support. Perhaps the reason that patients perceive the opportunity to discuss feelings, especially negative ones, as one of the most important types of support (see Wortman & Dunkel-Schetter, 1979, for a review) is that this specific kind of support is often unavailable (Mitchell & Glicksman, 1977). Patients often want to discuss worries and concerns regarding the illness, but network members believe talking about the illness is bad for patients and upsetting to themselves. In a study of support group attenders, 55% said that they wished they could talk more openly with family members (Taylor, Falke, Shoptaw, & Lichtman, 1986). Dunkel-Schetter (1984) found that 87% of patients said they coped with their illness by keeping thoughts and feelings to themselves. Patients were concerned about how others would react to their expression of feelings.

Although a lack of emotional support from family and friends is especially harmful, there are limits on the extent to which family and friends can provide certain kinds of emotional support. For example, reassurance ("Everything will work out") or empathy ("I know how you feel") may not be helpful and may be viewed as minimization of the problem when conveyed by family and friends (Rowland, 1989; Wortman & Lehman, 1985). These same responses, however, may be viewed as genuine and helpful when conveyed by peers—those facing a similar stressor. Wortman and Lehman (1985) suggested that peers are in a unique position to provide support because they do not share others' misconceptions about coping with cancer and they are not vulnerable to the anxiety and threat that discussing the illness poses for other network members.

Relations of Support to Adjustment

Although there is a great deal of literature linking social support to adjustment to cancer (see Lindsey, Norbeck, Carrieri, & Perry, 1981, and Rowland, 1989, for reviews), we include only studies that examined specific kinds of support. Many studies averaged over multiple kinds of social interactions. We describe the relations of three kinds of social interactions (emotional, informational, and instrumental) to cancer adjustment. We also distinguish between patients' perceptions of support availability (i.e., perceived support) and reports of support receipt (i.e., received support). In studies that compared the two, perceived support was more strongly related to adjustment (Cohen & Hoberman, 1983; Cohen & Wills, 1985; Wethington & Kessler, 1986). When applicable, we describe the source of support. The sources most often studied were close family, friends, and health care professionals. Unless otherwise noted, the studies reported below are cross-sectional and hence subject to third-factor explanations and reverse causation.

Six studies focused only on emotional support in examining adjustment to cancer. Each of these studies revealed a positive link between emotional support and good adjustment. For example, in a study of 41 women who had mastectomies an average of 22 months prior to the interview, those who perceived greater emotional support from spouse, physician, surgeon, nurses, or children rated themselves as having better emotional adjustment (Jamison, Wellisch, & Pasnau, 1978). Similarly, in a study of 86 women with advanced breast cancer who were interviewed an average of 28 months after diagnosis, Bloom and Spiegel (1984) found that perceived emotional support from family members (cohesion, expressiveness, low conflict) was associated with a favorable outlook (i.e., hope for the future). Greater levels of perceived emotional support also were found to be associated with better social and emotional adjustment (enhanced role functioning, self-esteem, and life satisfaction; reduced hostility) in 301 women with breast cancer with favorable prognoses (Stage I or II; Zemore & Shepel, 1989).

A longitudinal study also provided evidence of relations between perceived emotional support and adjustment. Northouse (1988) interviewed 50 women 3 days (Time 1) and 30 days (Time 2) postmastectomy. Emotional support was measured as the availability of five sources (spouse, family member, friend, nurse, physician) to listen, understand, express love and concern, encourage the patient to talk about problems, and allow the patient to be herself. A composite index of adjustment was computed from measures of mood, psychological distress, and psychosocial functioning. Positive associations of emotional support and adjustment emerged in cross-sectional analyses at both Time 1 and Time 2. Time 1 emotional support was similarly related to Time 2 adjustment, but Time 1 adjustment was not statistically controlled in this analysis.

The possibility that the relation between emotional support and adjustment is mediated by coping was investigated in a study by Bloom (1982). One hundred thirty-three women with nonmetastatic breast cancer were interviewed between 1 week and 2.5 years after surgery. An index of perceived emotional support (i.e., family cohesion), the presence of a confidant, and two aspects of social affiliation (perceptions of social contacts and leisure activities) were measured. None of the support variables was directly associated with any of the three adjustment indexes (self-concept, sense of power, and psychological distress), but the emotional support index and social contact variables were indirectly associated with all three adjustment indexes through their inhibiting effects on poor coping strategies. A second interview, conducted 2 months later on a portion of the same patients ($n = 112$), revealed the same cross-sectional pattern of findings.

Finally, a prospective study that focused on the perceived adequacy of emotional support showed beneficial effects on both adjustment and survival. Ell, Nishimoto, Mediansky, Mantell, and Hamovitch (1992) interviewed 294 people with breast, lung, or colorectal cancer within 3–6 months of initial diagnosis and followed them for approximately 3 months. Emotional support was correlated with reduced distress during the initial interview and predicted survival. Separate analyses revealed survival benefits only for women with breast cancer and only for those with localized disease. Thus, the site and stage of cancer may be important moderators of the association between social support and health.

Three studies measured multiple aspects of support. All three suggested links between emotional support and adjustment. For example, in a study of 58 women with breast cancer (mean length since diagnosis was 4 years), fibrocystic disease, or diabetes, five aspects of support receipt were measured (expression of positive affect toward patient, affirmation, extent patient confides to network member, reciprocity [extent network member discusses important problems with patient], and aid) from four sources (spouse, family, friends, and others; Primomo, Yates, & Woods, 1990). The first four kinds of support reflect emotional support as defined earlier. Two aspects of emotional support (affect and reciprocity) were associated with less depression in each of the three groups of women when the source was a partner or family member. Aid (i.e., instrumental support) from any source was not related to depression.

Perceived emotional support, professional support, and financial support were examined among 151 women who had mastectomies 3 to 12 months prior to the interview (Funch & Mettlin, 1982). Emotional support (i.e., the extent to which patients perceived they could rely on and talk to network members) was linked to all three adjustment measures (positive affect, negative affect, and index of well-being). Professional support (i.e., information from and satisfaction with physician) was linked to two of the three adjustment indexes (negative affect and well-being). Neither emotional support nor professional support was associated with any of five indexes of physical recovery. Instead, financial support (i.e., income, insurance) was associated with better physical recovery on all five indexes. Thus, the kinds of support that are associated with psychological and physical health may be distinct.

Perceived availability of emotional support (i.e., willingness to listen) and instrumental support (i.e., help) from spouse, family, friends, minister, physician, and nursing staff was examined among 49 women who had mastectomies (Woods & Earp, 1978). Neither kind of support was associated with depression for women with a high number of physical complications from surgery, but both were related to reduced depression among women with a low number of physical complications from surgery. The authors reasoned that social support was helpful only up to a given level of physical disability. The pattern of findings was stronger for instrumental than for emotional support.

Finally, two studies focused only on received informational support and only on one source—the physician. In studies of two separate samples of 50 patients undergoing radiation therapy, the majority of patients reported that their physicians had not prepared them for the treatments (Mitchell & Glicksman, 1977; Peck & Bowland, 1977). In both studies, the lack of information was associated with unnecessary and irrational fears.

In summary, few studies have distinguished among the kinds of support related to cancer adjustment, but among those that have, the strongest link between support and adjustment involved emotional support. Research has focused more on emotional than informational or instrumental support, reflecting the perception among the scientific and clinical communities—accurate or not—that emotional support is most important. Informational support seems to be helpful when the source is a health care professional. There is limited evidence for health benefits of instrumental support, but it has rarely been assessed. The effects of instrumental support may be limited to certain health outcomes (e.g., physical recovery) or to patients with a particular level of difficulties (e.g., Dakof & Taylor, 1990; Woods & Earp, 1978).

Limitations

The correlational research linking social support to adjustment to cancer is limited in two ways. First, the issue of causality cannot be addressed because the majority of the studies have been cross-sectional. Social support may enhance adjustment, better adjustment may lead to more supportive interactions, or some third variable may be responsible for the association between support and adjustment (e.g., patient neuroticism). Second, these studies have usually measured the perception of network members' behaviors rather than the actual behavior, and we do not know the basis for this perception. Intervention studies that manipulate the social environment remedy these two deficiencies.

Studies of Social Support Interventions for Cancer Patients

The intervention studies that have examined the influence of social interactions on adjustment to cancer largely focused on the role of social support provided by peers, that is, by others with cancer. This is in contrast to the correlational research, which has typically focused on close family, friends, or health care professionals. There are at least two reasons why interactions with peers have been the focus of intervention research. First, the correlational research suggests that there are some needs that are not met by naturally occurring social environments that may be met by peers (e.g., willingness to discuss illness, empathy, validation; Coates & Winston, 1983). To the extent that the naturally occurring social environment minimizes negative feelings, forces cheerfulness, and encourages patients to put the experience behind them before they are ready to do so, patients may feel further alienated from their social networks. Peers can provide validation for negative feelings. Second, because cancer can negatively affect existing social relationships, patients may turn to persons outside of their immediate network for support. One alternative source of support is what is commonly known as a support group, that is, a group of other persons experiencing the same stressor. In a study that compared patients who attended such groups with those who did not, attenders reported significantly more negative experiences with the medical community and marginally more difficulties communicating with family (Taylor et al., 1986).

The group interventions described below are diverse in nature, and the effects on a wide array of outcomes are not consistent. According to Holland (1991), over 20 intervention studies have been conducted that involved social interactions and behavioral techniques, the majority of which demonstrated improvement in psychological adjustment. The data on mortality, however, were more equivocal. Most of the intervention studies lacked theoretical frameworks and many had serious methodological flaws (e.g., lacked a control group, lacked randomization). In a review of the literature on psychosocial interventions with cancer patients, Taylor, Falke, Mazal, and Hilsberg (1988) concluded that participation in some form of group intervention reduces distress and helps patients resume daily activities but that the process by which these outcomes occur has rarely been investigated. We examined the nature of group interventions conducted to date to determine the kind of social interaction that leads to increased adjustment.

Taken collectively, there are two primary components of group interventions— discussion with peers and education. Group discussion ranges from unstructured conversation to focused discussions on psychological issues. In theory, the discussion takes place within an atmosphere of caring and acceptance, and the primary form of support fostered is emotional support, that is, listening, reassurance, comfort, and caring. Education involves providing information about the disease and how to manage it. Thus, the educational groups primarily foster informational support.

First, we review studies of interventions that integrated group discussion and education; second, studies of discussion-based interventions; third, studies of education-based interventions; and fourth, studies that distinguished and compared the two. The studies are listed in Table 1 in the order we discuss them. We include all intervention studies that were conducted with groups rather than individuals, used some type of comparison group, and were published in peer reviewed scientific journals. Unless otherwise stated, the control groups used in these studies were no-treatment controls.

Combined Education and Discussion

Most interventions have combined different kinds of social interactions. We report four studies, each of which showed an intervention effect on outcome variables. The first three suffer from a variety of methodological flaws, and all four are limited in that the effect of one intervention component cannot be distinguished from the effects of the others.

One study evaluated a group counseling intervention for patients with advanced cancer (variety of sites). The intervention began with education and ended with group

Table 1—*Characteristics of Group Intervention Studies*

Authors	Type	Prognosis	Site	Duration	Follow-Up
Ferlic et al. (1979)	Combined	Advanced	Variety	2 weeks	After
Vachon et al. (1982)	Combined	All stages	Breast	3 weeks	After
Morgenstern et al. (1984)	Combined	All stages	Breast	Unspecified	6 months to 3 years[a]
Fawzy et al. (1990)	Combined	Stages I, II	Melanoma	6 weeks	6 months, 6 years[a]
Houts et al. (1986)	Dyad discussion	All stages	Gynecologic	10 weeks	During, 2 weeks
Spiegel et al. (1981)	Group discussion	Advanced	Breast	1 year	During, after, 10 years[a]
Kriss & Kraemer (1986)	Group discussion	All stages	Breast	1 year	After
Lonnqvist et al. (1986)	Group discussion	All stages	Breast	8 weeks	4 to 5 years
Heinrich & Schag (1985)	Education	All stages	Variety	6 weeks	After
Cain et al. (1986)	Education	All stages	Gynecologic	8 weeks	1–2 weeks, 6 months
Johnson (1982)	Education	All stages	Variety	4 weeks	After
Berglund et al. (1994)	Education	Localized	80% Breast	7 weeks	After; 3, 6, 12 months
Manne et al. (1994)	Education	Stages I, III	Breast	2 hr	After
Gruber et al. (1993)	Education	Stage I	Breast	9 weeks	During, after, 3 months
Jacobs et al. (1983)	Education vs. group discussion	All stages	Hodgkins	8 weeks	Few weeks
Telch & Telch (1986)	Education vs. group discussion	All stages	Breast	6 weeks	After
Cunningham & Tocco (1989)	Combined vs group discussion	All stages	Variety	6 weeks	After; 2–3 weeks
Duncan & Cumbia (1987)	Education vs. group discussion	Advanced	Breast	5 weeks	2 weeks

Note. "Combined" represents interventions that involved both group discussion and education. "After" means that the follow-up was described as taking place after the intervention, presumably immediately after the intervention ended.

[a]The only outcome assessed at this follow-up period was survival or recurrence.

discussion (Ferlic, Goldman, & Kennedy, 1979). The education was intended to provide informational support, and the group discussion was intended to provide emotional support. The intervention groups met three times per week for 2 weeks; each session was 90 min; and each group consisted of about 8 patients. Patients were assigned to the intervention group ($n = 30$) or to a control group ($n = 30$) that was matched on age, sex, and education. (It is unclear if the assignment was random.) Self-concept (a measure of self-esteem) and what the authors broadly construed as psychosocial adjustment (reflecting confidence in communication with network members, health care professionals, and other cancer patients; knowledge of cancer; and understanding of death) were measured before and after group participation. Compared with the control group, intervention participants increased in self-esteem and psychosocial adjustment over the 2 weeks.

A second intervention provided informational and emotional support to women with breast cancer. The intervention consisted of educational meetings, advice on coping given by cancer survivors, and peer group discussion of fears and concerns (Vachon, Lyall, Rogers, Cochrane, & Freeman, 1982). The intervention took place in the hospital and was provided to patients who received radiation therapy as inpatients. The number of intervention groups was not specified. After radiation ended (approximately 3 weeks), the in-hospital intervention patients ($n = 64$) were less distressed than the in-home controls ($n = 104$). Unfortunately, the control group consisted of women who received radiation therapy on an outpatient basis; thus, the effect of the intervention cannot be distinguished from the effect of living in the hospital. The findings of this study also are limited in that patients were not randomized to condition.

Finally, two studies evaluated the effects of group interventions on survival. In a study of women with breast cancer, both informational and emotional support were provided in a set of weekly sessions of 90 min each (Morgenstern, Gellert, Walter, Ostfeld, & Siegel, 1984). Each session involved group discussion as well as training in mental imagery and meditation. Patients were followed between 6 months and 3 years (depending on the date they entered the study) for *survival*. Each participant ($n = 34$) was matched with three nonparticipants ($n = 102$) on age at diagnosis, stage of disease, and kind of surgery by tumor registries. Intervention groups consisted of 8 to 12 patients, which suggests that three or four separate groups were conducted. The goals of the group sessions were to promote acceptance of the disease, to instill hope, and to enhance control. Results revealed that group participation was associated with longer survival, but the time lag between diagnosis and study participation was longer for intervention participants than nonparticipants, which suggests that the sickest patients may have been selected out of the intervention group. The intervention effect was not statistically reliable when the time interval between diagnosis and study participation was controlled in the analysis. Patients also were not randomly assigned to conditions.

An elegant study that randomly assigned patients to an intervention ($n = 38$) or a control group ($n = 28$) was conducted with Stage I and II malignant melanoma patients (Fawzy et al., 1990). The intervention combined education, stress management, coping skills, and discussion with patients and facilitators. Thus, informational and emotional support were provided. The intervention consisted of six weekly 90-min sessions, and four separate intervention groups were conducted. Six months after the intervention had ended, patients in the intervention group had reduced psychological distress (Fawzy et al., 1990) and altered immune function (increased natural killer cell activity, decreased T cells, increased lymphocytes; Fawzy et al., 1993) compared with patients in the control group. The intervention decreased recurrence and increased survival 6 years later (Fawzy et al., 1993). Alterations in immune function, however, did not explain the intervention's effect on mortality.

Although all of these studies suggest that multifaceted interpersonal interventions positively influenced adjustment to cancer when compared with no-treatment control groups, several suffer from methodological flaws. In addition, none distinguished among the effects of individual intervention components.

Discussion With Peers

We divide the peer discussion interventions into two types: (a) dyadic discussion between a newly diagnosed cancer patient and a cancer survivor, sometimes referred to as peer counseling, and (b) group discussion among more than 2 cancer patients, usually at least 6, sometimes referred to as a support group.

Discussion With Former Patients

One form of discussion that has been fostered among cancer patients is that between newly diagnosed patients and cancer survivors. The assumption behind this type of intervention is that cancer survivors can provide a unique kind of emotional support. They can offer comfort and empathy by virtue of having gone through the experience; they can provide validation of feelings; and they can provide reassurance by demonstrating to newly diagnosed patients that it is possible to recover.

Only one study has compared the efficacy of the peer dyad intervention to a control group. Gynecological cancer patients were randomly assigned to a no-treatment control group ($n = 18$) or a group that received counseling by former cancer patients ($n = 14$; Houts, Whitney, Mortel, & Bartholomew, 1986). The former cancer patients were social workers. They called patients three times: prior to hospitalization, 5 weeks later, and 10 weeks later. The peer counselors offered encouragement, listened to patients' concerns, shared feelings, and provided advice on how to cope with cancer. No group differences in psychological distress appeared 6 weeks or 12 weeks after the intervention began. The length of the intervention may have been too brief (three phone calls) or the nature of the contact inadequate (by phone) for it to have had a significant impact on well-being. Some aspects of the intervention also may not have been appropriate (e.g., patients were advised to maintain normal routine). Although advice by peers could be considered to reflect informational support, informal (nonexpert) advice giving by peers is likely to occur to some extent in all peer support interventions. This kind of information presumably is not as accurate as that provided by experts in educational interventions.

Group Discussion

Many interventions have consisted of group discussions that were more or less structured by group leaders. We report three studies. In the first, metastatic breast cancer patients were randomized to a control group ($n = 24$) or a group discussion inter- vention ($n = 34$; Spiegel, Bloom, & Yalom, 1981). Three discussion groups were run. The intervention consisted of weekly 90-min meetings for 1 year. Meetings focused on problems involved in having a terminal illness and ways to improve relationships. Mood was measured at the beginning of the intervention and then 4, 8, and 12 months later. No group differences in adjustment appeared at 4 months or 8 months, but at 1 year the intervention group reported better adjustment (less de- pression, greater vigor, less fatigue, less confusion) compared with the control group. By 1 year, however, only half the patients remained in the intervention and control groups. Attrition was mostly due to death. Ten years later, this team of researchers found that the intervention increased survival by 18 months (Spiegel, Bloom, Krae- mer, & Gottheil, 1989).

A second long-term (12 months) intervention also found adjustment benefits from group discussion (Kriss & Kraemer, 1986). The intervention was provided to 62 women who had mastectomies; it consisted of 90-min meetings, weekly for the first 6 months and monthly for the next 6 months. There were six intervention groups, each consisting of 8 to 12 women. The group format was loosely structured, but the content focused on self-perception, body image, and sexuality. Group leaders at- tempted to create an atmosphere of acceptance and caring (i.e., emotional support) and used role playing, psychodrama, and guided imagery. At the end of the year, the intervention did not affect body image but increased positive affect and sexual ad- justment, the two variables on which the postmastectomy women fared poorly com- pared with a group of 51 healthy women before the study. The conclusions are limited in that the women were not randomized to condition (in fact, intervention participants were self-selected) and the controls were healthy women, not breast cancer patients who did not receive the intervention.

The remaining intervention evaluation (Lonnqvist, Halttunen, Hietanen, Sevila, & Heinonen, 1986) found no effects for group discussion, but the intervention was shorter in duration, had a high refusal rate (40%), and included only a single follow- up several years later. In addition, an inadequate description of the intervention makes it difficult to evaluate its actual content. An 8-week group psychotherapy program was provided to 32 newly diagnosed breast cancer patients in Helsinki. Patients formed five separate intervention groups, and each group was matched on age, sex, and illness with a separate control group ($n = 33$). Follow-up data were collected for intervention patients 6 months after the intervention and for both in- tervention and control patients 4 to 5 years after the onset of the illness. The authors did not report whether intervention patients showed changes in adjustment at 6 months, but there was no difference between the intervention and control groups on psychosocial adjustment 4 to 5 years later.

In summary, few evaluations of interventions compared discussion groups with no-treatment controls. Moreover, the interventions that have been evaluated differ widely in nature. Existing data do suggest, however, a positive effect for two 12- month interventions (Kriss & Kraemer, 1986; Spiegel et al., 1981).

Education

Educational interventions have involved providing information about cancer, cancer treatment, and how to manage the disease and its treatment. We review six studies that compared group education interventions with no-treatment controls. Each of these studies showed effects of education on at least one outcome variable, and each randomized patients to condition. The last study, however, suffers from problems associated with small sample sizes.

Heinrich and Schag (1985) developed a stress and activity management treatment program that involved education, relaxation, problem-solving, and exercise. The program consisted of six weekly 2-hr sessions. Groups of 5 to 10 patients (with a variety of cancer sites) were randomized to intervention or control groups. At the end of the program, intervention patients' ($n = 26$) knowledge of cancer increased compared with that of controls ($n = 25$), but there were no group differences in psychological adjustment or activity level.

A second study found that education influenced psychological adjustments as well as knowledge of cancer. Gynecological cancer patients were randomly assigned to individual counseling ($n = 21$), group counseling ($n = 28$), or a control group ($n = 31$; Cain, Kohorn, Quinlan, Latimer, & Schwartz, 1986). The counseling groups participated in eight weekly educational sessions that focused on information about cancer and positive health strategies (e.g., diet, exercise, relaxation). There were 4 to 6 patients in the group counseling intervention, which suggests that there were between five and seven separate groups. Anxiety, depression, and psychosocial adjustment to illness were evaluated by a social worker before patients were randomly assigned to condition and by a research assistant, blind to condition, at two follow-up periods (1 to 2 weeks after the intervention and 6 months after the intervention). One to 2 weeks after the intervention, the individual counseling patients were rated as less anxious than the group counseling patients or the control patients, but both intervention groups showed greater gains in knowledge compared with the control group. By 6 months, both individual and group counseling patients were rated as less anxious, less depressed, and better adjusted to the illness than were control patients. This study provides evidence that education delivered to an individual or a group increases knowledge of cancer and improves psychological adjustment. Although individual counseling had a greater impact on anxiety in the short run, over time the group intervention was equally successful in facilitating psychological adjustment.

A third study of patients with a variety of cancer sites also revealed effects of an educational intervention on knowledge of cancer and psychological adjustment (Johnson, 1982). Age, sex, and pretest scores on anxiety, meaningfulness of life, and knowledge of cancer were used to place patients into pairs. One member of each pair was randomized to one treatment group ($n = 22$) or one control group ($n = 22$). The treatment consisted of eight 90-min educational sessions that focused on informational support. These were administered over a 4-week period. At the end of the treatment, the intervention group showed significantly greater improvements on anxiety, meaningfulness of life, and knowledge of cancer than the control group.

A fourth study revealed psychological health benefits of an educational intervention but showed that some positive effects disappear over time (Berglund, Bolund, Gustafsson, & Sjoden, 1994). Patients (80% with breast cancer) were randomly assigned to an educational program that involved information, physical training, and coping skills ($n = 98$) or to a control group ($n = 101$). The intervention consisted of 11 meetings held over 7 weeks. Between 3 and 7 patients attended each session. Outcome variables were measured pre- and postintervention as well as 3 months, 6 months, and 12 months after the intervention. After the educational program, intervention patients had improved physical strength and "fighting spirit" (a subscale on a cancer adjustment scale) compared with controls, and these benefits were maintained over the 12 months. However, other short-term benefits derived by intervention patients compared with control patients (reduced depression, enhanced body image) disappeared by 12 months.

A recent study evaluated the effects of a brief educational program ("Look Good, Feel Better") aimed at enhancing cancer patients' physical appearance (Manne, Girasek, & Ambrosino, 1994). Women who had surgery for breast cancer (mostly Stage I and III) volunteered to participate in the program. After completing a baseline questionnaire in the morning, patients either attended the 2-hr program in the early afternoon (experimental group, $n = 45$) or waited to attend the program (control group, $n = 76$). After the 2-hr program, all patients (experimental and no-treatment controls) completed the follow-up questionnaire. The intervention had a positive effect on mood and perceptions of attractiveness. Self-esteem decreased in the control group but was maintained in the experimental group. The findings are limited, however, by the facts that (a) patients self-selected into the program and (b) the dependent variables were assessed immediately after the program (i.e., while patients' physical appearance was enhanced).

A final study revealed an effect of an educational intervention on immune function but not on psychosocial adjustment (Gruber et al., 1993). Stage I breast cancer patients were randomly assigned to an intervention that provided informational support ($n = 7$) or a wait-list control group ($n = 6$). The intervention involved a 9-week sequence of relaxation, guided imagery, and electromyographic biofeedback. It was conducted in a highly structured group setting to minimize peer supportive interactions. Immune measures were collected weekly: 3 weeks prior to the intervention, during the intervention, and 3 months after the intervention. After baseline levels of immune function were controlled for, intervention patients showed enhanced immune function (i.e., natural killer cell activity, concanavalin A responsiveness, mixed lymphocyte responsiveness) compared with controls. At the end of the intervention, no group differences appeared on any of the measures of psychosocial adjustment, including affect, mental adjustment to cancer, locus of control, or social support. Small cell sizes, however, severely limited the study's power to detect effects.

In summary, studies that have compared educational interventions to no-treatment controls show that education increases patients' knowledge of cancer and improves psychological and physical adjustment. Although the majority of follow-up assessments took place shortly after the interventions ended, two studies demonstrated that some positive effects lasted from 6 months to 1 year (Berglund et al., 1994; Cain et al., 1986). We now examine studies that compared the effects of group discussion, education, and no treatment.

Discussion Versus Education Interventions

Four studies attempted to distinguish the effects of group discussion from those of education on adjustment to cancer. The first three randomized patients to conditions and demonstrated the superiority of education over group discussion interventions. The fourth did not find effects for either group discussion or education but failed to randomize patients to conditions and suffers from a sample size insufficient for detecting effects.

Education was compared indirectly with discussion in a study of patients with Hodgkin's disease (Jacobs, Ross, Walker, & Stockdale, 1983). Two experiments were conducted. One randomly assigned patients either to an education group that received informational support in the form of booklets and newsletters ($n = 21$) or to a no-treatment control group ($n = 26$). The second randomly assigned patients either to a discussion group that provided emotional support through discussion of problems and common concerns ($n = 16$) or to a no-treatment control group ($n = 18$). The discussion group met for eight weekly 90-min sessions. It is not clear whether either of the interventions consisted of more than one subgroup. At the end of the study (approximately 3 months later), patients in the education group reported increased knowledge of Hodgkin's disease, fewer treatment problems, less anxiety, less depression, and less life disruption than patients in the corresponding control group. There were no differences in adjustment between patients in the discussion group and patients in the corresponding no-treatment control group. The education and discussion groups were not directly compared, however.

In a second study (Telch & Telch, 1986), education and group discussion were directly compared. The educational intervention was clearly superior to the discussion intervention. Cancer patients (with a variety of cancer sites) were randomly assigned to either an educational intervention that provided informational support in the form of expanded coping skills ($n = 13$), a nondirective group discussion intervention that provided emotional support and emphasized mutual sharing of feelings and concerns ($n = 14$), or a control group ($n = 14$). The interventions consisted of six weekly 90-min sessions. Each intervention consisted of three separate groups of about 5 patients each. Psychological distress, self-efficacy, and cancer-related problems (e.g., physical appearance, pain, activity restriction, relationships) were measured before and after the interventions. In addition, psychological adjustment (e.g., problems in daily living, medical concerns, relationship concerns) was rated by a therapist who interviewed the patient and by an independent judge, blind to condition, who listened to the audiotaped interview. At the end of the study (6 weeks later), participants in the educational intervention were better adjusted (i.e., showed reduced psychological distress and greater feelings of self-efficacy) than participants in the group discussion intervention. Group discussion patients were better adjusted than control patients. Pre-post comparisons of the dependent variables revealed an improvement for the educational group, no change for the discussion group, and a deterioration for the control group. In addition, the education group scored lower on the measure of cancer-related problems than did the discussion or control groups. The latter two groups did not significantly differ from each other. Finally, at the end of the intervention, patients in the educational intervention were rated as better adjusted than group discussion or control patients by both the therapist and the independent judge. There were no differences in psychological adjustment ratings for group discussion and control patients.

In a third study, the effects of education with group discussion were distinguished from the effects of group discussion alone. Cunningham and Tocco (1989) randomly assigned patients with a variety of cancer sites and prognoses to either an educational program that focused on coping skills (e.g., relaxation, mental imagery, lifestyle changes) with the addition of supportive discussion ($n = 28$) or to a supportive discussion group only ($n = 25$). Both interventions met for six weekly 2-hr sessions in groups of 7 to 10 patients. Mood and psychological symptoms were measured prior to the first meeting, at the end of the second meeting, and 2–3 weeks later. Both groups showed improvements over time, but the education with discussion group showed greater improvements. A nonrandomized wait-list control group ($n = 18$) showed no changes in psychological adjustment over a 6-week period.

Finally, a study of a small sample of patients ($n = 18$) compared an education-based intervention with a discussion-based intervention and found that neither influenced psychological adjustment (Duncan & Cumbia, 1987). Adult metastatic breast cancer patients were involved in either a nondirective discussion group aimed at providing emotional support through empathy and acceptance ($n = 6$), an educational group that focused on the provision of informational support in the form of teaching patients skills to cope with their disease ($n = 6$), or a control group ($n = 6$). The two intervention groups met for 90 min, twice a week for 5 weeks. Patients were interviewed within 2 weeks after the intervention. The authors reported no effect of either intervention on adjustment, but the specific dependent variables were not described, small sample size led to insufficient statistical power, and it is not clear whether patients were randomly assigned to conditions.

To the extent that the two kinds of interventions have been evaluated, education has been shown to have a greater effect on psychological adjustment than has group discussion. Again, the nature of the discussion-based interventions varied widely, which makes it difficult to draw strong conclusions about the kind of peer discussion that affects adjustment.

Summary

Although our review includes several studies that found effects of support interventions on mortality (Fawzy et al., 1993; Morgenstern et al., 1984; Spiegel et al., 1989), the number and scope of studies focusing on physical adjustment are not yet sufficient for us to assess the effectiveness of these interventions or to speculate seriously on responsible mechanisms (see Andersen, Kiecolt-Glaser, & Glaser, 1994; Cohen, 1988, for a discussion of how psychological and behavioral factors influence disease course). Consequently, our summary (and discussion) focuses on the role of social support interventions in psychological adjustment.

The group (peer) intervention studies we examined evaluated the effectiveness of group discussion, group education, or the combination of the two. We view group discussion interventions primarily as attempts to provide emotional support and educational interventions primarily as attempts to provide informational support. This literature is neither large enough nor methodologically sound enough for us to reach any definitive conclusions, but we feel it offers some strong hints. Overall, the evidence for the effectiveness of group discussion interventions is less than one would expect on the basis of descriptive and correlational research. Educational interventions, however, appear to be as effective as, if not more effective than, group discussion interventions. First, studies that compared group discussion with no-treatment controls and group education with no-treatment controls revealed more evidence for the effectiveness of education than group discussion. The only evidence for benefits of group discussion came from very long (12-month) interventions (Kriss & Kraemer,

1986; Spiegel et al., 1989). This is in contrast to educational interventions, which lasted no longer than 9 weeks and, in some cases, showed positive effects that lasted between 6 months and 1 year (see Table 1). Thus, at the very least, educational interventions are more cost-effective than group discussion interventions. Second, the two studies (with adequate sample sizes) that evaluated group discussion and education and included comparisons with no-treatment controls showed stronger effects of education than of group discussion on adjustment.

One difficulty that arises in comparing the two kinds of interventions is caused by the fact that they were probably not pure education or pure group discussion. Some informal discussion may have occurred in the educational interventions, and some informal information giving may have occurred in the group discussion interventions. At the very least, one may conclude that short-term interventions that attempt to provide education, regardless of whether informal discussion occurs, appear to have greater benefits for adjustment than do interventions that provide group discussion in the absence of education. It is worth noting that Meyer and Mark's (1995) recent meta-analytic review of all psychosocial interventions did not show differential effectiveness for different kinds of interventions (e.g., education, supportive therapy).

The lack of evidence for positive effects of group discussion is inconsistent with the correlational research on the kinds of support that facilitate adjustment to cancer and with descriptive studies on the kinds of support cancer patients say they desire. Descriptive and correlational studies suggest that the most important kind of support is emotional support, particularly the availability of someone with whom the patient can disclose worries and concerns. This is exactly the kind of emotional support supposedly fostered in peer discussion groups. Instead, intervention research does not provide strong evidence for the benefits of emotional support. Is the correlational research wrong, or is the conclusion from the intervention research faulty? We discuss both possibilities.

Reconciling Correlational and Intervention Research

In reconciling these contradictory findings, we need to ask why one would expect social support to facilitate adjustment. If we identify the mechanisms by which social interactions influence well-being, we can determine the kind of naturally occurring support and support intervention that should influence these mechanisms and influence adjustment to cancer. In the following discussion, we examine why past research may have shown group discussions to be less effective and educational interventions to be more effective in influencing some of these support processes.

Difficulties With Group Discussion Interventions

Theoretically, group discussion interventions benefit patients' adjustment to cancer by enhancing their self-esteem (Lieberman, 1988; Yalom & Greaves, 1977) through the provision of emotional support. Discussion with peers is intended to convey caring and acceptance, to reduce feelings of uniqueness, and to validate feelings through the sharing of experiences; that is, it is intended to encourage positive feelings toward the self or to diminish any feelings of personal inadequacy that may accompany cancer. Mutual support and encouragement also are intended to enhance patients' optimism about the future. Finally, the process of expressing the self in a warm and accepting environment may affect adjustment by increasing patients' awareness of previously unacknowledged emotions, permitting them access to new emotions, leading them to acceptance of emotions, or altering their emotions (Greenberg & Safran, 1989).

Then why have group discussion interventions been relatively unsuccessful? The failure to find a consistent positive effect of group discussion on adjustment to cancer could be due to methodological weaknesses that plague the literature (e.g., small sample sizes). However, there are some serious conceptual problems as well. Group discussion interventions have as much potential to adversely affect patients' illness reactions as they do to positively influence these reactions. Group discussion may reduce self-esteem, diminish perceptions of control, or focus on the wrong source of emotional support (peers).

1. Group Discussion Interventions Have the Potential to Negatively Affect Self-Esteem and Optimism About the Future

The content of peer group discussions varies widely. A peer group may consist of patients with different personalities and often different prognoses and kinds of cancer. These differences have a greater effect on the nature and content of discussion-based interventions than of education-based interventions. Group members can bring up uncomfortable and frightening topics that increase anxiety if not placed in proper perspective by trained leaders. Although the intention may be to have feelings validated, group members may learn that others do not share their feelings and thus may be left feeling more alone and isolated. Groups that consist of members with varying cancer sites may have greater difficulty validating each other's experiences. Thus, self-esteem may be damaged by harmful group interactions.

Talking to group members who are doing well (upward comparisons) may be inspiring, but talking to group members who are not doing well (downward comparisons) may be fear arousing. Although downward comparisons typically enhance self-esteem and lead patients to feel better about themselves, this is more likely to occur when patients have the opportunity to select their social comparisons (Helgeson & Mickelson, in press). In the context of a support group, multiple social comparisons are forced on patients. There is some evidence that participants in support groups feel uncomfortable in the presence of downward comparisons (Coates & Winston, 1983; Taylor et al., 1988; Vernberg & Vogel, 1993). The presence of others who are worse off may diminish patients' optimism about the future.

Finally, peer discussion groups have the potential to damage self-esteem by reinforcing the participant's identity as a member of a deviant or stigmatized group (Coates & Winston, 1983). To the extent that identification with the group interferes with integration into society, group participants may have increased difficulty obtaining support from their naturally occurring social environments.

Some of these problems can be addressed with structured formats and trained facilities (Dunkel-Schetter & Wortman, 1982; Lieberman, 1988). Structure does not imply that the dialogue of these groups is standardized. As Goldberg and Wool (1985) noted, it is difficult to standardize psychotherapeutic interventions because people present with different problems. Instead, structure implies that trained facilitators (a) keep group members on track and reduce chaotic conversation, (b) promote acceptance and feelings of commonality as opposed to uniqueness and deviance, (c) normalize and validate experiences, and (d) clarify misconceptions. Group discussion without this kind of structure may be just as likely to have a negative as a positive effect on well-being.

2. Group Discussion May (Temporarily) Reduce Perceived Control Among Some Patients

One way to maintain control over the illness experience is by denying its existence, and group discussion could break down denial—thus having the apparent effect of increasing distress. There are two groups of patients who appear "nondistressed" on most psychological instruments: the truly nondistressed and the deniers (Shedler, Mayman, & Manis, 1993). The combined effects of decreasing distress among patients who initially reported distress and increasing distress among deniers may result in an intervention's apparent ineffectiveness (Shedler et al., 1993). One may argue that this reasoning also should apply to the education-based interventions, which appear to be effective. However, an education-based intervention is not as likely to reduce denial because information about the disease and appropriate treatment is less likely than a discussion of personal feelings to threaten a patient's perception that he or she is coping well.

The idea that expressing negative feelings might temporarily increase distress but benefit health in the long run has been suggested by other researchers (Pennebaker, Colder, & Sharp, 1990), including those studying support groups for other problems (Coates & Winston, 1983; Cowan & Cowan, 1986). If one assumes that group discussions will eventually aid those who initially deny distress, longer term follow-ups may provide more sensitive evaluations. For example, in the Spiegel et al. (1989) group discussion intervention, beneficial effects on adjustment did not appear during the intervention (at 4 months and 8 months) but appeared immediately after the intervention ended (12 months).

3. Emotional Support Provided by Peers in an Intervention May Not Influence Well-Being

It may be that emotional support from existing network members—friends and family and physicians—has a greater influence on adjustment than does emotional support from other cancer patients. First, emotional support provided by peers is typically of shorter duration (finite time length of intervention) than emotional support provided by members of naturally occurring networks. Second, emotional support from peers may not be as effective in reducing distress as emotional support from other sources—either because the relationship is not as intimate or because the support is artificial in the context of an intervention (Rook & Dooley, 1985). The long-term peer support interventions may be effective because they foster "natural" friendships between peers, which changes an "artificial" relationship into a "natural" one.

Effectiveness of Educational Interventions

Education may directly influence adjustment to cancer because it helps patients restore control or find meaning in the experience. Education may indirectly influence adjustment to cancer by restoring patients' self-esteem and optimism about the future.

1. Educational Interventions Enhance Perceptions of Control

Educational interventions can help to restore patients' loss of control by providing them with information about the cause, course, and treatment of the illness and by teaching them ways to manage the illness and its side effects. Because of their expertise, health care professionals, not peers, are the most effective and accurate sources of information about the disease, disease course, treatment, and side effects.

2. Educational Interventions May Affect Self-Esteem and Optimism

To the extent that patients respond to the information provided in an educational intervention, self-esteem and optimism about the future may increase. For example, patients may gain information about how to enhance physical appearance during chemotherapy that will restore self-esteem if used. Information about the disease may increase hope and information about how to cope with side effects may lead to a more favorable outlook for the future if these coping strategies are implemented and effective.

In summary, educational interventions may be more effective than group discussion interventions because they meet the needs of a greater proportion of patients and because they are less likely to place patients at risk for negative outcomes. Educational interventions have the opportunity to restore lost control, provide meaning for the experience, restore self-esteem, and instill optimism about the future. Educational interventions also may appear more effective than group discussion interventions because patients receive both informational support and informal emotional support.

Future Directions

If we take our review seriously, we would recommend developing educational programs for cancer patients. Educational interventions have more consistent positive effects on adjustment and are easier and less costly to implement than group discussion interventions. The question remains, however, whether we should take the literature seriously enough to guide clinical practice. We believe that given the correlational literature and the theoretical arguments regarding the importance of emotional support, discarding the hypothesis that group-based emotional support interventions are beneficial to patients is premature. In view of this conclusion, we suggest two directions for future intervention research: (a) more methodologically sound evaluations of controlled peer discussion interventions, and (b) evaluation of interventions focused on improving emotional support provision from members of naturally occurring support networks.

Methodological Improvements of Group Discussion Intervention

Studies should use no-treatment control groups, randomize patients to conditions, structure and monitor group discussions, and measure the mechanisms by which the intervention is expected to achieve its effects (e.g., enhancement of self-esteem). Researchers should consider measuring denial, other coping styles, and individual difference variables (e.g., gender, prognosis) that may determine who benefits the most from discussion-based interventions. Discussion-based interventions should be structured and portable so that they can be implemented by trained facilitators. It also would be advantageous to include more diverse classes of people, because past intervention research has involved mostly White, middle- to upper-class women (Meyer & Mark, 1995; Taylor et al., 1988).

Adjustment should be measured before, during, and after the intervention. Both short-term and long-term (at least 1 year) follow-ups should be included. Short-term effects of an intervention may dissipate over time, or it may take a longer period of time for health benefits of an intervention to appear. The latter effect is consistent with discussion-based support groups in other areas (e.g., Cowan & Cowan, 1986).

Researchers should consider the effect of combining cancer patients with different cancer sites and prognoses in a single intervention. These differences may interfere with the empathy and shared experiences that are expected to normalize and validate patients' feelings. The presence of a good-prognosis patient and a poor-prognosis patient in the same discussion group not only influences the nature of the discussion but may mask any differential effectiveness of the intervention with respect to prognosis.

Multiple groups should be used to evaluate the interventions. In the literature reviewed in this article, the numbers of groups within each intervention were generally small with a mode of one. Groups vary substantially in their response to an intervention, and optimal designs would treat groups (as opposed to individual patients) as the unit of analysis. At the very least, a large enough number of groups should be used so that group differences within each treatment can be statistically controlled.

More studies of peer dyad interventions are needed because this intervention is not vulnerable to some of the problems that plague group discussion interventions. Cancer role models can be selected on the basis of their optimism, psychological stability, and positive response to disease. The American Cancer Society's "Reach to Recovery" program, in which women who have surgery for breast cancer are visited in the hospital by a former cancer patient, is based on this idea.

Interventions to Improve Naturally Occurring Support Networks

Descriptive and correlational research focused on support provided by existing network members, whereas the intervention research focused on support provided by new network members. Future intervention research may benefit from altering existing social relationships rather than creating new social relationships to meet patients' needs for emotional support.

Family and Friends

Interventions that involve family and friends could be aimed at dispelling myths (e.g., it is bad for the patient to talk about the illness), improving communication, and facilitating both patients' and family members' expressions of needs and feelings. For example, after surgery, spouses often perceive patients as fragile and are afraid that physical closeness will be harmful. Patients perceive spouses' lack of physical closeness as withdrawal and respond in kind. Improving communication helps both patients and spouses to understand each others' actions.

Interventions that address the patient-spouse relationship would seem to be particularly important because spouse support is critical to adjustment (Jamison et al., 1978). Two studies were designed to improve communication among women with breast cancer and their spouses. In one, postmastectomy patients and their spouses were randomly assigned to communication counseling or a no-treatment control group (Christensen, 1983). There was a decrease in depression among patients and an increase in sexual satisfaction among patients and spouses assigned to the intervention group compared with those assigned to the control group. In a second, Samarel and Fawcett (1992) added a "coach" component to a support group to help family members become aware of patients' needs and how to provide emotional support. Unfortunately, the effectiveness of the intervention has not been evaluated.

Physicians

Interventions could focus on training physicians to provide emotional support to patients. Physicians must learn to convey information in a caring and accepting manner as well as in a way that patients are able to understand. Patients are more likely to return to an empathic physician than a physician who is competent but not understanding (Korsch & Negrete, 1972). Moreover, increasing the emotional support from physicians to patients will increase patient trust, openness, confidence, and feelings of control and will enable patients to elicit the information they need.

There are barriers to implementing interventions that alter the existing social environment. Chapman and Pancoast (1985) discussed a number of obstacles, three of which are relevant to our discussion. First, it is difficult to change the content of exchanges that occur in established relationships. Second, caregivers are overburdened and may not be receptive to participating in an intervention. Third, some relationships are nonsupportive or conflicted and not amenable to a support intervention.

An alternative approach to altering the social environment is equipping the patient with skills to influence the social network (Cohen et al., 1988). Such training might focus on general social skills (e.g., assertiveness) that will help patients communicate their needs and be able to distinguish helpful from unhelpful social resources. Educating patients about how their illness affects relationships (e.g., places a burden on caregivers) may reduce miscommunications and increase understanding of social interactions.

Conclusion

The descriptive and correlational literatures suggest that the support most desired by cancer patients and most strongly linked to adjustment is emotional support—specifically, the availability of someone with whom to discuss illness-related concerns and worries. The intervention research, however, offers little evidence that short-term peer discussion groups aimed at providing emotional support influence cancer adjustment. Instead, educational interventions aimed at providing informational support appear to have an equal, if not greater, impact on adjustment. To reconcile these divergent findings, we examined (a) the mechanisms by which one would expect social interactions to influence psychological and physical adjustment to cancer, and (b) the extent to which educational versus group discussion interventions address these mechanisms. We suggest five psychological mechanisms: enhancement of self-esteem, restoration of perceived control, instilling of optimism about the future, provision of meaning for the experience, and fostering of emotional processing. The current state of the literature leads us to conclude that previous educational interventions have a greater potential than group discussion interventions to affect more of these mechanisms. Because the evaluations of group discussion interventions reviewed in this article are limited by methodological flaws and conceptual weaknesses, we suggest that better tests of this intervention should be conducted before discarding the hypothesis that discussion with peers is an effective vehicle for providing the emotional support cancer patients desire.

References

American Cancer Society. (1992). *Cancer facts and figures.* Atlanta, GA: Author.

Andersen, B. L., Kiecolt-Glaser, J. K., & Glaser, R. (1994). A biobehavioral model of cancer stress and disease course. *American Psychologist, 49,* 389–404.

Berglund, G., Bolund, C., Gustafsson, U. L., & Sjoden, P. O. (1994). One-year follow-up of the 'Starting Again' group rehabilitation programme for cancer patients. *European Journal of Cancer, 30A,* 1744–1751.

Bloom, J. R. (1982). Social support, accommodation to stress and adjustment to breast cancer. *Social Science and Medicine, 16,* 1329–1338.

Bloom, J. R., & Kessler, L. (1994). Emotional support following cancer: A test of the stigma and social activity hypotheses. *Journal of Health and Social Behavior, 35,* 118–133.

Bloom, J. R., & Spiegel, D. (1984). The relationship of two dimensions of social support to the psychological well-being and social functioning of women with advanced breast cancer. *Social Science and Medicine, 19,* 831–837.

Cain, E. N., Kohorn, E. I., Quinlan, D. M., Latimer, K., & Schwartz, P. E. (1986). Psychosocial benefits of a cancer support group. *Cancer, 57,* 183–189.

Chapman, N., & Pancoast, D. L. (1985). Working with the informal helping networks of the elderly: The experiences of three programs. *Journal of Social Issues, 41,* 47–63.

Christensen, D. N. (1983). Postmastectomy couple counseling: An outcome study of a structured treatment protocol. *Journal of Sex and Marital Therapy, 9,* 266–275.

Coates, D., & Winston, T. (1983). Counteracting the deviance of depression: Peer support groups for victims. *Journal of Social Issues, 39,* 169–194.

Cohen, S. (1988). Psychosocial models of social support in the etiology of physical disease. *Health Psychology, 7,* 269–297.

Cohen, S., & Hoberman, H. M. (1983). Positive events and social supports as buffers of life change stress. *Journal of Applied Social Psychology, 13,* 99–125.

Cohen, S., Lichtenstein, E., Mermelstein, R., Kingsolver, K., Baer, J. S., & Kamarck, T. W. (1988). Social support interventions for smoking cessation. In B. H. Gottlieb (Ed.), *Marshaling social support: Formats, processes, and effects* (pp. 211–240). Newbury Park, CA: Sage.

Cohen, S., & Wills, T. A. (1985). Stress, social support, and the buffering hypothesis. *Psychological Bulletin, 98,* 310–357.

Cowan, C., & Cowan, P. A. (1986). A preventive intervention for couples becoming parents. In C. F. Z. Boukydis (Ed.), *Research on support for parents and infants in the postnatal period* (pp. 225–251). New York: Ablex.

Cunningham, A. J., & Tocco, E. K. (1989). A randomized trial of group psychoeducational therapy for cancer patients. *Patient Education and Counseling, 14,* 101–114.

Dakof, G. A., & Taylor, S. E. (1990). Victims' perceptions of social support: What is helpful from whom? *Journal of Personality and Social Psychology, 58,* 80–89.

Duncan, J. A., & Cumbia, G. G. (1987). Lessons learned while providing group counseling for adult patients with metastatic cancer. *Journal for Specialists in Group Work, 12,* 70–75.

Dunkel-Schetter, C. (1984). Social support and cancer: Findings based on patient interviews and their implications. *Journal of Social Issues, 40,* 77–98.

Dunkel-Schetter, C., & Wortman, C. B. (1982). The interpersonal dynamics of cancer: Problems in social relationships and their impact on the patient. In H. S. Friedman & M. R. DiMatteo (Eds.), *Interpersonal issues in health care* (pp. 69–100). New York: Academic Press.

Ell, K., Nishimoto, R. H., Mediansky, L., Mantell, J. E., & Hamovitch, M. B. (1992). Social relations, social support and survival among patients with cancer. *Journal of Psychosomatic Research, 36,* 531–541.

Fawzy, F. I., Cousins, N., Fawzy, N. W., Kemeny, M. E., Elashoff, R., & Morton, D. (1990). A structured psychiatric intervention for cancer patients: I. Changes over time in methods of coping and affective disturbance. *Cancer Intervention, 47,* 720–725.

Fawzy, F. I., Fawzy, N. W., Hyun, C. S., Elashoff, R., Guthrie, D., Fahey, J. L., & Morton, D. L. (1993). Malignant melanoma: Effects of an early structured psychiatric intervention, coping, and affective state on recurrence and survival 6 years later. *Archives of General Psychiatry, 50,* 681–689.

Ferlic, M., Goldman, A., & Kennedy, B. J. (1979). Group counseling in adult patients with advanced cancer. *Cancer, 43,* 760–766.

Funch, D. P., & Mettlin, C. (1982). The role of support in relation to recovery from breast surgery. *Social Science and Medicine, 16,* 19–98.

Glantz, K., & Lerman, C. (1992). Psychosocial impact of breast cancer: A critical review. *Annals of Behavioral Medicine, 14,* 204–212.

Goldberg, R. J., & Wool, M. S. (1985). Psychotherapy for the spouses of lung cancer patients: Assessment of an intervention. *Psychotherapy Psychosomatics, 43,* 141–150.

Greenberg, L. S., & Safran, J. D. (1989). Emotion in psychotherapy. *American Psychologist, 44,* 19–29.

Gruber, B. L., Hersh, S. P., Hall, N. R., Waletzky, L. R., Kunz, J. F., Carpenter, J. K., Kverno, K. S., & Weiss, S. M. (1993). Immunological responses of breast cancer patients to behavioral interventions. *Biofeedback and Self Regulation, 18,* 1–22.

Heinrich, R. L., & Schag, C. C. (1985). Stress and activity management: Group treatment for cancer patients and spouses. *Journal of Consulting and Clinical Psychology, 53,* 439–446.

Helgeson, V. S., & Mickelson, K. D. (in press). Coping with chronic illness among the elderly. In S. Manuck, R. Jennings, & B. Rabin (Eds.), *Perspectives in behavioral medicine.* Hillsdale, NJ: Erlbaum.

Holland, J. C. (1991). Psychosocial variables: Are they factors in cancer risk or survival? In J. C. Holland, L. M. Lesko, & M. J. Massie (Eds.), *Current concepts in psycho-oncology IV* (pp. 25–34). New York: Memorial Sloan-Kettering Cancer Center.

House, J. S. (1981). *Work stress and social support.* Reading, MA: Addison-Wesley.

House, J. S., & Kahn, R. L. (1985). Measures and concepts of social support. In S. Cohen & L. Syme (Eds.), *Social support and health* (pp. 83–108). Orlando, FL: Academic Press.

Houts, P. S., Whitney, C. W., Mortel, R., & Bartholomew, M. J. (1986). Former cancer patients as counselors of newly diagnosed cancer patients. *Journal of the National Cancer Institute, 76,* 793–796.

Jacobs, C., Ross, R. D., Walker, I. M., & Stockdale, F. E. (1983). Behavior of cancer patients: A randomized study of the effects of education and peer support groups. *American Journal of Clinical Oncology, 6,* 347–353.

Jamison, K. R., Wellisch, D. K., & Pasnau, R. O. (1978). Psychosocial aspects of mastectomy: I. The woman's perspective. *American Journal of Psychiatry, 135,* 432–436.

Janoff-Bulman, R., & Frieze, I. H. (1983). A theoretical perspective for understanding reactions to victimization. *Journal of Social Issues, 39,* 1–17.

Johnson, J. (1982). The effects of a patient education course on persons with a chronic illness. *Cancer Nursing, 5,* 117–123.

Kahn, R. L., & Antonucci, T. C. (1980). Convoys over the life course: Attachments, roles, and social support. In P. B. Baltes & O. Brim (Eds.), *Life-span development and behavior* (Vol. 3, pp. 253–286). New York: Academic Press.

Korsch, B. M., & Negrete, V. F. (1972). Doctor–patient communication. *Scientific American, 227,* 66–74.

Kriss, R. T., & Kraemer, H. C. (1986). Efficacy of group therapy for problems with post-mastectomy self-perception, body image, and sexuality. *Journal of Sex Research, 22,* 438–451.

Lesko, L. M., Ostroff, J., & Smith, K. (1991). Life after cancer treatment: Survival and beyond. In J. C. Holland, L. M. Lesko, & M. H. Massie (Eds.), *Current concepts in psycho-oncology IV* (pp. 47–53). New York: Memorial Sloan-Kettering Cancer Center.

Lieberman, M. A. (1988). The role of self-help groups in helping patients and families cope with cancer. *Cancer, 38,* 162–168.

Lindsey, A. M., Norbeck, J. S., Carrieri, V. L., & Perry, E. (1981). Social support and health outcomes in postmastectomy women: A review. *Cancer Nursing 4*(5), 377–384.

Lonnqvist, J., Halttunen, A., Hietanen, P., Sevila, A., & Heinonen, M. (1986). Subjective symptoms of breast cancer patients: A controlled follow-up study on the effects of group psychotherapy to support the adaptation of the new consecutive breast cancer patients. *Psychiatria Fennica Supplementum,* Suppl., 187–197.

Manne, S. L., Girasek, D., & Ambrosino, J. (1994). An evaluation of the impact of a cosmetics class on breast cancer patients. *Journal of Psychosocial Oncology, 12,* 83–99.

Meyer, T. J., & Mark, M. M. (1995). Effects of psychosocial interventions with adult cancer patients: A meta-analysis of randomized experiments. *Health Psychology, 14,* 101–108.

Mitchell, G. W., & Glicksman, A. S. (1977). Cancer patients: Knowledge and attitudes. *Cancer, 40,* 61–66.

Morgenstern, H., Gellert, G. A., Walter, S. D., Ostfeld, A. M., & Siegel, B. S. (1984). The impact of a psychosocial support program on survival with breast cancer: The importance of selection bias in program evaluation. *Journal of Chronic Disability, 37,* 273–282.

National Cancer Institute. (1984, November 26). Surveillance Epidemiology and End Results Program (SEER) cancer patient survival statistics. In *Update: Annual cancer statistics review* (pp. 1–8). Bethesda, MD: Author.

Neuling, S. J., & Winefield, H. R. (1988). Social support and recovery after surgery for breast cancer: Frequency and correlates of supportive behaviors by family, friends, and surgeon. *Social Science and Medicine, 27,* 385–392.

Northouse, A. L. (1988). Social support in patients' and husbands' adjustment to breast cancer. *Nursing Research, 37,* 91–95.

Peck, A., & Bowland, J. (1977). Emotional reactions to radiation treatment. *Cancer, 40,* 180–184.

Pennebaker, J. W., Colder, M., & Sharp, L. K. (1990). Accelerating the coping process. *Journal of Personality and Social Psychology, 58,* 528–537.

Peters-Golden, H. (1982). Breast cancer: Varied perceptions of social support in the illness experience. *Social Science and Medicine, 16,* 483–491.

Primomo, J., Yates, B. C., & Woods, N. F. (1990). Social support for women during chronic illness: The relationship among sources and types to adjustment. *Research in Nursing and Health, 13,* 153–161.

Reynolds, P., & Kaplan, G. A. (1990). Social connections and risk for cancer: Prospective evidence from the Alameda County study. *Behavioral Medicine, 16,* 101–110.

Rook, K. S., & Dooley, D. (1985). Applying social support research: Theoretical problems and future directions. *Journal of Social Issues, 41,* 5–28.

Rose, J. H. (1990). Social support and cancer: Adult patients' desire for support from family, friends, and health professionals. *American Journal of Community Psychology, 18,* 439–464.

Rowland, J. H. (1989). Developmental stage and adaptation: Adult model. In J. C. Holland, & J. H. Rowland (Eds.), *Handbook of psychooncology: Psychological care of the patient with cancer* (pp. 25–43). New York: Oxford University Press.

Samarel, N., & Fawcett, J. (1992). Enhancing adaptation to breast cancer: The addition of coaching to support groups. *Oncology Nursing Forum, 19,* 591–596.

Scott, D. W., & Eisendrath, S. J. (1986). Dynamics of the recovery process following initial diagnosis of breast cancer. *Journal of Psychosocial Oncology, 3*(4), 53–67.

Shedler, J., Mayman, M., & Manis, M. (1993). The illusion of mental health. *American Psychologist, 48,* 1117–1131.

Spiegel, D., Bloom, J. R., Kraemer, H. C., & Gottheil, E. (1989). Effect of psychosocial treatment on survival of patients with metastatic breast cancer. *Lancet, 2,* 888–891.

Spiegel, D., Bloom, J., & Yalom, I. (1981). Group support for patients with metastatic cancer —A prospective randomized outcome study. *Archives of General Psychiatry, 38,* 527–533.

Taylor, S. E. (1983). Adjustment to threatening events: A theory of cognitive adaptation. *American Psychologist, 38,* 1161–1173.

Taylor, S. E., Falke, R. L., Mazal, R. M., & Hilsberg, B. L. (1988). Sources of satisfaction and dissatisfaction among members of cancer support groups. In B. H. Gottlieb (Ed.), *Marshaling social support: Formats, processes and effects* (pp. 187–208). Newbury Park, CA: Sage.

Taylor, S. E., Falke, R. L., Shoptaw, S. J., & Lichtman, R. R. (1986). Social support, support groups, and the cancer patient. *Journal of Consulting and Clinical Psychology, 54,* 608–615.

Telch, C. F., & Telch, M. J. (1986). Group coping skills instruction and supportive group therapy for cancer patients: A comparison of strategies. *Journal of Consulting and Clinical Psychology, 54,* 802–808.

Thoits, P. A. (1985). Social support and psychological well-being: Theoretical possibilities. In I. G. Sarason & B. R. Sarason (Eds.), *Social support: Theory, research, and applications* (pp. 51–72). Dordrecht, The Netherlands: Martinus Nijhoff.

Vachon, M. L. S., Lyall, W. A. L., Rogers, J., Cochrane, J., & Freeman, S. J. J. (1982). The effectiveness of psychosocial support during post-surgical treatment of breast cancer. *International Journal of Psychiatry in Medicine, 11,* 365–372.

Vernberg, E. M., & Vogel, J. M. (1993). Psychological responses of children to natural and human-made disasters: II. Interventions with children after disasters. *Journal of Clinical Child Psychology, 22,* 485–498.

Wethington, E., & Kessler, R. C. (1986). Perceived support, received support, and adjustment to stressful life events. *Journal of Health and Social Behavior, 27,* 78–89.

Woods, N. F., & Earp, J. L. (1978). Women with cured breast cancer: A study of mastectomy patients in North Carolina. *Nursing Research, 27,* 279–285.

Wortman, C. B., & Conway, T. L. (1985). The role of social support in adaptation and recovery from physical illness. In S. Cohen & S. L. Syme (Eds.), *Social support and health* (pp. 281–302), Orlando, FL: Academic Press.

Wortman, C. B., & Dunkel-Schetter, C. (1979). Interpersonal relationships and cancer: A theoretical analysis. *Journal of Social Issues, 35,* 120–155.

Wortman, C. B., & Dunkel-Schetter, C. (1987). Conceptual and methodological issues in the study of social support. In A. Baum & J. E. Singer (Eds.), *Handbook of psychology and health: Vol. V. Stress* (pp. 63–108). Hillsdale, NJ: Erlbaum.

Wortman, C. B., & Lehman, D. R. (1985). Reactions to victims of life crises: Support attempts that fail. In I. G. Sarason & B. R. Sarason (Eds.), *Social support: Theory, research and applications* (pp. 463–489). Dordrecht, The Netherlands: Martinus Nijhoff.

Yalom, I. D., & Greaves, C. (1977). Group therapy with the terminally ill. *American Journal of Psychiatry, 134,* 396–400.

Zemore, R., & Shepel, L. F. (1989). Effects of breast cancer and mastectomy on emotional support and adjustment. *Social Science and Medicine, 28,* 19–27.

Chapter 4
PSYCHOLOGICAL ADJUSTMENT IN ADULTS
WITH CANCER:
The Self as Mediator

Susan M. Heidrich, Cynthia A. Forsthoff, and Sandra E. Ward

Understanding positive adjustment to cancer is an important aspect of research aimed at enhancing quality of life for patients. It has been noted that although the initial, short-term response to cancer may include significant depression, anxiety, and other symptoms of distress and impaired social functioning, the majority of individuals with cancer adjust successfully and, over time, are no different on most psychological outcome measures from individuals with benign disease (Andersen, Anderson, & deProsse, 1989; Cassileth, Lusk, Brown, & Cross, 1986; Felton, Revenson, & Hinrichsen, 1984; Krouse & Krouse, 1982; Vinokur, Threatt, Caplan, & Zimmerman, 1989). However, empirical research investigating theoretical explanations of how individuals manage to maintain or regain their psychological well-being when faced with the diagnosis or treatment of cancer is lacking. The purpose of this study was to examine the role of self-discrepancies in adjustment to cancer.

Conceptual Model

Rosenberg and Taylor (Rosenberg, 1986; Taylor, 1983; Taylor & Brown, 1988; Taylor, Lichtman, & Wood, 1984) offered theoretical perspectives regarding the adaptive capacity of the self that are useful in examining how expectations regarding the self are related to adjustment to illness. Rosenberg's conceptualization of the self-concept as dynamic and multidimensional provides a meaningful approach to investigating differences in adaptation. In his view, there are multiple aspects of the self that develop through both internal self-evaluations and interpersonal experiences. The self is dynamic because, in response to external events, different aspects of one's self may be changed or modified. Rosenberg also proposed that the self is multidimensional; two of those dimensions are the ideal self and the actual self. *Ideal self* refers to aspirations as to who one could potentially be, whereas *real self* refers to conceptions of who one really is. Individuals are motivated to achieve a match between the ideal self and the actual self because a discrepancy results in psychological tension or discomfort, experienced as either depression or anxiety (Higgins, 1987; Higgins, Bond, Klein, & Strauman, 1986). Thus, when external events threaten a person's self-conception, different aspects of the self-concept are altered in an attempt to maintain an actual-ideal self match and thereby reduce psychological distress. In this sense, achieving a match among different aspects of the self is a process of psychological adjustment.

Reprinted from *Health Psychology, 13*(5), 346–353. (1994). Copyright © 1994 by the American Psychological Association. Used with permission of the author.

The diagnosis of cancer can be particularly threatening because it is associated with fears of pain and death due to the disease and fears of painful, debilitating, or disfiguring treatment (Levin, Cleeland, & Dar, 1985; Ward, Heidrich, & Wolberg, 1989; Weisman, 1979). Therefore, a diagnosis of cancer may be a particularly potent motivation for engaging in adjustments related to the self (Curbow, Somerfield, Legro, & Sonnega, 1990). In fact, alterations in self-concept might help explain the paradoxical findings that although persons with cancer initially experience high levels of distress, over time they are as well adjusted as others and, in fact, may perceive themselves as being better adjusted than they were before their illness (Wood, Taylor, & Lichtman, 1985; Zenmore, Rinholm, Shepel, & Richards, 1989).

On the basis of her studies of women with cancer, Taylor (1983) argued that one way individuals adjust to threatening events is by altering their views of the self in such a way that self-esteem is enhanced. Heidrich and Ward (1992) found that elderly women with cancer had lower actual and ideal self-ratings than women without cancer but were no different in terms of self-discrepancies and adjustment. They suggested that women with cancer lowered their expectations concerning their ideal self to align their ideal and actual self-conceptions, thus reducing self-discrepancies and psychological distress. Thus, if Rosenberg (1986) and Taylor are correct, adjustment to cancer can occur by reducing the discrepancy between one's ideal and actual self-concepts. Neither Rosenberg nor Taylor, however, discussed specific factors that might make an event such as cancer particularly threatening to the self.

Previous empirical research identified a number of factors that predict adjustment to cancer and other chronic illnesses, but little is known about how these factors may also influence the self or be mediated by the self. Three such factors are symptoms, functional health, and the perceived time line of the illness.

In terms of adjustment, a number of studies have demonstrated that more severe symptoms, whether due to disease or to treatments such as chemotherapy or radiotherapy, are associated with higher levels of psychological distress (Christman, 1990; Herr, Kornblith, & Ofman, 1993; McCorkle & Quint-Benoliel, 1983; Ward, Viergutz, Tormey, DeMuth, & Paulen, 1992). Functional health is also associated with adjustment. When individuals experience difficulties with activities of daily living due to health problems, higher levels of psychological distress and lower levels of psychological well-being are reported (Heidrich, 1993; Heidrich & Ryff, 1993a, 1993b). Finally, perceived time line of the illness, that is, whether individuals perceive their illness to be an acute or chronic problem, is related to psychological outcomes (Meyer, Leventhal, & Gutmann, 1985). In women with cancer, the perception of illness as chronic, regardless of the actual stage of the disease, has been associated with increased depression (Ward et al., 1992).

These three factors, although associated with psychological adjustment to cancer, have not been sufficiently examined for their relationship with self-conceptions. Symptoms, functional health, and time line might influence a person's sense of self in a number of ways. For instance, more severe symptoms and declines in functional ability might impair a person's ability to carry out important social roles, such as wife, parent, or employee. In turn, relationships with significant others may be altered and influence the person's conceptions of him- or herself as a supportive spouse, good parent, or breadwinner. Time line, or perceiving one's illness as chronic, might influence one's sense of possible future selves because aspirations and ideals may be altered on the basis of beliefs about the course of one's illness and future physical, cognitive, or social capabilities. Thus, both actual self and ideal self-conceptions may be altered in response to these three health status perceptions.

This study was conducted to determine whether self-discrepancies are related to psychological well-being and psychological distress in cancer patients. According to the conceptual model presented here, a person's perceptions regarding his or her physical health status—that is, symptoms due to cancer or side effects of treatment, functional health, and perceived time line of the disease—are hypothesized to have direct effects on psychological well-being and psychological distress. Furthermore, we hypothesized that self-discrepancies (discrepancies between ideal and actual self) mediate the relationship between physical health status perceptions and psychological well-being and distress.

Method

Participants

One hundred and ten persons with cancer were invited to participate in this study. Of these, 2 declined, and 108 (98%) agreed. They were recruited over a 15-month period from a large oncology clinic that serves a middle- and lower income, ethnically diverse, metropolitan area in southern California. Patients over 18 years of age who could read and write English were informed of the study by their physician, if the physician judged they were physically capable of completing a 30-min questionnaire. In general, those individuals with an extremely poor prognosis (i.e., less than 1 month survival anticipated) were excluded. The average age of participants was 62 years, with a range of 26 to 86 years. There were 35 men and 68 women (5 did not specify gender). The majority were White (86%), married (62%), had some college or postgraduate education (76.8%), and had incomes over $30,000 (53%). The participants were relatively advantaged in terms of education and occupation.

Measures

Physical Health Variables

Perceptions of physical health status were assessed by self-report measures covering three dimensions of health: symptom bother, instrumental activities of daily living, and time line. We developed a 12-item symptom-bother scale for this study. It consisted of 12 physical symptoms—for example, pain, nausea, and fatigue—commonly experienced by cancer patients due to illness or treatment. The content validity of the scale was assessed by having the items reviewed by oncologists, nurse researchers in the area of cancer, and three cancer patients. Participants rated how much they were bothered by each symptom on a scale ranging from *do not have this symptom* (0) to *a lot* (3), and a mean score was computed. The reliability (alpha) coefficient in this sample was .73.

A revised version of the Older American Resource Services ADL measure (Duke University Center for the Study of Aging and Human Development, 1978) was used to measure instrumental activities of daily living. The Instrumental Activities of Daily Living (IADL) scale consists of five items reflecting different activities of daily living. Participants rated how much help they needed in carrying out each activity on a 3-point scale ranging from *no help* (0) to *can't do at all* (2), and a mean score was computed. The IADL scale has been shown to be related to other measures of functional status, depression, anxiety, and life satisfaction (Duke University Center for the Study of Aging and Human Development, 1978). The reliability (alpha) coefficient in this sample was .87.

Time line was assessed with the following question:

> People think about illness and diseases in different ways. Some illnesses we see as acute—we get them, they get treated and they're gone. Some illnesses we see as episodic—they come and go. We're sick for a while, get better, get sick again, get better. Some illnesses we think of as chronic—we become ill and more or less learn to live with the illness; it doesn't go away. Would you describe your cancer as acute, episodic, or chronic?

Because few people (*n* = 19) described their cancer as episodic, their data were collapsed with those who viewed their disease as chronic, and only two categories, acute and chronic, were used in analyses. A similar item has been used in previous research and has been found to have theoretically predicted relationships with other variables (Ward et al., 1992).

Participants were also asked their diagnosis (what kind of cancer), years since diagnosis, current treatment (chemotherapy, radiotherapy, or other), and whether their disease was local or metastatic. Participants were also asked to rate their present health (*excellent* to *poor* on a 5-point scale), present compared with past health, present compared with future health, and ideal compared with present health (*much worse* to *much better than present* on a 5-point scale for each). Higher scores better perceived health.

Self-Discrepancy

A 20-item self-discrepancy scale was developed for this study. Before completing the scale, participants read a description and example of actual self, ideal self, and a match between actual and ideal self and then were asked to take a few minutes to think about their personal qualities, goals, and dreams about themselves. They then were asked to indicate the extent of their agreement (*strongly agree* to *strongly disagree* on a 6-point scale) with the statement "My actual self and ideal self are a very close match," in each of 20 life domains. Examples of domains include "my physical health," "coping with change," and "pursuing my leisure interests and hobbies." Mean ratings across the 20 domains were computed; higher scores indicate higher levels of self-discrepancy (i.e., little match between actual and ideal self).

Before the scale's use in the present study, its content validity was assessed by asking 11 doctoral students in nursing to examine the items and the instructions for clarity, relevance, validity, and inclusiveness of the domains assessed. After revision, three patients with cancer were asked to review and complete the instrument. On the basis of their suggestions, minor revisions in wording were made.

Table 1—*Correlations Between Physical Health, Self-Discrepancy,*
and Self-Esteem

Physical health	Self-discrepancy	Self-esteem
Present health	−.41*	.28*
Past health	−.34*	−.02
Future health	−.34*	.14
Ideal health	−.48*	.02
Symptoms	.32*	−.26
IADL	.31*	−.21
Time line	.45*	−.14
Years since diagnosis	.24	.18
Local-metastatic	.35*	−.09

Note. N = 108. IADL = Instrumental Activities of Daily Living.
*p < .01.

The scale was then used in the present study. The average interitem correlation was .37, and Cronbach's alpha was .92. Construct validity was tested by examining the correlations among the self-discrepancy measure; self-esteem (measured with Rosenberg's, 1986, Self-Esteem Scale); and physical health variables. According to Rosenberg and others (Higgins, Klein, & Strauman, 1985), high self-esteem should be related to low self-discrepancy. In the present data, this hypothesis was supported; there was a significant inverse correlation between self-discrepancy and self-esteem ($r = -.44$, $p < .01$). In addition, because self-discrepancies were assessed across multiple domains, this measure should be more highly related to physical health than is self-esteem—a more global, undifferentiated measure. As expected, the correlations between self-discrepancy and the health measures were of greater magnitude and were more often statistically significant than were the correlations between self-esteem and the health measures (see Table 1).

Adjustment

Three scales were used to assess positive adjustment or psychological well-being: purpose in life, personal growth, and positive relations with others (Ryff, 1989). Each scale consists of 15 items, divided approximately equally between positively and negatively keyed items. The items from each scale are randomly mixed into a single self-report instrument. Subjects were asked to respond to each item on a 6-point scale ranging from *strongly disagree* (1) to *strongly agree* (6), with higher scores indicating higher levels of well-being.

These well-being scales have previously been used in research on adult personality development and were originally derived from concepts of adult mental health and development (Erikson, 1959; Jahoda, 1958; Rogers, 1961; Ryff, 1989). In initial psychometric testing, reliability of the scales (alpha coefficients) ranged from .86 to .91, and test-retest reliability ranged from .81 to .88 (Ryff, 1989). In the present sample, the alpha coefficients were purpose in life, .87; personal growth, .74; and positive relations with others, .83. Evidence for validity of the scales were found in prior research by comparing them with commonly used measures of positive functioning and negative functioning; for example, correlations between the scales and a measure of life satisfaction ranged from .38 to .59 (Ryff, 1989).

One measure of poor adjustment or psychological distress was included. Depression was measured by the Center for Epidemiological Studies Depression Scale (CES–D), a 20-item self-report scale designed to assess depressive symptomatology (Radloff, 1977). This measure was selected because the emphasis is on depressed mood or affect rather than somatic symptoms. Respondents answer each item on the basis of how often they felt or behaved that way in the past week (on a 0 to 3 scale), and a summary score is computed. The CES–D has had extensive psychometric testing and has been shown to discriminate between clinically depressed and nondepressed groups and to be positively correlated with other measures of depression (George, 1989; Radloff, 1977). Reliability (Cronbach's α) in this sample was .88.

Procedure

Participants were informed of the study and invited to participate by their oncologist during routine clinic visits. Informed consent was obtained by the physician or nurse. The self-report measures and a demographic questionnaire were completed while waiting for an exam or treatment in the clinic.

Results

Results are presented in two parts. Descriptive statistics about physical health status perceptions, self-discrepancies, and adjustment are presented first, followed by the analyses related to the mediating effects of self-discrepancies.

Descriptive Statistics

The most frequently reported diagnoses were breast cancer (27%), colorectal cancer (20%), lung cancer (13%), and lymphomas (12%). Five persons reported not knowing their diagnosis, although all of the participants had been informed of their diagnosis by their physician. Table 2 includes descriptive statistics concerning the remaining physical health variables. The sample was somewhat evenly divided among those who described their cancer as local (45%) versus metastatic (36%) and acute (51%) versus chronic (43%). Of those who described their cancer as local, 80% described their illness as acute and 20% as chronic. Of those who described their cancer as metastatic, 71% described their illness as chronic and 29% as acute. Of those who did not know their status, 59% described their illness as chronic and 41% as acute. Thus, individuals' self-reports of their disease status (local vs. metastatic; an indication of the severity of their illness) corresponded in a meaningful way with their perceptions regarding the time line of the illness. Current treatment included chemotherapy (61%) and radiotherapy (10%). The average number of years since diagnosis was 3.4 ($SD = 4.6$).

The symptom and IADL ratings indicated that the majority of participants reported low levels of symptoms and had little difficulty with IADLs. Because these

Table 2—*Descriptive Statistics for Measures of Physical Health*

Measure	Freq	%	M	SD	Range
Local versus metastatic					
Local	49	45%			
Metastatic	39	36%			
Don't know	20	18%			
Time line					
Acute	55	51%			
Chronic	46	43%			
Current treatment					
Chemotherapy	66	61%			
Radiotherapy	11	10%			
Other	9	8%			
Years since diagnosis			3.41	4.63	1–37
IADL			0.20	0.39	0–1.6
Symptoms			9.49	5.43	0–22

Note. Freq = frequency. IADL = Instrumental Activities of Daily Living.

ratings can be affected by treatment (e.g., chemotherapy) and diagnosis (breast, colorectal, lung, lymphoma, and other), patients currently undergoing chemotherapy (n = 66) were compared to patients not currently receiving chemotherapy (n = 42) on the above measures using t tests. There were no significant differences. Analyses of variance (ANOVAs) and chi-square tests were conducted to determine whether there were differences by diagnosis on any of the demographic, physical health perception, or adjustment measures. The only significant ($p < .05$) difference was age. Individuals with a diagnosis of breast cancer or lymphoma were younger than other individuals.

As expected, higher levels of self-discrepancy were significantly related to a greater degree of bothersome symptoms, worse functional health, and perceptions of cancer as a chronic rather than an acute illness (see Table 1 correlations). A higher level of self-discrepancy was also related to more years since diagnosis ($r = .24$, $p < .05$) but not to current treatment.

Descriptive statistics and correlations among the self-discrepancy and adjustment ratings are presented in Table 3. Higher levels of self-discrepancy were related to lower levels of psychological well-being and higher levels of depression. Preliminary

Table 3—*Means, Standard Deviations, and Correlations of Self-Discrepancy and Adjustment Measures*

Measure	M	SD	2	3	4	5
1. Self-discrepancy	2.54	0.89	−.54*	−.25	−.47*	.45*
2. Purpose in life	4.61	0.95	—	—	—	—
3. Personal growth	4.80	0.67	.62*	—	—	—
4. Positive relations	4.97	0.78	.54*	.46*	—	—
5. Depression	12.67	9.78	−.49*	−.31*	−.27*	—

*$p < .01$.

analyses were performed to determine whether the demographic variables (age, gender, education, income, and martial status) were related to the physical health, self-discrepancy, and adjustment measures, using t tests (for gender and marital status) and correlations (for age, education, and income). There were no significant gender or marital status differences. There were significant correlations ($p < .05$) between age and years since diagnosis ($r = .24$), purpose in life ($r = -.24$), and positive relations ($r = -.28$). Therefore, age and years since diagnosis were controlled in the remaining analyses.

Mediating Effects of Self-Discrepancies

To test the hypothesis that self-discrepancies mediate the relationship between cancer and adjustment, a series of multiple regression analyses were performed following the procedures suggested by Baron and Kenny (1986). Mediating effects are those that account for the relationship between a predictor (physical health perception) and a criterion (adjustment). Mediating effects are inferred when the following conditions are met: (a) The predictor (physical health perception) is significantly related to the mediator (self-discrepancy), (b) the mediator is significantly related to the criterion (adjustment), and (c) when the relationships in the first two conditions are controlled, a previously significant relationship between the predictor and the criterion is reduced or no longer significant. Mediating effects were tested separately for each physical health perception measure (symptoms, IADLs, time line) and for each psychological outcome (purpose in life, personal growth, positive relations, and depression). Age and years since diagnosis were controlled in each regression, and alpha was set at $p < .01$.[1]

Condition a was met. After we controlled for age and years since diagnosis, the direct relationship between each physical health measure and the mediator (self-discrepancy) was significant; symptoms ($\beta =.34$), IADLs ($\beta = .27$), and time line ($\beta = .42$). Condition b was met for three of the outcome measures and was in the predicted direction of the fourth. That is, after we controlled for age and years since diagnosis, self-discrepancy was a significant predictor of purpose in life ($\beta = -.49$), positive relations ($\beta = -.44$), and depression ($\beta = .45$), but for personal growth the results were not significant at the .01 level ($\beta = -.26$, $p < .02$). Because self-discrepancy was not significantly related to personal growth, this outcome variable was not tested further.

Condition c is the test of mediating effects. The results related to these effects are in Table 4. The first two columns display the standardized beta coefficients and change in R^2 for the direct path between physical health perceptions and adjustment without the mediator, self-discrepancy, included in the model. The last two columns contain the standardized beta coefficients and change in R^2 reflecting the path between physical health perceptions and adjustment with self-discrepancy included. Self-discrepancy was a significant mediator of the effect of symptoms, IADLs, and time line on purpose in life. The effect of all three physical health variables on purpose in life became nonsignificant (in terms of beta) when self-discrepancy was

---

[1] For exploratory purposes, the interaction of self-discrepancy and physical health was tested in each regression. Only one of nine interactions was significant (Self-Discrepancy × Symptoms in predicting purpose in life), so these effects are not reported.

Table 4—*Standardized Beta Coefficients and Change in R^2 for Paths From Physical Health to Adjustment With and Without Mediating Effects*

Criterion/ predictor	Without self-discrepancy		With self-discrepancy		
	β	R^2	β	R^2	F change
Purpose in life					
Symptoms	−.35*	.12*	−.21	.14*	20.61*
IADL	−.31*	.09*	−.19	.17*	24.11*
Time line	−.26*	.06*	−.07	.17*	22.56*
Positive relations					
Symptoms	−.08	.00	−.08	.18*	22.80*
IADL	.06	.00	.06	.18*	23.09*
Time line	−.28*	.07*	−.11	.12*	15.31*
Depression					
Symptoms	.41*	.16*	.28*	.10*	12.75*
IADL	.34*	.11*	.24	.13*	16.02*
Time line	.28*	.07*	.11	.13*	14.93*

Note. Age and years since diagnosis are controlled in all analyses. IADL = Instrumental Activities of Daily Living.
*$p < .01$.

added to the prediction. Figure 1 illustrates how self-discrepancy mediated the relationship between time line and purpose in life. Self-discrepancy was a significant mediator of the effect of time line on positive relations. However, neither symptoms nor IADLs had significant direct effects on positive relations so mediating effects could not occur. However, the indirect effects of self-discrepancy on positive relations were significant in both cases and added 18% to the explained variance.

Self-discrepancy also mediated the effects of IADLs and time line on depression. The effect of symptoms on depression was reduced (in terms of beta), but the direct effects remained significant. For symptoms, the indirect effect of self-discrepancy was significant, adding 10% to the explained variance in depression.

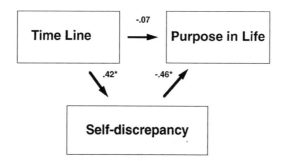

Figure 1. Mediating effect of self-discrepancy on relationship between time line and purpose in life. Age and years since diagnosis were controlled. *$p < .01$.

Discussion

Regardless of the level of symptoms, difficulty with IADLs, or perceptions of cancer as a chronic illness, individuals with less self-discrepancy had higher levels of purpose in life and positive relations with others and lower levels of depression. Conversely, individuals with more self-discrepancy had higher levels of depression and lower levels of psychological well-being. As predicted, perceptions about physical health status had a direct effect on adjustment, but this effect was mediated through self-discrepancy. We suggest, albeit cautiously given the cross-sectional nature of the data, that self-discrepancy theory has potential as a meaningful framework for understanding the role of self-perceptions in psychological adaptation to serious illness. Although the self has not been neglected in research on quality of life in cancer patients (Anderson, 1992), the role of the self has more often been empirically, rather than theoretically, described.

An important aspect of this study was the multidimensional assessment of psychological adaptation, investigating both well-being and distress. Numerous empirical studies of adjustment to cancer have operationalized adjustment in terms of low levels of psychological distress or psychosomatic symptoms (e.g., see reviews by Glanz & Lerman, 1992; Irvine, Brown, Crooks, Roberts, & Browne, 1991). Such an approach fails to consider evidence that positive and negative affect may be independent dimensions of well-being (Heidrich & Ryff, 1993a), sheds limited light on other important dimensions of well-being that reflect quality of life, and ignores how psychological well-being, not just distress, is related to physical health. The results of this study suggest that self-discrepancies mediate multiple dimensions of adjustment to cancer. Additionally, self-discrepancies have differential relationships with different aspects of physical health perceptions, psychological well-being, and psychological distress.

Purpose in life may be an especially meaningful aspect of adjustment for those facing a life-threatening illness. Self-discrepancy was more important than perceptions about physical health status (symptoms, IADLs, and time line) in participants' sense of having meaning or purpose in life. This suggests that individuals whose ideal and actual selves are in alignment have higher levels of purpose in life, regardless of the severity of their disease.

Positive relations with others, another measure of adjustment, taps the perception that one has warm, satisfying, trusting relationships with others; that one is capable of strong empathy and affection; and that one understands the give and take of human relationships (Ryff, 1989). Note that unlike purpose in life and depression, there was no direct effect of symptoms or functional health on positive relations. However, self-discrepancies added significantly to the explained variance in positive relations over and above these two physical health variables and significantly mediated the effects of time line. Thus, self-discrepancy was more important than physical health perceptions in patients' perceptions of their relations with others. Although social support is seen as important in interventions aimed at enhancing quality of life of cancer patients (Anderson, 1992), research examining how social support is related to an individual's sense of self and subsequent psychological well-being has been neglected. Because there is conceptual similarity between perceived social support and positive relations with others, these results suggest that further work in this area may be fruitful.

A somewhat different pattern emerged in relation to psychological distress or depression. In contrast to the findings for well-being, symptoms continued to have a significant direct effect on depression after self-discrepancies were added to the equation, although the increase in explained variance due to self-discrepancies was significant. A similar pattern of findings was reported by Heidrich and Ryff (1993a) in a study of the self-system of elderly women with chronic illnesses. Self-conceptions may be more powerful in determining well-being than depression, or alternatively, perceptions about physical health may have a greater impact on psychological distress than on psychological well-being.

There is further work needed, however, in the area of self-discrepancy and adjustment to illness. Perhaps most striking is the need to disentangle direction of causality and to clarify the distinctions made between self-discrepancy and psychological well-being or depression. Higgins's (1987) self-discrepancy theory posits that depression, or dejection-related negative affect, is the outcome of actual–ideal self-discrepancies. Support for this view has been found in a number of short-term longitudinal studies of undergraduate students indicating that self-discrepancies are associated with subsequent negative affect or depression (Cantor, Norem, Brower, Niedenthal, & Langston, 1987; Forston & Stanton, 1992; Strauman & Higgins, 1988) and physical symptoms (Higgins, Vookles, & Tykocinski, 1992). Heidrich and Ryff (1993a), using confirmatory factor analysis, found that self-discrepancy, psychological well-being, and psychological distress constituted three distinct factors. In this study, correlations between self-discrepancy and the various dimensions of psychological well-being and distress were moderate ($r = .27 - .54$), indicating that self-discrepancy and psychological well-being are not equivalent. However, longitudinal designs are necessary to determine if it is most correct to view depression and well-being as outcomes that are mediated by self-discrepancy (as tested in this study) or whether it is more accurate to see such variables as driving the system. That is, perhaps persons who are depressed are those who are at risk for experiencing large self-discrepancies when faced with the challenge of physical illness. There is no direct evidence to support this latter view, but longitudinal studies have shown that persons with initially high levels of depression are more likely to encounter disease- and treatment-related distress than are persons with initially low levels of depression (Ell, Nishimoto, Morvay, Mantell, & Hamovitch, 1989; Ward et al., 1992). These studies did not, however, take self-discrepancies into account. Another possible interpretation is that individuals with high levels of self-discrepancy are more apt to either experience or report symptomatology, functional difficulties, or label their illness as chronic and, in addition, experience lower levels of psychological well-being.

It is likely that there is a substantial amount of nonrecursiveness in the model, yet it is clinically important to distinguish which variables have the greatest causal influence because selection of intervention approaches would be guided by such findings. For instance, if depression (or well-being) is driving the system, then a search for interventions could be directed toward those that have been helpful in dealing with depression in non-physically ill populations. For example, Nezu's problem-solving approach might prove useful (Nezu & Perri, 1989). On the other hand, if self-discrepancy is driving the system, then new interventions that target the self-system need to be tested. One possibility would be to build on the work of Johnson and Leventhal, who demonstrated that the provision of accurate sensory information facilitates coping with noxious physical experiences (Johnson, Lauver,

& Nail, 1989; Leventhal & Johnson, 1983). By analogy, perhaps presenting persons with accurate information about the likely consequences of diagnosis and treatment could arm them to expect changes in their capabilities. These accurate expectations might, in turn, prevent the development of discrepancies between what persons ideally think they should be or would like to be and how they presently see themselves.

Another potentially fruitful avenue of investigation would be to examine persons who begin with and maintain low levels of self-discrepancy when faced with the diagnosis of serious illness. What could we learn about their approach to life? Although numerous theories of the self maintain that the self is dynamic, there may also be consistency in some aspects of the self that results in low levels of self-discrepancy. Research on the relationship between personality (i.e., dispositional optimism), health, and self-discrepancies would be useful in clarifying these processes (Costa & McCrae, 1984).

Other contributions of this study deserve mention. The measurement of self-discrepancies reported here differs from previous studies. Previous studies have relied on difference scores that are based on ideal and actual self measures (Heidrich & Ryff, 1993a) or have utilized the Selves Questionnaire, which derives self-discrepancy scores from a content analysis of self-descriptors (Heidrich & Ryff, 1993a; Higgins et al., 1985; Higgins et al., 1992). The use of difference scores is problematic because of their unreliability. The Selves Questionnaire is an idiographic measure, making comparisons between subjects difficult; its reliability has not been established; and its usefulness in older adults has been questioned (Heidrich & Ryff, 1993a). The self-discrepancy measure developed for this study is face valid, easy to administer and score, and, most important, taps a wide variety of domains deemed salient to adults of all ages. Initial evidence of discriminant and construct validity and of reliability is promising, although further psychometric testing in larger, more heterogeneous, samples is necessary.

A variety of perceptions about physical health status that impact on the self were also assessed in this study. More bothersome symptoms (whether from the disease or treatment), a lower level of functional abilities, and perceptions of cancer as a chronic disease were all significant predictors of higher levels of discrepancy between the actual and ideal self and lower levels of psychological well-being. These findings support our intuitive notions about how physical health affects the self. For instance, symptoms, beyond causing discomfort, interfere with one's abilities to carry out meaningful roles or maintain relationships with others and make it less likely that one's ideals can be achieved. Declines in functional health, a direct assessment of one's ability to carry out activities of daily living, may influence self-perceptions in a similar manner by increasing the distance between one's actual behavior and the self one ideally wishes to be. Time line may influence self-conceptions because one's view of an illness as chronic changes one's sense of future possibilities, possible selves, or achievable goals and may cause one to redefine specific aspects of the self.

Caution is in order in interpreting these results, however. In addition to the cross-sectional nature of the data, there were a number of other limitations in this study that need to be addressed before the role of self-discrepancies in adjustment is understood; particularly sampling bias and generalizability and the lack of objective measures of physical health status.

Although we attempted to sample a socioeconomically diverse group, we were not successful. The majority of individuals in this study were White and advantaged in terms of education and income. Therefore, these results cannot be generalized to other ethnic or socioeconomic groups.

In addition, as is true of many efforts to understand psychological adjustment to illness, there was a bias in the present study toward including persons who were doing relatively well. Because questionnaire completion for this investigation required 30 min of time, persons who were very ill were not able to participate. This is a most vexing issue because persons unable to complete a 30-min self-report questionnaire are also unable to be interviewed for any length of time. It would be useful to develop and validate very short forms of the questionnaires used in this study, so that persons who were quite ill could participate. Similarly, non-English-speaking persons were excluded from this study. The growing numbers of Hispanic and Southeast Asian persons in the United States behoove us to develop instrumentation that will allow such persons to participate in investigations.

Finally, we used perceptions of physical health status rather than objective measures, such as medical record data regarding disease and treatment status, which might be considered more reliable. Different results might have been obtained if more objective physical health measures had been used. However, self-assessments of physical health and functional abilities have been shown to be reliable and valid and are, in fact, more predictive of morbidity and mortality than many objective indicators or physician's ratings (Diener, 1984; Idler & Kasl, 1991; Mossey & Shapiro, 1982; Myers, Holliday, Harvey, & Hutchinson, 1993).

In spite of such limitations, demonstrating that self-discrepancy mediates the relationship between physical health perceptions and adjustment sets the stage for understanding how persons who face a life-threatening illness manage to maintain or regain well-being over time. The data suggest a process in which ideals are aligned to match present capabilities. This line of reasoning is consistent with patients' observations that the diagnosis of a life-threatening illness leads them to reevaluate what is most important in life (Northouse & Northouse, 1987; O'Connor, Wicker, & Germino, 1990).

References

Andersen, B., Anderson, B., & deProsse, C. (1989). Controlled prospective longitudinal study of women with cancer: II. Psychological outcomes. *Journal of Consulting and Clinical Psychology, 57*, 692–697.

Anderson, B. (1992). Psychological interventions for cancer patients to enhance the quality of life. *Journal of Consulting and Clinical Psychology, 60*, 552–568.

Baron, R., & Kenny, D. (1986). The moderator–mediator variable distinction in social psychological research: Conceptual, strategic, and statistical considerations. *Journal of Personality and Social Psychology, 51*, 1173–1182.

Cantor, N., Norem, J. K., Brower, A. M., Niedenthal, P. M., & Langston, C. A. (1987). Life tasks, self-concept ideals, and cognitive strategies in a life transition. *Journal of Personality and Social Psychology, 53*, 1178–1191.

Cassileth, B., Lusk, E., Brown, L., & Cross, P. (1986). Psychosocial status of cancer patients and next-of-kin: Normative data from the Profile of Mood States. *Journal of Psychosocial Oncology, 3*, 99–105.

Christman, N. (1990). Uncertainty and adjustment during radiotherapy. *Nursing Research, 39*, 17–20.

Costa, P. T., & McCrae, R. R. (1984). Personality as a lifelong determinant of well-being. In C. Z. Malatesta & C. E. Izard (Eds.), *Emotion in adult development* (pp. 141–155). Beverly Hills, CA: Sage.

Curbow, B., Somerfield, M., Legro, M., & Sonnega, J. (1990). Self-concept and cancer in adults: Theoretical and methodological issues. *Social Science and Medicine, 31*, 115–128.

Diener, E. (1984). Subjective well-being. *Psychological Bulletin, 95*, 542–575.

Duke University Center for the Study of Aging and Human Development. (1978). *Multidimensional functional assessment: The OARS methodology.* Durham, NC: Duke University.

Ell, K., Nishimoto, R., Morvay, T., Mantell, J., & Hamovitch, M. (1989). A longitudinal analysis of psychological adaptation among survivors of cancer. *Cancer, 63*, 406–413.

Erikson, E. (1959). Identity and the life cycle: Selected papers. *Psychological Issues, 1*, 1–171.

Felton, B. J., Revenson, T. A., & Hinrichsen, G. A. (1984). Stress and coping in the explanation of psychological adjustment among chronically ill adults. *Social Science and Medicine, 18*, 889–898.

Forston, M. T., & Stanton, A. L. (1992). Self-discrepancy theory as a framework for understanding bulimic symptomatology and associated distress. *Journal of Social and Clinical Psychology, 11*, 103–118.

George, L. K. (1989). Stress, social support and depression over the life course. In M. S. Markides & C. L. Cooper (Eds.), *Aging, stress and health* (pp. 241–267). New York: Wiley.

Glanz, K., & Lerman, C. (1992). Psychosocial impact of breast cancer: A critical review. *Annals of Behavioral Medicine, 14*, 204–212.

Heidrich, S. M. (1993). The relationship between physical health and psychological well-being in elderly women. *Research in Nursing and Health, 16*, 123–130.

Heidrich, S. M., & Ryff, C. D. (1993a). Physical and mental health in later life: The self-system as mediator. *Psychology and Aging, 8*, 327–328.

Heidrich, S. M., & Ryff, C. D. (1993b). The role of social comparison processes in the psychological adaptation of elderly adults. *Journal of Gerontology: Psychological Sciences, 48*, P127–P136.

Heidrich, S. M., & Ward, S. E. (1992). The role of the self in adjustment to cancer in elderly women. *Oncology Nursing Forum, 19*, 1491–1496.

Herr, H., Kornblith, A., & Ofman, U. (1993). A comparison of the quality of life of patients with metastatic prostate cancer who received or did not receive hormonal therapy. *Cancer, 71*, 1143–1150.

Higgins, E. T. (1987). Self-discrepancy: A theory relating self and affect. *Psychological Review, 94*, 319–340.

Higgins, E. T., Bond, R. N., Klein, R., & Strauman, T. (1986). Self-discrepancies and emotional vulnerability: How magnitude, accessibility, and type of discrepancy influence affect. *Journal of Personality and Social Psychology, 51*, 5–15.

Higgins, E. T., Klein, R., & Strauman, T. (1985). Self-concept discrepancy theory: A psychological model for distinguishing among different aspects of depression and anxiety. *Social Cognition, 3*, 51–76.

Higgins, E. T., Vookles, J., & Tykocinski, O. (1992). Self and health: How "patterns" of self-beliefs predict types of emotional and physical problems. *Social Cognition, 10*, 125–150.

Idler, E. L., & Kasl, S. (1991). Health perceptions and survival: Do global evaluations of health status really predict mortality? *Journal of Gerontology: Social Sciences, 46*, S55–S65.

Irvine, D., Brown, B., Crooks, D., Roberts, J., & Browne, G. (1991). Psychosocial adjustment in women with breast cancer. *Cancer, 67*, 1097–1117.

Jahoda, M. (1958). *Current concepts of positive mental health.* New York: Basic Books.

Johnson, J., Lauver, D., & Nail, L. (1989). Process of coping with radiation therapy. *Journal of Consulting and Clinical Psychology*, *57*, 358–364.

Krouse, H., & Krouse, J. (1982). Cancer as crisis: The critical elements of adjustment. *Nursing Research*, *31*, 96–101.

Leventhal, H., & Johnson, J. (1983). Laboratory and field experimentation: Development of a theory of self-regulation. In P. Wooldridge, M. Schmitt, & J. Skipper (Eds.), *Behavioral science and nursing theory* (pp. 189–262). St. Louis, MO: Mosby.

Levin, D., Cleeland, C., & Dar, R. (1985). Public attitudes toward cancer pain. *Cancer*, *56*, 2337–2339.

McCorkle, R., & Quint-Benoliel, J. (1983). Symptom distress, current concerns and mood disturbance after diagnosis of life-threatening disease. *Social Science and Medicine*, *17*, 431–438.

Meyer, D., Leventhal, H., & Gutmann, M. (1985). Common-sense models of illness: The example of hypertension. *Health Psychology*, *4*, 115–135.

Mossey, J. M., & Shapiro, E. (1982). Self-rated health: A predictor of mortality among the elderly. *American Journal of Public Health*, *72*, 800–808.

Myers, A. M., Holliday, P. J., Harvey, K. A., & Hutchinson, K. S. (1993). Functional performance measures: Are they superior to self-assessments? *Journal of Gerontology: Medical Sciences*, *48*, M196–M206.

Nezu, A., & Perri, M. (1989). Social problem-solving therapy for unipolar depression: An initial dismantling investigation. *Journal of Consulting and Clinical Psychology*, *57*, 408–413.

Northouse, P., & Northouse, L. (1987). Communication and cancer: Issues confronting patients, health professionals, and family members. *Journal of Psychosocial Oncology*, *5*, 17–46.

O'Connor, A., Wicker, C., & Germino, B. (1990). Understanding the cancer patient's search for meaning. *Cancer Nursing*, *13*, 167–175.

Radloff, L. (1977). The CES–D Scale: A self-report depression scale for research in the general population. *Applied Psychological Measurement*, *1*, 385–401.

Rogers, C. R. (1961). *On becoming a person*. Boston: Houghton Mifflin.

Rosenberg, M. (1986). *Conceiving the self*. Malabar, FL: Krieger.

Ryff, C. D. (1989). Happiness is everything, or is it? Explorations on the meaning of psychological well-being. *Journal of Personality and Social Psychology*, *57*, 1069–1081.

Strauman, T. J., & Higgins, E. T. (1988). Self-discrepancies as predictors of vulnerability to distinct syndromes of chronic emotional distress. *Journal of Personality*, *56*, 685–707.

Taylor, S. E. (1983). Adjustment to threatening events: A theory of cognitive adaptation. *American Psychologist*, *38*, 1161–1173.

Taylor, S. E., & Brown, J. (1988). Illusion and well-being: A social psychological perspective on mental health. *Psychological Bulletin*, *103*, 193–210.

Taylor, S., Lichtman, R., & Wood, J. (1984). Attributions, beliefs about control, and adjustment to breast cancer. *Journal of Personality and Social Psychology*, *44*, 489–502.

Vinokur, A., Threatt, B., Caplan, R., & Zimmerman, B. (1989). Physical and psychosocial functioning and adjustment to breast cancer. *Cancer*, *63*, 394–405.

Ward, S. E., Heidrich, S., & Wolberg, W. H. (1989). Factors women take into account when deciding upon type of surgery for breast cancer. *Cancer Nursing*, *13*, 191–196.

Ward, S. E., Viergutz, G., Tormey, D., DeMuth, J., & Paulen, A. (1992). Patients' reactions to completion of adjuvant breast cancer therapy. *Nursing Research*, *41*, 362–366.

Weisman, A. (1979). *Coping with cancer*. New York: McGraw-Hill.

Wood, J. V., Taylor, S. E., & Lichtman, R. R. (1985). Social comparison in adjustment to breast cancer. *Journal of Personality and Social Psychology*, *49*, 1169–1183.

Zenmore, R., Rinholm, J., Shepel, L., & Richards, M. (1989). Some social and emotional consequences of breast cancer and mastectomy: A content analysis of 87 interviews. *Journal of Psychosocial Oncology*, *7*, 33–45.

Chapter 5
HOW COPING MEDIATES THE EFFECT OF OPTIMISM ON DISTRESS:
A Study of Women With Early Stage Breast Cancer

Charles S. Carver, Christina Pozo, Suzanne D. Harris, Victoria Noriega,
Michael F. Scheier, David S. Robinson, Alfred S. Ketcham,
Frederick L. Moffat, Jr., and Kimberley C. Clark

A good deal of research now indicates that the personality dimension of optimism–pessimism plays an important role in a wide range of behavioral and psychological outcomes when people confront adversity (reviewed in Scheier & Carver, 1992). What is less clear is the mechanism (or mechanisms) by which the beneficial effects of optimism take place. One possibility is that optimists do better than pessimists because they cope more effectively.[1] There is an abundance of evidence that they at least cope *differently*. Optimists and pessimists differ from one another in reports of their general coping tendencies (Carver, Scheier, & Weintraub, 1989) and in the coping responses they bring to mind when considering hypothetical situations (Scheier, Weintraub, & Carver, 1986), recalling a stressful situation from the recent past (Scheier et al., 1986), dealing with infertility problems (Litt, Tennen, Affleck, & Klock, 1992), managing a life transition (Aspinwall & Taylor, 1992), coping with a serious disease (Friedman et al., 1992), and dealing with worries about specific health threats (Stanton & Snider, 1993; Taylor et al., 1992).

Far less information is available, however, concerning the hypothesis that these differences in coping serve as the vehicle by which optimists experience better eventual outcomes. Three studies in the literature are relevant to the question. One of them (Scheier et al., 1989) examined men undergoing coronary artery bypass surgery. These subjects did not complete a full measure of coping but indicated their use of several cognitive–attentional strategies before and after the surgery. Although optimism was related to several of these strategies, there was scant evidence that the strategies mediated the beneficial effect of optimism on subsequent outcomes. The second study (Aspinwall & Taylor, 1992) assessed optimism and coping in a group of students entering college and assessed well-being 3 months later. In this case, the beneficial effects of optimism appeared to operate at least in part through differences in both active coping and avoidance coping.

Both of these studies have an important limitation, however. Neither included an initial measure of the variables that served as the later outcome measure. Thus,

Reprinted from *Journal of Personality and Social Psychology, 65*(2), 375–390. (1993). Copyright © 1993 by the American Psychological Association. Used with permission of the author.

Collection of the data was supported in part by National Science Foundation Grant BNS 8717783. Preparation of the article was supported by National Science Foundation Grants BNS 9011653 and BNS 9010425, Grant PBR-56 from the American Cancer Society, and National Heart, Lung, and Blood Institute Grant HL44436-01A1.

[1]In most research on this topic, subjects are not divided into groups; rather, the continuous dimension of optimism versus pessimism is related to the outcome measure. For convenience, however, we will refer to people who are less optimistic on this continuous dimension as pessimists.

although the pattern of relationships found by Aspinwall and Taylor (1992) is consistent with the mediation hypothesis, the data cannot distinguish whether coping predicted shifts in well-being over time or whether coping mediated basal well-being, which was maintained across time. The findings from the third relevant study are limited in a different way. Stanton and Snider (1993) found that avoidance coping mediated the effect of optimism on concurrent distress among women awaiting the results of a biopsy. However, they found no evidence that optimism predicted distress prospectively, which made tests of prospective mediation irrelevant. Thus, although there is evidence that the relation between optimism and subjective well-being at a given time is mediated by coping, there is at present no clear evidence that prospective effects on well-being (independent of earlier well-being) are mediated by coping.

Coping

Much of the broader literature of coping per se is subject to limitations similar to those just noted. Far more is known about concurrent associations between coping and distress than is known about how coping influences distress prospectively. Several recent studies have used prospective designs, but sometimes no prospective analyses are reported (e.g., Folkman & Lazarus, 1985). Most of the studies of this group do not examine coping with specific stressful events, but rather coping with life in general (e.g., Aldwin & Revenson, 1987; Glyshaw, Cohen, & Towbes, 1989; Holahan & Moos, 1987; Menaghan, 1982; Menaghan & Merves, 1984; L. W. Smith, Patterson, & Grant, 1990; Vitaliano, Russo, Young, Teri, & Maiuro, 1991), although the life situations examined in some of these studies do involve a chronic disease or another serious burden (e.g., Felton & Revenson, 1984; Vitaliano et al., 1991). Although the information provided by such research is important, it is limited in an important way. The studies may reveal the consequences of various aspects of coping with ordinary life events or with chronic strain, but there is no way of knowing whether the aspects of coping that matter most in these periods are the same as those that matter when one is coping with a crisis. Very few studies have examined the latter type of situation using prospective designs.

    One very recent project that did so (Stanton & Snider, 1993) studied women undergoing a biopsy for breast cancer, some of whom proved to have positive diagnoses. Among women diagnosed with cancer, the use at prebiopsy of cognitive avoidance (wishful thinking and turning the situation over to others) predicted higher levels of distress after the positive diagnosis and after surgery. Another recent study (Litt et al., 1992) examined the reactions of women who failed in an attempt at in vitro fertilization. Earlier reports of escape as a coping tactic were associated with greater distress after the failure. A third study found that earlier reports of wishful thinking were prospective predictors of increases in anxiety during the final anticipation of a major examination (Bolger, 1990).

    Although these studies represent a promising beginning, more information is needed. For example, all three of these studies used the Ways of Coping Checklist (Lazarus & Folkman, 1984) to assess coping. As noted elsewhere (Carver et al., 1989), this instrument measures many but not all coping reactions that might be important in stressful circumstances. It seems important to broaden the available knowledge base by testing the prospective effects of coping with a variety of measures.

Purposes of the Present Research

The study reported here had four purposes, three of which correspond to the issues discussed in the preceding sections. One purpose was to examine individual differences in optimism–pessimism as a prospective predictor of well-being during the period surrounding a crisis. A second was to learn more about what aspects of people's coping reactions have prospective effects—either good or bad—on well-being over the course of such a stressful transaction. Our third purpose was to examine whether coping reactions constitute a mechanism by which optimism–pessimism exerts its effects.

A final, more general purpose of the study was to examine the pattern of various aspects of coping as they occur over the course of a crisis. Surprisingly little information is available concerning such fundamental questions as what coping reactions are most common and least common at various stages of stressful transactions of various types (for exceptions, see Bolger, 1990; Folkman & Lazarus, 1985; Stanton & Snider, 1993). We addressed these four research questions in the context of a health crisis: the diagnosis of, and surgery for, breast cancer.

Breast Cancer

The diagnosis of breast cancer, which strikes one in every nine American women, is threatening on many levels (cf. Derogatis, 1986; Sinsheimer & Holland, 1987; Taylor, 1983). Most obvious are the fact that the patient's life is placed in jeopardy by the disease and the fact that surgical intervention for the disease is disfiguring. The diagnosis also holds further implications for social relations and emotional well-being (e.g., fear of being stigmatized and rejected once people know the diagnosis, worry over whether the cancer has spread, uncertainty about the future of one's children if the cancer does not respond to treatment, the issue of whether to have reconstructive surgery, and financial issues). Given the wide range of repercussions, it is clear that the diagnosis of breast cancer and subsequent treatment constitute a serious crisis in the lives of the women affected.

Early research on breast cancer suggested that severe emotional reactions such as depression, anxiety, and anger were the norm (for reviews, see Meyerowitz, 1980, or Miller, 1980). More recent studies paint a more positive picture, finding that women with no prior psychiatric disorder are unlikely to develop severe psychological symptoms (Bloom et al., 1987; Penman et al., 1987; see also Gordon et al., 1980; Lansky et al., 1985). Although responses are not as severe as in the past, this should not obscure the fact that the experience remains a major stressor. Furthermore, the experience is worse for some patients than for others. There is every reason to believe that differences in personality and coping play a role in the success with which patients adapt to the experience (cf. Andersen, 1992; Holland & Rowland, 1987; Sinsheimer & Holland, 1987).

To find out, we conducted a prospective, longitudinal study in which optimism was measured initially and coping and distress were assessed repeatedly, both in the early stages of the crisis (the period surrounding the surgery) and in its later stages (at 3, 6, and 12 months postsurgery). Coping was measured with a self-report inventory called the COPE (Carver et al., 1989). The COPE assesses a broad range of coping responses, some of which are not measured by other widely used instruments such as the Ways of Coping Checklist (e.g., denial, acceptance, behavioral disengagement, and use of humor). We examined the pattern of coping across the phases of the transaction, and we examined coping both as a correlate of emotional adjustment and as a prospective influence on adjustment. Finally, we assessed whether the effect of optimism on adjustment over time would be mediated by these coping reactions.

Method

Subjects

Subjects were 59 private patients of the University of Miami Oncology Clinic who were diagnosed with either Stage I ($n = 42$) or Stage II ($n = 17$) breast cancer.[2] Subjects who showed evidence of cancer in axillary lymph nodes (Stage II) had an average of 2.52 positive nodes ($SD = 1.58$). Some of the women had come to the clinic for a second opinion after a prior diagnosis of cancer ($n = 41$). Others had not yet been diagnosed and were at the clinic either for a routine checkup or because of a change in the breast noted by themselves or by their physician ($n = 18$). All were English speakers, none had a previous psychiatric history, none had had a prior cancer, and none had a major concurrent disease.

The women ranged in age from 33 to 72 years ($M = 58.02$, $SD = 10.83$). Forty-two were married or in an equivalent relationship, 7 were divorced, 6 were widowed, and 4 were single. Fifty-two of the women were White, 4 were Black, and 3 were Hispanic. Twenty-nine of the women worked outside the home, and 30 did not. The women had completed an average of 14.15 ($SD = 2.49$) years of education. Forty-three said they considered themselves religious, and 16 did not. Forty of the women underwent modified radical mastectomies, 5 had bilateral mastectomies, and 14 had lumpectomies (tumor excision). Twelve subsequently underwent radiation therapy, 12 had chemotherapy, and 21 had tamoxifen therapy.

---

[2]The sample used for the analyses reported in this article is a subset of a somewhat larger sample (Pozo et al., 1992). We included here all women from that sample who completed both presurgery and postsurgery interviews plus at least two of the three follow-ups. Of those included, 3 could not be reached for the 3-month follow-up, 7 for the 6-month follow-up, and 7 for the 12-month follow-up. Rather than analyze nonidentical subsets of subjects at different points in the prospective design, we substituted for these missing data points values generated by standard estimation procedures involving both group data at that time point and the subject's data at other time points (e.g., Kirk, 1982). To assess whether this data substitution affected the findings materially, associations between variables were reassessed in two ways: using only subjects who had no missing data and using all subjects from the larger sample who had data pertinent to the association in question. These subsidiary analyses revealed a pattern of effects that was quite similar in form and magnitude to the findings reported here. Comparisons between subjects included in this sample and those excluded revealed only one difference between the groups: Those included were less distressed at postsurgery than were those not included.

Data Collection Procedure

The project was conducted as a series of interviews. We chose to use interviews (reading items aloud and collecting oral responses) rather than self-administering questionnaires to maximally engage subjects in the data collection process and to provide a full opportunity to clarify any aspect of the instrumentation that might be ambiguous or confusing. For each participant, the interviews took place during a period of slightly over a year.

Subjects were recruited during their diagnostic office visit. The physician introduced the study to the women and referred them to the (female) interviewer, who described what participation would entail. Virtually all women to whom the physician introduced the study spoke with the interviewer, and approximately 85% of them chose to participate. After informed consent was obtained, an initial interview took place, incorporating demographic and personality measures. The presurgery interview took place on the day before the surgery. The measures administered at this time focused on more labile psychological qualities (e.g., mood level and coping) as they existed before surgery. The postsurgery interview took place approximately 7–10 days after surgery. This interview focused on coping and mood disturbance in the immediate postoperative period. Follow-up interviews took place at the time of the women's 3-month, 6-month, and 12-month medical follow-ups. These interviews included readministrations of the measures of mood and coping. In each case, the interviewer was blind to the results of previous assessments.

Psychological Measures

Optimism–Pessimism

The personality disposition of optimism versus pessimism was assessed at the initial interview by the Life Orientation Test (LOT; Scheier & Carver, 1985). The LOT is an eight-item scale (plus four fillers) that yields a continuous distribution of scores. Example items are "In uncertain times, I usually expect the best" and "I hardly ever expect things to go my way." The response choices used in this study ranged from *I agree a lot* (1) to *I disagree a lot* (4), as opposed to the more commonly used scale of 1–5. Scheier and Carver (1985) reported a Cronbach's alpha of .76 and a test–retest reliability coefficient of .79 (over a 4-week interval) for a college sample using the 5-point range. Alpha reliability in the present sample was .87, and test–retest reliability (over a 12-month interval) was .74. The distribution of scores in this sample ($M = 25.63$, $SD = 5.34$) tended toward the optimistic (which is also typical among college students), but not extremely so.[3]

---

[3]Marshall, Wortman, Kusulas, Hervig, and Vickers (1992) have suggested that the optimistically and pessimistically phrased items of the LOT may measure distinct psychological qualities. For this reason, the analyses reported in this article were repeated separately for the two item sets. In general, the positively phrased item set tended to be more closely associated with distressed and coping outcomes than did the negatively phrased item set, but the differences were neither large nor very consistent. For this reason, and because the results of this study are already complex, this article is restricted to analyses treating the LOT as a unitary scale.

Coping

Coping was assessed by the COPE (Carver et al., 1989), an inventory of coping responses with a range of conceptually distinct scales (scales and sample items are presented in the Appendix). Responses assessed by the COPE range from aspects of problem-focused coping (e.g., active coping, planning), to the use of social support, to turning to religion as a coping device, to positive reframing of the situation, to aspects of avoidance coping (e.g., denial, behavioral disengagement). Because of time constraints (the data reported here come from a more extensive project incorporating additional measures), the situational version of the COPE was reduced to three items per scale (the items of each scale that seemed most clearly worded). Instructions asked subjects to indicate how they had been responding to the full range of stressors imposed by diagnosis and surgery. Response choices ranged from *I have not been doing this at all* (1) to *I have been doing this a lot* (4). Instructions for the COPE also referred to a specific time frame. At presurgery, subjects indicated the extent to which they had experienced each coping response since finding out the surgery was necessary. At postsurgery, they reported their coping since the surgery. At each follow-up, they were asked to report on their responses during the preceding month.

Internal reliability of most COPE scales was adequate (alphas averaged across the administrations ranged from .65 to .90). There were three exceptions, however: the scales measuring active coping, denial, and mental disengagement. Further examination revealed that one item on each scale reduced that scale's reliability, and did so consistently at each point of administration. Consequently, these three items were dropped, yielding two-item scales to assess active coping, denial, and what might be better labeled self-distraction, with alphas averaging .69, .79, and .58, respectively. It will be noted that reliabilities of some scales are at the lower end of the acceptable range. The possibility should not be discounted that failure of these variables to be involved in important relationships in the study would be attributable to low reliabilities. The lowest reliabilities were those of self-distraction (.58), restraint (.65), acceptance (.68), and active coping (.69).

Distress

Mood disturbance was assessed by the Profile of Mood States (POMS; McNair, Lorr, & Droppelman, 1971). The POMS, an instrument widely used in research, is designed to assess a range of moods (e.g., depression, anger, and anxiety). It consists of a series of adjectives, each of which is a mood descriptor. Respondents indicate the extent to which they have had that feeling for a specified time period using response choices that range from *not at all* (1) to *a lot* (5). At presurgery, the women were asked to indicate how they had been feeling since they found out they needed to have surgery. At postsurgery, they were asked to indicate how they had felt since the operation. At the 3-month, 6-month, and 12-month follow-ups, they were asked to report their feelings over the preceding month. Abbreviated scales, each composed of three to four items, were used. The focus in this report is on anxiety (tense, nervous, and anxious), depression (helpless, unhappy, worthless, and hopeless), and anger (angry, resentful, and grouchy). These scales were all highly reliable (alphas across administrations averaged from .77 to .87). Preliminary analyses determined that they were also highly interrelated at each measurement (alphas for an index incorporating the three totals averaged .87). For this reason, they were combined into an index of distress, which constitutes the study's primary outcome variable.

Results

Before proceeding to the main analyses, we assessed the extent to which demographic and treatment variables were related to the study's outcome measures, thus determining the need to control for these variables in the main analyses. Examined for this purpose were age, employment status, marital status, education, extent of surgery, stage of disease, number of positive nodes, tamoxifen therapy, radiation therapy, and chemotherapy (the last two were analyzed as present vs. absent during each of the periods assessed). Three significant associations with distress emerged from these analyses, two involving age and one involving chemotherapy. Age correlated inversely with distress at the 3-month and 6-month follow-ups. Although chemotherapy was not related to concurrent mood, postsurgical distress correlated with chemotherapy in the next phase of treatment (perhaps reflecting anticipation of the chemotherapy). Given these associations, analyses of postoperative distress incorporated a control for 3-month chemotherapy, and analyses of 3-month and 6-month distress incorporated a control for age.

Well-Being and Coping Across Time

The first aspect of data analysis was descriptive: What was the nature of subjects' experience across time? Table 1 shows means and standard deviations at each measurement point in the study for the POMS-derived index of distress and for the COPE scales. These measures are displayed as per-item scores (i.e., totals divided by the number of items contributing to the score), thereby permitting easy comparison with the response ranges used in administering the items (1–5 for the POMS and 1–4 for the COPE).

The data in Table 1 make several points. First, the distress reported by patients was not extreme at any point during the course of the study, consistent with findings from other recent studies (e.g., Cella et al., 1989; Stanton & Snider, 1993). Mood disturbance was greatest before surgery, and it diminished significantly from pre- to postsurgery, $t(58) = 5.07$, $p < .001$. Further shifts across each subsequent interval of the study did not approach significance.

A second point is that many coping reactions were more prominent early in the crisis than later. Repeated measures analyses yielded significant overall effects for eight scales. In some cases, responses fell off quickly, either immediately after surgery or by 3 months postsurgery. For example, active coping fell significantly from presurgery to the 3-month point, $t(55) = 2.24$, $p < .05$, with no further change from then on. Planning fell marginally significantly from presurgery to postsurgery, $t(58) = 1.93$, $p < .06$, fell further from postsurgery to 3-month follow-up, $t(55) = 2.17$, $p < .05$, and then stabilized. Use of religion as a coping response declined from pre- to postsurgery, $t(58) = 2.62$, $p < .02$, and then stabilized.

Table 1—Means on Distress (Profile of Mood States Composite) and on COPE Scales at Each Measurement Point

| Scale | Presurgery | | Postsurgery | | Follow-Up | | | | | | p^a |
| | | | | | 3-month | | 6-month | | 12-month | | |
	M	SD	M	SD	M	SD	M	SD	M	SD	
Distress	2.35	0.93	1.98	0.84	1.91	0.85	1.97	0.84	1.89	0.71	.001
Active Coping	2.81	1.08	2.60	1.07	2.51	1.08	2.42	0.97	2.24	1.11	.002
Suppression of Competing Activities	2.17	0.92	2.17	0.98	1.78	0.86	1.77	0.72	1.63	0.66	.0001
Planning	2.75	1.10	2.48	0.94	2.21	1.03	2.17	0.98	2.00	1.01	.0001
Restraint	1.98	0.81	2.07	0.76	1.92	0.78	1.87	0.72	1.67	0.61	.005
Use of Social Support	2.97	0.98	2.76	0.92	2.34	0.99	2.45	0.97	1.97	0.83	.0001
Positive Reframing	2.68	0.97	2.71	0.91	2.67	0.92	2.56	0.84	2.64	0.85	ns
Religion	2.84	0.99	2.67	1.11	2.61	1.01	2.59	0.98	2.56	1.03	.009
Acceptance	3.48	0.75	3.55	0.60	3.44	0.75	3.58	0.58	3.70	0.59	.06
Denial	1.88	1.07	1.53	0.77	1.40	0.77	1.43	0.78	1.29	0.67	.001
Behavioral Disengagement	1.24	0.61	1.13	0.45	1.20	0.49	1.21	0.45	1.07	0.28	ns
Use of Humor	1.92	1.08	1.83	1.07	2.09	1.04	1.99	1.12	1.89	0.45	ns
Self-Distraction	2.62	1.04	2.46	0.84	2.35	1.07	2.31	0.99	2.10	1.02	.007

[a]Significance levels for overall F values across repeated measurements.

In contrast to this pattern of relatively quick change followed by stability, several responses showed more gradual, sustained decreases across time. Efforts to suppress attention to competing activities fell from postsurgery to the 3-month follow-up, $t(55)$ = 3.48, $p < .002$, and fell once again from the 6-month to the 12-month follow-up, $t(44)$ = 2.05, $p < .05$. Use of social support fell from presurgery to postsurgery at a marginal level ($p < .07$), fell significantly from postsurgery to the 3-month follow-up, $t(55)$ = 3.83, $p < .001$, and fell yet again during the period from 3 to 12 months postsurgery, $t(48)$ = 3.20, $p < .01$. Denial also fell from presurgery to postsurgery, $t(58)$ = 2.93, $p < .006$, with a further, more gradual drop from postsurgery to the 12-month follow-up, $t(51)$ = 3.01, $p < .01$. Self-distraction decreased significantly from presurgery to the 1-year follow-up, $t(51)$ = 2.93, $p < .01$, but not at any intermediate step along the way. Restraint formed a slightly different pattern, with reduction primarily between 6 and 12 months postoperatively, $t(44)$ = 2.32, $p < .05$.

Different in form from any other scale was the pattern for acceptance, which tended to drift upward across the span of the year, although this upward drift was only marginally significant.

One kind of consistency in coping concerns the consistency in mean levels across the span of the study. A different kind of consistency concerns how well correlated coping reactions were across time. That is, means can be identical from one assessment to the next, but the appearance of stability would be illusory if the correlation across assessments was low. Examination of correlations between adjacent measurements (presurgery vs. postsurgery, postsurgery vs. 3-month follow-up, etc.) revealed a good deal of consistency, but also some interesting exceptions. Most closely correlated across time were use of religion and use of humor, with average correlations of .81 and .79, respectively. Excluding them, three fourths of the remaining correlations fell between .5 and .7. There was only one clear deviation from this picture of consistent moderate stability. Behavioral disengagement, after associations of .50 to .54, correlated only .12 from 6- to 12-month follow-up, a difference that was significant, $T(56)$ = 4.98, $p < .01$ (Steiger, 1980).

Prevalence of Aspects of Coping

A third point made by the data in Table 1 is that some kinds of coping reactions occurred more than others. Two scales are particularly noteworthy in this regard: At each measurement point, reports of acceptance were significantly higher than any other scale and reports of behavioral disengagement were significantly lower than any other scale. These findings reflect the fact that the women of this sample generally retained an orientation that kept them engaged with their lives, rather than giving up.

The rankings of the other scales varied somewhat across measurement points, but there was also a considerable degree of consistency. At presurgery, active coping, planning, the use of social support, positive reframing, religion, and self-distraction all formed a second tier of coping responses (behind acceptance), not differing from one another (except that self-distraction occurred significantly less than social support). All these were reported significantly more than suppression of competing activities, restraint, use of humor, and denial, which formed another tier of scale rankings that did not differ from one another.

At postsurgery, active coping, planning, use of social support, positive reframing, religion, and self-distraction fell again in a second tier behind acceptance, all differing significantly from scales with lower means. This second tier was somewhat less cohesive than at presurgery, however, with both planning and self-distraction reported less than use of social support. The lower tier changed slightly as well. Denial (having fallen from presurgery levels) was now reported significantly less than the others of that group (although still more than behavioral disengagement). In the 3-month and later follow-ups, the relative rankings again shifted somewhat, as coping in general continued to fall off.

Correlations Among Coping Reactions

How were the coping reactions interrelated? Table 2 displays mean correlations among COPE scales, averaged from correlations at each of the five assessments. As can be seen there, several positive reactions formed an interrelated cluster: positive reframing, active coping, suppression of competing activities, planning, restraint coping, and use of social support. Denial and behavioral disengagement were moderately related to one another, forming a cluster uncorrelated with the first one. The existence of these clusters is quite consistent with earlier findings (e.g., Carver et al., 1989) and with the notion that people's coping reactions can be seen, in general terms, as reflecting either efforts to move forward toward their goals or an impulse to disengage from such efforts (Carver, Scheier, & Pozo, 1992). Not surprisingly, denial and behavioral disengagement were inversely related to acceptance, which was relatively unrelated to any other scale except positive reframing.

Although the correlations shown in Table 2 provide a general sense of the interrelations among coping reactions, some of the values shown there are also misleading because of variation across assessments. By far the largest number of atypical correlations occurred at presurgery. Presurgical self-distraction was virtually unrelated to positive reframing, active coping, denial, restraint, suppression of competing activities, or planning, thereby reducing the correlations shown in Table 2. On the other hand, several presurgical correlations were atypically high: active coping with acceptance and the use of humor ($rs = .32$ and $.33$, $ps < .02$), and the inverse relation of acceptance to behavioral disengagement ($r = -.67$, $p < .001$). At other measurement points, these associations were weaker than they appear in Table 2.

Optimism and Distress

The next step in data analysis was to examine hypothesized associations between optimism and distress. Table 3 displays correlations of the LOT with the distress index. Recall that the postsurgery correlation incorporates a control for upcoming chemotherapy, and that the 3- and 6-month correlations incorporate a control for age. The final column lists the results of an additional test, in which a further control was instituted in each case for the previously assessed level of distress.

The figures in Table 3 reveal that optimism, as measured in the initial interview, was inversely and strongly related to distress at each assessment point. What is more noteworthy is that optimism was a good prospective predictor of relative distress.

Table 2—Mean Correlations Among COPE Scales (Averaged From Correlations at Each of the Five Measurement Points)

Scale	1	2	3	4	5	6	7	8	9	10	11	12
1. Active Coping	—	.57**	.76**	.40**	.50**	.48**	.30*	.14	.10	-.20	.10	.37**
2. Suppression of Competing Activities		—	.65**	.57**	.50**	.35**	.27*	.11	.17	.09	.00	.39**
3. Planning			—	.43**	.53**	.46**	.26*	.11	.16	.02	.02	.34**
4. Restraint				—	.31*	.28*	.22	.02	.14	.17	.01	.34**
5. Use of Social Support					—	.29*	.24	.11	.20	.02	.07	.30*
6. Positive Reframing						—	.35**	.34**	-.17	-.14	.30*	.21
7. Religion							—	.18	.06	-.05	.23	.16
8. Acceptance								—	.34**	-.33	.15	.05
9. Denial									—	.34**	-.17	.29*
10. Behavioral Disengagement										—	-.09	.08
11. Use of Humor											—	-.01
12. Self-Distraction												—

*p < .05.
**p < .01.

Table 3—*Associations of Optimism With Distress Index (From the Profile of Mood States)*

Time	Control (if any)	r	r controlling also for prior level
Presurgery	—	−.56***	—
Postsurgery	Chemotherapy at 3 months	−.57***	−.24*
3-month follow-up	Age	−.62***	−.42***
6-month follow-up	Age	−.61***	−.31**
12-month follow-up	—	−.57***	−.32**

*p < .07.
**p < .05.
***p < .01.

That is, even after controlling for the distress reported at the prior assessment, optimism was significantly associated with the distress index at each measurement point except postsurgery, at which the effect was only marginal (p < .07, two-tailed). The LOT's prospective prediction is especially remarkable given the strong association of the distress index from one measurement point to the next. Presurgical distress correlated .80 with postsurgical distress; postsurgical distress correlated .62 with distress at the 3-month follow-up, which correlated .71 with distress at 6 months, which in turn correlated .68 with the final distress measure.

Optimism and Coping

How did optimism relate to coping? The correlations are shown in Table 4. The picture they present is generally consistent with that emerging from previous studies. Optimism was linked to active coping efforts and planning early in the crisis period— before the surgery took place. Optimism was also associated with acceptance of the reality of the situation and with the use of humor as a coping tactic at every measurement point except the 1-year follow-up. A similar association with positive reframing diminished so that it was no longer significant at the 6-month follow-up.

In contrast to these positive correlates, the inverse correlates of the LOT largely reflect avoidance coping. Optimism was inversely related to reports of overt denial and to the experience of behavioral disengagement throughout the study period. Optimism was inversely linked to one further coping reaction at the 1-year mark, the tendency to suppress attention to competing activities in order to cope with the situation. This association came as a surprise. It may be that at this point pessimists were belatedly trying to deal with the dimensions of a crisis that they had put off for nearly a year.

The overall picture that emerges from this pattern of associations is one of optimists as engaged copers, planful and active during the period when there are plans to be made and actions to engage in, trying to make the best of a situation that they are also trying to accept as real. People at the other end of the optimism dimension, in contrast, show evidence of trying to escape from the reality of the situation and of tending to experience a disengagement from their other life goals.

Table 4—*Correlations Between Optimism and COPE Scales at Each Measurement Point*

Scale	Presurgery	Postsurgery	Follow-Up 3-month	Follow-Up 6-month	Follow-Up 12-month
Active Coping	.33*	.13	.16	.07	−.11
Suppression of Competing Activities	.03	.00	.08	−.12	−.30*
Planning	.46**	.02	.11	.01	−.07
Restraint	.12	−.19	.04	−.04	−.24
Use of Social Support	.00	−.06	.01	.14	−.00
Positive Reframing	.41**	.36**	.26*	.25	.15
Religion	.03	−.03	.00	.00	−.01
Acceptance	.56**	.37**	.38**	.33*	.14
Denial	−.39**	−.50**	−.37**	−.35**	−.40**
Behavioral Disengagement	−.46**	−.30*	−.34**	−.28*	−.29*
Use of Humor	.40**	.48**	.38**	.42**	.25
Self-Distraction	.07	−.06	−.06	−.23	−.18

*$p < .05$.
**$p < .01$.

Coping and Concurrent Distress

How did the coping reactions relate to distress? Correlations between COPE scales and the distress index are shown in Table 5. (Analyses of postsurgery data were also repeated, controlling for 3-month chemotherapy, and analyses of the 3- and 6-month data were repeated, controlling for age; those partial correlations did not differ appreciably from the correlations shown in Table 5.)

The picture presented by the associations shown in Table 5 is, in many respects, consistent across the repeated assessments. Distress was positively related to denial and disengagement responses at all measurements, inversely related to acceptance at all measurements, and inversely related to positive reframing at all but the last measurement. In contrast to this relative consistency, associations between distress and several other coping responses differed across the period of the study. Distress was inversely related to the use of humor at postsurgery and 6-month follow-up, but not significantly so at other times. Distress was related to restraint coping at pre- and postsurgery, but at no other point. Distress was positively related to use of social support at presurgery and the 3-month follow-up, but not at other measurements. Distress was linked with active attempts at self-distraction in the 6-month data, but not at other times. With the exception of restraint coping, these inconsistent relations shown no discernible pattern.

It should also be noted that the correlations of these various coping responses with distress are not entirely independent of one another. That is, the coping reactions are intercorrelated, in some cases fairly substantially so. To assess the extent to which specific coping reactions were uniquely related to distress, multiple regression analyses were conducted in which all coping responses that were significant at the bivariate level were entered simultaneously as predictors.

Table 5—*Correlations Between COPE Scales and Distress at Each Measurement Point*

Scale	Presurgery	Postsurgery	Follow-Up		
			3-month	6-month	12-month
Active Coping	−.03	.16	.04	.18	.04
Suppression of Competing Activities	.20	.17	.02	.15	.28*
Planning	−.01	.29*	.18	.24	.11
Restraint	.26*	.27*	−.07	.16	.24
Use of Social Support	.33*	.22	.27*	.09	−.08
Positive Reframing	−.48**	−.26*	−.27*	−.30*	−.14
Religion	.04	−.04	.00	.06	.03
Acceptance	−.68**	−.47**	−.29*	−.43**	−.27*
Denial	.70**	.66**	.46**	.39**	.42**
Behavioral Disengagement	.55**	.53**	.40**	.37**	.30*
Use of Humor	−.20	−.34**	−.20	−.41**	−.13
Self-Distraction	.20	.14	.25	.31*	.17

*$p < .05$.
**$p < .01$.

At presurgery, four coping reactions made significant unique contributions—denial ($\beta = .34$), use of social support ($\beta = .27$), acceptance ($\beta = -.27$), and positive reframing ($\beta = -.22$)—with a total adjusted R^2 for the equation of .66. At postsurgery, after entering upcoming chemotherapy three coping reactions made unique contributions to predicting distress—acceptance ($\beta = -.33$), denial ($\beta = .44$), and behavioral disengagement ($\beta = .22$)—with a total adjusted R^2 of .73. Overall prediction was not as good at the 3-month follow-up, with an adjusted R^2 of .32 and only two variables contributing uniquely: positive reframing ($\beta = -.30$) and denial ($\beta = .28$). At 6 months, the adjusted R^2 was .37, with unique contributions from use of humor ($\beta = -.26$) and positive reframing ($\beta = -.26$) and the effect of acceptance nearly significant ($\beta = -.23$, $p < .07$). At 12 months, two variables made unique contributions—denial ($\beta = .31$) and suppression of competing activities ($\beta = .26$) —with an adjusted R^2 of .24.

These multivariate analyses suggest several conclusions. First, it is apparent that a relatively large amount of variance is shared among the coping reactions. Second, it is clear that the overall association between distress and coping becomes weaker across the 1-year period. Finally, there was evidence of both diversity and consistency across the multivariate analyses. The clearest consistency was the frequent (although not inevitable) appearance of both acceptance and denial as significant contributors to the regression equations.

Coping and Distress: Prospective Prediction

The patterns of associations between distress and coping reactions just outlined are all concurrent in nature and thus are inherently ambiguous about causality. One way to gain a better sense of whether coping influences distress is to test prospective prediction from the one to the other, in much the same way as was done with regard to optimism earlier. In these analyses, coping at one time point was used to predict distress at the next time point, while controlling for earlier distress levels.

The first analyses examined how coping reactions reported presurgically related to postoperative distress, after controlling for preoperative distress. Because postoperative distress was also influenced by upcoming chemotherapy, the latter variable was also controlled. Only one coping reaction emerged as a significant prospective predictor of postsurgical distress: Higher levels of acceptance presurgery were associated with less postsurgical distress, $r(55) = -.35$, $p < .04$. That is, accepting the reality of the situation before surgery predicted better emotional adjustment immediately afterward. Prediction of relative distress at the 3-month follow-up from postsurgical coping was less successful. After adjusting for postoperative distress level and age (which was correlated with 3-month distress), no coping reaction was even marginally significant as a predictor.

In contrast to this poor prediction from postsurgical coping, three coping reactions at the 3-month point were significant prospective predictors of distress at the 6-month follow-up (controlling for age and 3-month distress): Denial and behavioral disengagement were positively related to subsequent distress, $rs(45) = .31$ and $.35$, $ps < .05$, and the use of humor was inversely related to subsequent distress, $r = -.32$, $p < .05$. Multiple regression analysis, entering all three variables simultaneously (after age and previous distress), revealed that each made a unique contribution to prediction, betas for denial, disengagement, and humor being $.21$, $.22$, and $-.21$, respectively, total adjusted $R^2 = .61$ (which considerably exceeded the variance accounted for by concurrent coping).

In the final prospective test of this group, no coping reaction at the 6-month point was a significant predictor of distress at the 12-month follow-up.

We also examined the question of reverse causality, using analyses in which distress at one time point was used to predict subsequent coping reactions, controlling for previous levels of that same coping reaction. These analyses yielded evidence that distress induces several responses during the early phases of this crisis. Distress before surgery was associated with higher levels of denial at postsurgery, $r(56) = .36$, $p < .01$, and with higher levels of planning postsurgery, $r(56) = .28$, $p < .04$. Postoperative distress was associated with higher levels of three responses at the 3-month follow-up, all of which reflect avoidance coping. These were denial, $r(53) = .27$, $p < .05$, behavioral disengagement, $r(53) = .34$, $p < .01$, and self-distraction, $r(53) = .32$, $p < .03$. Distress at the 3-month level predicted one coping reaction at 6 months, but at only a marginal level. Specifically, 3-month distress tended to predict lower levels of acceptance, $r(46) = -.25$, $p < .08$. Finally, distress at 6 months predicted subsequent tendencies to suppress competing activities to focus more on this stressor, $r(42) = .30$, $p < .05$.

In sum, the prospective tests provided evidence of reciprocal influence between coping and distress. In general, the variables that emerged from the analyses tended to be the ones that were important in concurrent analyses. Indeed, the findings hint at a spiral of distress and dysfunctional avoidance coping. That is, lower levels of acceptance at presurgery led to higher postoperative distress; postoperative distress led to denial and disengagement at the 3-month follow-up; and denial and disengagement at 3 months led to higher levels of distress at 6 months.

Flexibility of Coping and Distress

On the basis of suggestions from reviewers, we undertook additional analyses to examine the possibility that flexibility in coping might be related to emotional adjustment (cf. Pearlin & Schooler, 1978). Flexibility here refers to the use of multiple aspects of coping, rather than restricting oneself to one or two. Two very different possibilities were suggested. One is that greater flexibility in coping may relate to better emotional adjustment, as the woman uses whatever coping reaction works best at the moment, shifting as needed. Alternatively, the occurrence of multiple coping reactions within any given time period may reflect ineffectiveness of the various coping reactions. As the woman finds that one response fails to help, she tries others in a fruitless search for greater peace of mind. To examine these possibilities, we computed indices of flexibility at each time point and related these indices to distress.

Flexibility was operationalized in two different ways for these tests. One operationalization was idiographic: Subjects' coping reports were summed across all scales; the contribution of each coping scale to this sum was then computed as a percentage.[4] A given coping reaction was defined as being ''in use'' if it accounted for 10% or more of the sum (cf. Dunkel-Schetter, Feinstein, Taylor, & Falke, 1992). For each subject, the coping reactions that satisfied this criterion were counted. The total from this count was the subject's flexibility score. This procedure was done separately for each time point (means ranged from 4.46 to 5.78).

Flexibility, as operationalized in this manner, proved not to be significantly related to concurrent distress (or to distress at the preceding or subsequent measurement point). (Nor did the sums of coping responses relate to distress.) Recall, however, that some coping reactions apparently are dysfunctional. It might be argued that if flexibility is beneficial, its effect would be obscured by including dysfunctional reactions in the index. For this reason, the analyses were repeated omitting behavioral disengagement, denial, and self-distraction from all computations. Although no concurrent association was significant, flexibility at 3 months was related both to earlier (postoperative) distress, $r = .40$, $p < .01$, and to subsequent (6-month) distress, $r = .34$, $p < .01$. This pattern suggests that postoperative distress may have induced flexibility, but that the flexibility was not helpful in reducing distress in the longer term. Note, however, that these are the only significant associations to emerge from a relatively large number of tests. They should therefore be interpreted with considerable caution.

The other operationalization of flexibility was nomothetic: A given coping response was defined as having been used to a relatively high degree if it was reported at a level above the group median on that response. The scales for which this criterion was satisfied were counted, and the total from this count was the subject's flexibility score. This procedure was done separately for each time point, and the results were correlated with distress. Once again, no significant association emerged, nor did any emerge when the analyses were repeated without the dysfunctional scales.

---

[4]Before conducting these analyses, we adjusted the response range from a 1–4 range to a 0–3 range; this adjustment was necessary so as to not overweight the contribution of infrequent coping responses.

Optimism, Coping, and Distress

Analyses reported earlier in this section indicated that dispositional optimism is a strong inverse correlate of distress at each measurement point in the study, and that optimism is a prospective predictor of lower distress levels, even after controlling for prior distress. Analyses reported in later sections indicated that optimism was systematically related to certain aspects of coping, and that certain aspects of coping themselves were related to distress. The final question to be addressed here concerns the extent to which the effects of optimism are mediated by coping.

This issue was examined by means of path analyses, examining direct paths and indirect paths (through coping) between optimism and distress. Only coping variables associated both with LOT scores and with distress were examined as mediators. At all stages of the study up to the 12-month follow-up, the relevant variables included positive reframing, acceptance, denial, and behavioral disengagement. Use of humor was also included for analyses bearing on postsurgery and 3-month follow-ups. At the 12-month point, the relevant variables were denial, disengagement, and suppression of competing activities.

Potential mediators were first tested individually in path models. If more than one variable showed significant evidence of mediation with respect to a given measure of distress, these individual tests were followed by tests of models in which the significant mediators were tested simultaneously in separate paths between optimism and distress. In some cases, the several mediators made independent contributions to the model; in other cases, what had seemed to be mediators (in individual models) failed to contribute uniquely. The models reported here are those in which the largest number of mediating variables are represented, omitting variables that did not contribute uniquely to the model.

At presurgery, the results of the analyses suggested mediational roles for both acceptance and denial. Figure 1A displays the model in which the effects of these two coping reactions and optimism were tested simultaneously.[5] As can be seen there, taking these two coping reactions into account reduced the direct effect of optimism quite substantially, although it remained significant. Each of the coping reactions also retained a significant unique association with distress. Although a separate analysis hinted at a mediating effect for behavioral disengagement as well, entering that variable into a model along with acceptance and denial indicated that it did not have a unique effect.

The postsurgery results involved the same coping responses as at presurgery but yielded even stronger evidence of mediation. Figure 1B displays the model in which the effects of acceptance, denial, behavioral disengagement, and optimism were tested simultaneously. Taking these three coping reactions into account resulted in a nonsignificant effect for optimism. Each of the coping reactions, in contrast, retained a significant unique association with distress.

By the 3-month point, the evidence of mediation was diminishing, with only the test involving denial causing a reduction in the direct effect of optimism, and the

---

[5]For simplicity in presentation, the path diagrams presented here do not include the control variables mentioned earlier (i.e., upcoming chemotherapy with respect to postoperative distress and age with respect to 3- and 6-month distress). In subsidiary analyses in which those variables were included, the direct and indirect paths for optimism were essentially the same as indicated here.

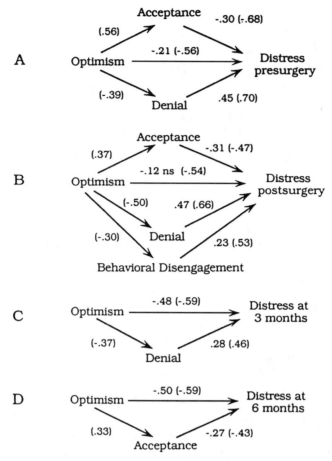

Figure 1. Path diagrams for models testing direct and indirect effects of optimism on distress. (Coping was assessed concurrently with distress. Models predicted distress [A] at presurgery, [B] 10 days postsurgery, [C] at 3-month follow-up, and [D] at 6-month follow-up. Values inside parentheses are simple correlations, and values outside parentheses are standardized regression coefficients. All relationships are significant unless indicated otherwise.)

effect being rather weak (Figure 1C). At 6 months, the only evidence of indirect effect was for acceptance, and the evidence of mediation was even weaker (Figure 1D). At 12 months, there was no indication that the effect of optimism was mediated by any of the coping reactions measured in the study.

Optimism, Coping, and Changes in Distress

The path analyses just described concern associations among optimism, coping, and the experience of distress. It is also possible to ask whether the effects of optimism on *change* in distress are mediated by coping. This requires taking prior level of distress into account in the path model. The tests undertaken to address this question resemble in general form the tests just reported, except that the immediately previous distress measure was also included in the path models.

In all but one case, these tests tended to indicate that the effect of optimism on change in distress is mediated by coping. When presurgical distress was added to prediction of postsurgical distress, the already-weakened direct relation between optimism and postsurgical distress was eliminated altogether (Figure 2A). The failure occurred when postsurgical distress was entered into prediction of 3-month distress: In this case, the only coping reaction that had previously played a role in prediction was no longer significant, leaving only a direct effect of optimism (Figure 2B). When 3-month distress was considered in predicting 6-month distress, use of humor made a significant contribution and acceptance made a marginal contribution ($p < .06$), with the direct effect of optimism no longer significant (Figure 2C). When 6-month distress was used in predicting 12-month distress, behavioral disengagement entered the model, and the optimism direct effect was no longer significant (Figure 2D).

In sum, evidence from the path analyses suggests rather strongly that the effects of optimism on distress and change in distress were mediated by aspects of subjects' coping reactions. Particularly important as mediators are acceptance, denial, and behavioral disengagement, the same variables that were prominent as correlates of distress in earlier, simpler analyses.

Discussion

The study described here makes several points. Some bear on the broad question of whether coping plays an important role in people's adjustment to stressful events. Others are more specific to the experience of early stage breast cancer patients. Yet others concern the nature of optimism and the mechanisms by which this personality quality seems to confer benefits. These questions are considered, in turn, in the following sections.

Does Coping Help?

Fifteen years ago, most researchers interested in stress and coping would probably not have seriously questioned the assumption that coping is an important determinant of people's emotional well-being during the various phases of stressful transactions. Today, in contrast, people are asking more frequently whether coping helps, is epiphenomenal (McCrae & Costa, 1986), or even interferes with outcomes such as good emotional adjustment (e.g., Aldwin & Revenson, 1987). This study found that some coping reactions were linked to good outcomes and others were linked to poor outcomes.

Beneficial Effects

Three coping responses are notable for their positive effects. Acceptance was consistently linked to low levels of concurrent distress and was a prospective predictor of low distress at postsurgery (cf. Coyne, Aldwin, & Lazarus, 1981, who found a

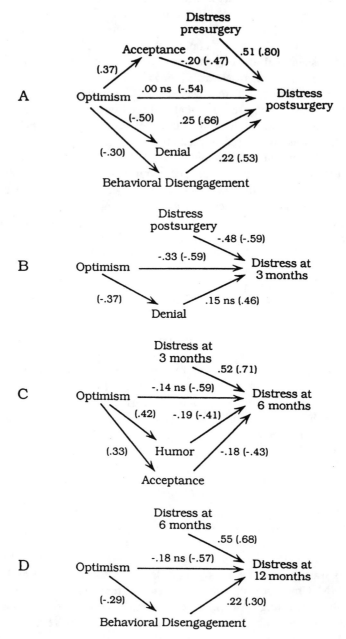

Figure 2. Path diagrams for models testing direct and indirect effects of optimism on distress, adjusting for previously assessed distress. (Coping was assessed concurrently with distress. Models predicted distress [A] 10 days postsurgery, [B] at 3-month follow-up, [C] at 6-month follow-up, and [D] at 12-month follow-up. Values inside parentheses are simple correlations, and values outside parentheses are standardized regression coefficients. All relationships are significant unless indicated otherwise.)

concurrent link between depression and a tendency not to appraise stressors as requiring acceptance). The use of humor was linked to low concurrent distress at postsurgery and at the 6-month follow-up and was a prospective predictor of low distress at the 6-month follow-up (cf. Nezu, Nezu, & Blissett, 1988). Positive reframing was related to low concurrent distress at all assessments until the final one, but it did not play a role in prospective tests.

There have been a few prior instances in which coping reactions had beneficial prospective effects on emotional adjustment, but such findings are more rare than is often assumed. In several cases, task-focused coping predicted better outcomes across spans of time that did not necessarily include specific stressors (Aldwin & Revenson, 1987; Aspinwall & Taylor, 1992; Glyshaw et al., 1989). In one case, a type of positive reframing predicted a better outcome across a similar span of time (Menaghan & Merves, 1984). As far as we know, the study reported here is the first in which situational reports of acceptance and the use of humor were shown to have beneficial prospective effects on subjective well-being. Indeed, somewhat surprisingly, these findings appear to be among the first instances in which any coping reaction has been shown to have a beneficial prospective effect on adjustment to a specific stressor.

It is worth pointing out that these findings could not possibly have been obtained using many existing measures of coping. Although scales for acceptance and the use of humor are included in the instrument used here, they are not part of most other measures. These findings illustrate how important it can be to assess a diverse range of coping reactions in one's studies.

Harmful Effects

Although certain coping reactions were helpful to these patients, others predicted poorer adjustment. Overt denial was consistently related to higher levels of concurrent distress, and denial predicted distress prospectively at the 6-month follow-up. A comparable but statistically independent pattern also emerged for behavioral disengagement (thoughts of giving up). These findings appear to complement and extend those of other studies in the literature. A wealth of data indicate that avoidance coping is positively tied to concurrent distress (Aldwin & Revenson, 1987; Billings & Moos, 1984; Cronkite & Moos, 1984; Felton, Revenson, & Hinrichsen, 1984; Folkman & Lazarus, 1985; Holahan & Moos, 1985; Rohde, Lewinsohn, Tilson, & Seeley, 1990; Vaillant, 1977; Wills, 1986), and the available data suggest that avoidance coping is also a prospective predictor of distress when confronting a major stressor or chronic burden (Bolger, 1990; Felton & Revenson, 1984; Litt et al., 1992; Stanton & Snider, 1993). Our findings add further substance to this conclusion.

Reciprocal Influences

In addition to evidence that coping had an influence on distress, there was also evidence of reverse causality, that is, that distress had an influence on coping. Higher levels of distress tended to promote higher levels of denial (at postsurgery and at 3 months), disengagement, and self-distraction. When this pattern of reciprocal influence is considered as a whole, it suggests a spiral in which a relative absence of acceptance presurgically led to postoperative distress, which in turn led to denial and disengagement at the 3-month follow-up, both of which led to higher relative levels of distress at the 6-month follow-up. This spiral of influence between distress and coping reactions across the stages of the transaction has never been observed in previous research, at least in part because it is very rare to have as many distinct measurement points as there were in this study. The pattern is quite intriguing, however, and it would seem to merit additional research attention.

Although some coping reactions appeared to play an important role in the adjustment process, the effects of others were negligible. For example, although active coping and planning were reported at relatively high levels early in the transaction, they were not tied to lower levels of distress. Similarly, subjects reported elevated use of their social support resources early in the transaction, but the data did not reveal any positive effect of doing so. As always, it is hard to interpret these null findings. It is impossible to know how distressed subjects would have been if they had not engaged in active coping and used social support to the extent they did. A possibility that cannot be discounted is that different people require different amounts of such responses to gain their benefits. If so, such differences in requirement would have obscured real relationships. Thus, we are reluctant to conclude from these null effects that these responses do not matter.

Limitations

Any broad conclusions to be drawn from this study about the role of coping are, of course, subject to limitations on the study's nature. Most important, the situation encountered by these women can be characterized best as one that they had to endure (cf. Lazarus & Folkman, 1984), with active efforts at problem management being possible only in limited respects. Given this, it may be unreasonable to expect active coping to play a major role in adjustment here. This line of thought also raises another question: whether the critical role of acceptance as a coping reaction may be limited to situations of the sort examined in this study. Perhaps acceptance matters less in situations that call primarily for active coping. There is at least some evidence that fits this picture from a study of how students cope with a college exam (Carver & Scheier, 1993). Although acceptance was the most-reported coping reaction at all stages of the transaction in that study, acceptance had absolutely no relation to emotional responses. The general notion implied here—that adjustment is best when coping reactions match the needs of the situation—is one that obviously deserves further attention (cf. Mattlin, Wethington, & Kessler, 1990; Pearlin & Schooler, 1978).

One more limitation on the generality of our findings should also be noted. The women who served as subjects in this study all had early stage disease, with a good prognosis. The distress levels they reported reflect the experience of a crisis that, overall, is being handled relatively well. These limitations are typical of research on breast cancer (see Irvine, Brown, Crooks, Roberts, & Browne, 1991), but they should not be discounted in evaluating the generality of the findings. For example, we cannot conclude from these results that optimism would confer benefits among patients with advanced cancers (cf. Tennen & Affleck, 1987), although there are certainly reasons to advance that hypothesis for study. In the same fashion, we cannot conclude that this pattern of results would generalize to any other population experiencing stressors of comparable severity. Examining that question will be an important task for future research.

Breast Cancer

Our findings complement and extend a small but growing literature concerning the impact of psychosocial variables in the adjustment of breast cancer patients. Much of that literature focuses on social support (see Irvine et al., 1991), but a few studies have dealt with personality. Two previous studies found associations between neuroticism and poorer emotional adjustment at approximately a 2-year follow-up (Jamison, Wellisch, & Pasnau, 1978; Morris, Greer, & White, 1977). To the extent that neuroticism and pessimism are similar (see later discussion), our findings extend those earlier ones. That is, using a fully prospective design, we found that pessimism is associated with distress throughout the 1st postoperative year, including the period just before and after surgery.

Our findings also provide a picture of the coping responses that are part of the phenomenology of adjusting to breast cancer. What is perhaps most striking about this picture is the prominent role played by acceptance. Acceptance was the most-reported coping response at each measurement point; indeed, it tended to become more common across the course of the year. The fact that acceptance predicted less distress is consistent with the assertion that cancer patients must accept the reality of their situation to adjust to it (Klein, 1971; Weisman & Worden, 1976/1977). The data contradict the argument that denial is the more beneficial resposne as long as it does not interfere with the seeking of treatment (see Meyerowitz, 1980). Indeed, to the extent that the COPE's denial scale reflects the denial construct as it is commonly used, the study provides no support at all for the idea that denial is adaptive.

We also found that aspects of avoidance coping, although not common in these patients, are problematic. Disengagement and denial were among the least-reported reactions, yet they remained strongly related to distress throughout the period of the study, and their levels at 3 months prospectively predicted distress at 6 months. These findings complement and extend those of Bloom (1982), who found an index of several aspects of avoidance coping to be associated with distress in breast cancer patients, and Stanton and Snider (1993), who found that cognitive avoidance was associated with postoperative distress in breast cancer patients.

Optimism and Its Mediators

We turn now to the personality variable of optimism. The findings of this study indicate that differences in dispositional optimism play an important role in the experiences of breast cancer patients, both in terms of their adjustment and in terms of their coping reactions. The pattern of relationships was also consistent with the idea that the differences in coping serve as a mediating mechanism by which differences in optimism influence subjective well-being (see also Aspinwall & Taylor, 1992).

Three reactions were particularly prominent here as mediators: acceptance, denial, and behavioral disengagement. Optimistic women were more likely than women who were less optimistic to accept the reality of the situation they were facing; they were less likely to make conscious efforts to try to put it aside and refuse to deal with it. Optimists were also less likely to experience the feelings of giving up that characterize a helpless response to an unmanageable situation. Path analyses indicated that these three reactions served as mediating routes through which optimism was related to distress at various points in the study and to changes in distress from one point to the next.

These mediational findings can be seen to fit reasonably well with the view of optimism that lies behind this research, although not all aspects of the fit may be obvious at first glance. Scheier and Carver's (1985) conception of optimism stems from a traditon of expectancy-value models of motivation and behavior. In line with this tradition, the LOT measures optimism as positive versus negative expectancies for the future. By construing the optimism dimension in this way, Scheier and Carver tied it most explicitly to predictions about overt action. That is, optimists should respond to difficulty with continued effort, whereas pessimists should be more likely to give up (cf. Wortman & Brehm, 1975). These behavioral predictions, by implication, focus on situations in which active coping is relevant to the stressor. What is less obvious from that theoretical analysis is how expectancies should influence reactions when the situation is one that has to be endured.

We suggest that the findings from this study fit a picture in which optimists make every effort to stay engaged with the important goals that give structure to their lives (an idea that complements the view just outlined, in which positive expectancies promote active striving). Remaining engaged with the important goals of one's life means realizing the reality of threats to those goals. It means not trying to wish problems away. One cannot cope with a new challenge until one has accepted its existence. The optimist seems to be the one who is most ready to move forward in this respect, saying, in effect, "Let me take on this new reality and deal with it." The pessimist says, in effect, "This new reality is too much for me to deal with," and tries (in vain) to define it out of existence. Because the new reality seems too much to deal with, the result is also a sense of helplessness and passivity, the same passivity that pessimistic doubt produces in situations where active coping is more critical.

How is it that optimists are more able than pessimists to engage in this acceptance? The answer may rest on optimists' overall positive expectancies for the future. Optimists believe that things will work out successfully in their lives. Although the diagnosis of cancer is a blow, the optimist tends to assume that the situation can be dealt with and that a good outcome awaits. This positive view of the future may make it easier to accept—and thereby to deal with—the threat in the present.

Less has been written about the accommodating side of the optimist as coper than about the active striving side. Yet ultimately the accommodating side may prove to be fully as important, or even more important. Many of the critical stresses of life involve threats and losses about which little can be done but adjust. When taken together with previous results, the findings reported here suggest a picture of the optimist not too different from the ideal of the well-known "serenity prayer." That is, the optimist appears to accept the things that cannot be changed, as well as exerting efforts to change those that can.

Third Variable Issue

Although the findings are consistent with this model of optimism, some attention must be given to the "third variable" issue, the idea that the effects depended on a variable that was not measured in the research. It has recently been suggested that optimism is less distinct from other constructs than had previously been assumed, and that results attributed to optimism may derive instead from related variables (e.g., Marshall & Lang, 1990; T. W. Smith, Pope, Rhodewalt, & Poulton, 1989). Because the study reported here was begun well before this issue was raised, we cannot address all aspects of it with data from this sample. There are, however, reasons for not concluding too quickly that optimism–pessimism was not the operative factor in this study.

The third variable that is of greatest concern at present is neuroticism. There are two distinct reasons for concern about neuroticism. The first derives from the association between neuroticism and the outcome variable (distress). It is sometimes argued that neuroticism is a nuisance variable, which influences ambient levels of distress and is of no further consequence (see, e.g., McCrae, 1990; McCrae & Costa, 1986; Watson & Pennebaker, 1989). From this perspective, the question is whether the predictor variable accounts for any variance in the dependent variable beyond that accounted for by neuroticism. If neuroticism is completely responsible for variations in the dependent variable, controlling for neuroticism will cause the effect under study to evaporate.

As just noted, there was no measure of neuroticism in this study. But if neuroticism acts to predispose people to experience distress, it follows that the best proxy for neuroticism is distress itself. In the study reported here, even after controlling for previous distress, pessimism predicted relative distress at the next assessment. Thus, it appears that the quality measured by the LOT bears on relative vulnerability to feelings of distress, rather than simply reflecting ambient distress.

This is not the only possible conceptualization of the role of neuroticism, however. One may construe neuroticism as a dynamic variable in its own right. Indeed, Bolger and Schilling (1991) found that neuroticism predicted not just ambient distress but reactivity to events (although they acknowledged that their subjects were in a period of "relative equilibrium" [p. 381] during the period of the study, rather than being stressed by a particular event). Perhaps, then, neuroticism acted in this dynamic fashion in the present research, and optimism–pessimism is irrelevant.

We are disinclined to draw this conclusion for two reasons, one empirical, the other conceptual. In a large data set collected to address issues of overlap and uniqueness between optimism and other constructs (Scheier & Carver, 1993), factor analyses of combined item sets (LOT items plus items of other scales, including measures of neuroticism and trait anxiety) yielded distinct factors composed of LOT items. These factors had unique relations to depression and to aspects of coping (see Scheier & Carver, 1992, for further discussion). In another study, Mroczek, Spiro, Ozer, Aldwin, and Bossé (in press) also found a unique link between optimism and distress after taking neuroticism into account. Thus, empirically there is reason to believe that optimism and neuroticism are not interchangeable.

The conceptual issue concerns the fact that neuroticism is conventionally viewed as a multifaceted construct, which consists partly (although not entirely) of pessimism. The broad scope of this construct means that it combines pessimism with several other qualities, such as emotional lability and worry. Combining qualities in this way can create problems of clarity of interpretation (Carver, 1989). Thus, to ask whether an effect of pessimism is really an effect of neuroticism begs in return the question of whether all facets of neuroticism are important to the effect, or only that part of neuroticism that is pessimism (which, in the case of the present study, we know is involved). Indeed, considering this issue raises the further question of whether dynamic effects previously shown for neuroticism (e.g., Bolger, 1990; Bolger & Schilling, 1991) depend on neuroticism in toto, or only that part of neuroticism that is pessimism.

In sum, it would not seem reasonable to assume that the present effects derive from a variable other than optimism. The questions raised here are important, however, and should be addressed in future research. Answering such questions would seem important for practical reasons, as well as for theoretical clarity. For example, if one were planning an intervention among patients of the sort studied here, should one focus on pessimism or on all the facets of neuroticism?

Implications

We close this article by briefly considering the applied relevance of the findings. Some readers will ask whether these findings have implications for interventions: whether there is a basis here for promoting certain kinds of coping reactions and orientations and for avoiding others. Our position in this regard is a cautious one. This was not an intervention study. We do not know whether inducing a particular coping response will have the same effect as that following from the spontaneous occurrence of the same response. It is easy, however, to suggest that some reactions are problematic, even if it is harder to be sure that others will invariably be beneficial.

In particular, it seems counterproductive to try to deny a reality that cannot be ignored. An attempt to deny the cancer cannot be effective when one is confronted repeatedly with evidence of its existence. Moreover, being caught up in an effort to hold onto one's life as it was represents a failure to move forward and adapt constructively to the new situation. Both the inability to define the threat out of existence and the failure to move forward in one's life can create a sense of helplessness and giving up. The more fully one's forward movement is suspended, the more the distress (cf. Carver & Scheier, 1990). We are not in a position to say that all patients should be urged to accept the reality of their situation as quickly as possible. We simply do not know whether acceptance can be fostered in an adaptive way for everyone, any more than we know that pessimists can be readily turned into optimists. We believe, however, that these are questions worth investigating.

References

Aldwin, C. M., & Revenson, T. A. (1987). Does coping help? A reexamination of the relation between coping and mental health. *Journal of Personality and Social Psychology, 53*, 337–348.

Andersen, B. L. (1992). Psychological interventions for cancer patients to enhance the quality of life. *Journal of Consulting and Clinical Psychology, 60*, 552–568.

Aspinwall, L. G., & Taylor, S. E. (1992). Modeling cognitive adaptation: A longitudinal investigation of the impact of individual differences and coping on college adjustment and performance. *Journal of Personality and Social Psychology, 63*, 989–1003.

Billings, A. G., & Moos, R. H. (1984). Coping, stress, and social resources among adults with unipolar depression. *Journal of Personality and Social Psychology, 46*, 877–891.

Bloom, J. R. (1982). Social support, accommodation to stress, and adjustment to breast cancer. *Social Science & Medicine, 16*, 1329–1338.

Bloom, J. R., Cook, M., Fotopoulos, S., Flamer, D., Gates, C., Holland, J. C., Muenz, L. R., Murawski, B., Penman, D., & Ross, R. D. (1987). Psychological response to mastectomy: A prospective comparison study. *Cancer, 59*, 189–196.

Bolger, N. (1990). Coping as a personality process: A prospective study. *Journal of Personality and Social Psychology, 59*, 525–537.

Bolger, N., & Schilling, E. A. (1991). Personality and the problems of everyday life: The role of neuroticism in exposure and reactivity to daily stressors. *Journal of Personality, 59*, 355–386.

Carver, C. S. (1989). How should multifaceted personality constructs be tested? Issues illustrated by self-monitoring, attributional style, and hardiness. *Journal of Personality and Social Psychology, 56*, 577–585.

Carver, C. S., & Scheier, M. F. (1990). Origins and functions of positive and negative affect: A control-process view. *Psychological Review, 97*, 19–35.

Carver, C. S., & Scheier, M. F. (1993). *Situational coping and coping dispositions in a stressful transaction.* Manuscript submitted for publication.

Carver, C. S., Scheier, M. F., & Pozo, C. (1992). Conceptualizing the process of coping with health problems. In H. S. Friedman (Ed.), *Hostility, coping, and health* (pp. 167–199). Washington, DC: American Psychological Association.

Carver, C. S., Scheier, M. F., & Weintraub, J. K. (1989). Assessing coping strategies: A theoretically based approach. *Journal of Personality and Social Psychology, 56*, 267–283.

Cella, D. F., Tross, S., Orav, E. J., Holland, J. C., Silberfarb, P. M., & Rafla, S. (1989). Mood states of patients after the diagnosis of cancer. *Journal of Psychosocial Oncology, 7*, 45–54.

Coyne, J. C., Aldwin, C., & Lazarus, R. S. (1981). Depression and coping in stressful episodes. *Journal of Abnormal Psychology, 90*, 439–447.

Cronkite, R. C., & Moos, R. H. (1984). The role of predisposing and moderating factors in the stress–illness relationship. *Journal of Health and Social Behavior, 25*, 372–393.

Derogatis, L. R. (1986). The unique impact of breast and gynecologic cancers on body image and sexual identity in women: A reassessment. In J. M. Vaeth (Ed.), *Body image, self-esteem, and sexuality in cancer patients* (2nd ed., pp. 1–14). Basel, Switzerland: Karger.

Dunkel-Schetter, C., Feinstein, L. G., Taylor, S. E., & Falke, R. L. (1992). Patterns of coping with cancer. *Health Psychology, 11*, 79–87.

Felton, B. J., & Revenson, T. A. (1984). Coping with chronic illness: A study of illness controllability and the influence of coping strategies on psychological adjustment. *Journal of Consulting and Clinical Psychology, 52*, 343–353.

Felton, B. J., Revenson, T. A., & Hinrichsen, G. A. (1984). Stress and coping in the explanation of psychological adjustment among chronically ill adults. *Social Science & Medicine, 18*, 889–898.

Folkman, S., & Lazarus, R. S. (1985). If it changes it must be a process: Study of emotion and coping during three stages of a college examination. *Journal of Personality and Social Psychology, 48*, 150–170.

Friedman, L. C., Nelson, D. V., Baer, P. E., Lane, M., Smith, F. E., & Dworkin, R. J. (1992). The relationship of dispositional optimism, daily life stress, and domestic environment to coping methods used by cancer patients. *Journal of Behavioral Medicine, 15*, 127–142.

Glyshaw, K., Cohen, L. H., & Towbes, L. C. (1989). Coping strategies and psychological distress: Prospective analyses of early and middle adolescents. *American Journal of Community Psychology, 17*, 607–623.

Gordon, W. A., Freidenbergs, I., Diller, L., Hibbard, M., Wolf, C., Levine, L., Lipkins, R., Ezrachi, O., & Lucido, D. (1980). Efficacy of psychosocial intervention with cancer patients. *Journal of Consulting and Clinical Psychology, 48*, 743–759.

Holahan, C. J., & Moos, R. H. (1985). Life stress and health: Personality, coping, and family support in stress resistance. *Journal of Personality and Social Psychology, 49*, 739–747.

Holahan, C. J., & Moos, R. H. (1987). Risk resistance and psychological distress: A longitudinal analysis with adults and children. *Journal of Abnormal Psychology, 96*, 3–13.

Holland, J. C., & Rowland, J. H. (1987). Psychological reactions to breast cancer and its treatment. In J. R. Harris & S. Hellman (Eds.), *Breast disease* (pp. 632–647). Philadelphia: Lippincott.

Irvine, D., Brown, B., Crooks, D., Roberts, J., & Browne, G. (1991). Psychosocial adjustment in women with breast cancer. *Cancer, 67*, 1097–1117.

Jamison, K. R., Wellisch, D. K., & Pasnau, R. O. (1978). Psychosocial aspects of mastectomy. I: The woman's perspective. *American Journal of Psychiatry, 135*, 432–436.

Kirk, R. E. (1982). *Experimental design: Procedures for the behavioral sciences* (2nd ed.). Monterey, CA: Brooks/Cole.

Klein, R. A. (1971). A crisis to grow on. *Cancer, 28*, 1660–1665.

Lansky, S. B., List, M. A., Herrmann, C. A., Ets-Hokin, E. G., Das-Gupta, T. K., Wilbanks, G. D., & Hendrickson, F. R. (1985). Absence of major depressive disorder in female cancer patients. *Journal of Clinical Oncology, 3*, 1553–1559.

Lazarus, R. S., & Folkman, S. (1984). *Stress, appraisal, and coping*. New York: Springer.

Litt, M. D., Tennen, H., Affleck, G., & Klock, S. (1992). Coping and cognitive factors in adaptation to *in vitro* fertilization failure. *Journal of Behavioral Medicine, 15*, 171–187.

Marshall, G. N., & Lang, E. L. (1990). Optimism, self-mastery, and symptoms of depression in women professionals. *Journal of Personality and Social Psychology, 59*, 132–139.

Marshall, G. N., Wortman, C. B., Kusulas, J. W., Hervig, L. K., & Vickers, R. R., Jr. (1992). Distinguishing optimism from pessimism: Relations to fundamental dimensions of mood and personality. *Journal of Personality and Social Psychology, 62*, 1067–1074.

Mattlin, J. A., Wethington, E., & Kessler, R. C. (1990). Situational determinants of coping and coping effectiveness. *Journal of Health and Social Behavior, 31*, 103–122.

McCrae, R. (1990). Controlling neuroticism in the measurement of stress. *Stress Medicine, 6*, 237–241.

McCrae, R. R., & Costa, P. T., Jr. (1986). Personality, coping, and coping effectiveness in an adult sample. *Journal of Personality, 54*, 385–405.

McNair, D., Lorr, M., & Droppelman, L. (1971). *Profile of Mood States manual*. San Diego, CA: EDITS.

Menaghan, E. (1982). Measuring coping effectiveness: A panel analysis of marital problems and coping efforts. *Journal of Health and Social Behavior, 23*, 220–234.

Menaghan, E., & Merves, E. (1984). Coping with occupational problems: The limits of individual efforts. *Journal of Health and Social Behavior, 25*, 406–423.

Meyerowitz, B. E. (1980). Psychosocial correlates of breast cancer and its treatments. *Psychological Bulletin, 87*, 108–131.

Miller, P. J. (1980). Mastectomy: A review of psychosocial research. *Health and Social Work, 4*, 60–65.

Morris, T., Greer, H. S., & White, P. (1977). Psychological and social adjustment to mastectomy: A 2-year follow-up study. *Cancer, 40*, 2381–2387.

Mroczek, D. K., Spiro, A., III, Ozer, D. J., Aldwin, C. M., & Bossé, R. (in press). Personality, optimism, and health: Findings from the normative aging study. *Health Psychology*.

Nezu, A. M., Nezu, C. M., & Blissett, S. E. (1988). Sense of humor as a moderator of the relation between stressful events and psychological distress: A prospective analysis. *Journal of Personality and Social Psychology, 54*, 520–525.

Pearlin, L. I., & Schooler, C. (1978). The structure of coping. *Journal of Health and Social Behavior, 19*, 2–21.

Penman, D. T., Bloom, J. R., Fotopoulos, S., Cook, M. R., Holland, J. C., Gates, C., Flamer, D., Murawski, B., Ross, R., Brandt, U., Muenz, L. R., & Pee, D. (1987). The impact of mastectomy on self-concept and social function: A combined cross-sectional and longitudinal study with comparison groups. *Women and Health, 11*, 101–130.

Pozo, C., Carver, C. S., Noriega, V., Harris, S. D., Robinson, D. S., Ketcham, A. S., Legaspi, A., Moffat, F. L., Jr., & Clark, K. C. (1992). Effects of mastectomy vs lumpectomy on emotional adjustment to breast cancer: A prospective study of the first year postsurgery. *Journal of Clinical Oncology, 10*, 1292–1298.

Rohde, P., Lewinsohn, P. M., Tilson, M., & Seeley, J. R. (1990). Dimensionality of coping and its relation to depression. *Journal of Personality and Social Psychology, 58*, 499–511.

Scheier, M. F., & Carver, C. S. (1985). Optimism, coping, and health: Assessment and implications of generalized outcome expectancies. *Health Psychology, 4*, 219–247.

Scheier, M. F., & Carver, C. S. (1992). Effects of optimism on psychological and physical well-being: Theoretical overview and empirical update. *Cognitive Therapy and Research, 16*, 201–228.

Scheier, M. F., & Carver, C. S. (1993). *Differentiating optimism from related constructs.* Manuscript in preparation.

Scheier, M. F., Matthews, K. A., Owens, J. F., Magovern, G. J., Sr., Lefebvre, R. C., Abbott, R. A., & Carver, C. S. (1989). Dispositional optimism and recovery from coronary artery bypass surgery: The beneficial effects on physical and psychological well being. *Journal of Personality and Social Psychology, 57*, 1024–1040.

Scheier, M. F., Weintraub, J. K., & Carver, C. S. (1986). Coping with stress: Divergent strategies of optimists and pessimists. *Journal of Personality and Social Psychology, 51*, 1257–1264.

Sinsheimer, L. M., & Holland, J. C. (1987). Psychological issues in breast cancer. *Seminars in Oncology, 14*, 75–82.

Smith, L. W., Patterson, T. L., & Grant, I. (1990). Avoidant coping predicts psychological disturbance in the elderly. *Journal of Nervous and Mental Disease, 178*, 525–530.

Smith, T. W., Pope, M. K., Rhodewalt, F., & Poulton, J. L. (1989). Optimism, neuroticism, coping, and symptom reports. *Journal of Personality and Social Psychology, 56*, 640–648.

Stanton, A. L., & Snider, P. R. (1993). Coping with a breast cancer diagnosis: A prospective study. *Health Psychology, 12*, 16–23.

Steiger, J. H. (1980). Tests for comparing elements of a correlation matrix. *Psychological Bulletin, 87*, 245–251.

Taylor, S. E. (1983). Adjustment to threatening events: A theory of cognitive adaptation. *American Psychologist, 38*, 1161–1173.

Taylor, S. E., Kemeny, M. E., Aspinwall, L. G., Schneider, S. G., Rodriguez, R., & Herbert, M. (1992). Optimism, coping, psychological distress, and high-risk sexual behavior among men at risk for acquired immunodeficiency syndrome (AIDS). *Journal of Personality and Social Psychology, 63*, 460–473.

Tennen, H., & Affleck, G. (1987). The costs and benefits of optimistic explanations and dispositional optimism. *Journal of Personality, 55*, 377–393.

Vaillant, G. E. (1977). *Adaptation to life.* Boston: Little, Brown.

Vitaliano, P. P., Russo, J., Young, H., Teri, L., & Maiuro, R. D. (1991). Predictors of burden in spouse caregivers of individuals with Alzheimer's disease. *Psychology and Aging, 6*, 392–402.

Watson, D., & Pennebaker, J. W. (1989). Health complaints, stress, and distress: Exploring the central role of negative affectivity. *Psychological Review, 96*, 234–254.

Weisman, A. D., & Worden, J. W. (1976/1977). The existential plight in cancer: Significance of the first 100 days. *International Journal of Psychiatry in Medicine, 7*, 1–15.

Wills, T. A. (1986). Stress and coping in early adolescence: Relationships to substance use in urban high schools. *Health Psychology, 5*, 503–529.

Wortman, C. B., & Brehm, J. W. (1975). Responses to uncontrollable outcomes: An integration of reactance theory and the learned helplessness model. In L. Berkowitz (Ed.), *Advances in experimental social psychology* (Vol. 8, pp. 277–336). San Diego, CA: Academic Press.

Appendix

Sample Items From Each COPE Scale

Active Coping

I've been concentrating my efforts on doing something about the situation I'm in.

Suppression of Competing Activities

I've been putting aside other activities in order to concentrate on this.

Planning

I've been trying to come up with a strategy about what to do.

Restraint

I've been making sure not to make matters worse by acting too soon.

Use of Social Support

I've been getting sympathy and understanding from someone.

Positive Reframing

I've been looking for something good in what is happening.

Religion

I've been putting my trust in God.

Acceptance

I've been accepting the reality of the fact that it happened.

Denial

I've been refusing to believe that it has happened.

Behavioral Disengagement

I've been giving up the attempt to cope.

Use of Humor

I've been making jokes about it.

Self-Distraction

I've been going to movies, watching TV, or reading, to think about it less.

Part III

Interventions and Outcomes

Chapter 6
PSYCHOLOGICAL INTERVENTIONS FOR CANCER PATIENTS TO ENHANCE THE QUALITY OF LIFE

Barbara L. Andersen

In 1989, approximately 985,000 Americans developed cancer, and 494,000 Americans died of the disease (Silberberg & Lubera, 1989). However disturbing these figures were, they were juxtaposed by a startling *Lancet* report of the long-term (10-year) follow-up of participants in a psychotherapy outcome study. David Spiegel, Joan Bloom, and their colleagues (Spiegel, Bloom, Kraemer, & Gottheil, 1989) reported mortality data for 36 no-treatment control and 50 intervention women with metastatic breast cancer who had participated in a group support intervention to enhance adjustment and reduce disease symptoms, such as pain. Their original reports (Spiegel, Bloom, & Yalom, 1981; Spiegel & Bloom, 1983; or Spiegel & Yalom, 1978, and others) had documented adjustment outcomes during the year-long intervention. These and related reports had suggested that gains could be achieved with psychological therapy, even as life ebbed away (Linn, Linn, & Harris, 1982). However, it would require a leap of faith to hypothesize a psychological or behavioral mechanism to effect any disease endpoint. Thus, when Spiegel reported an *18-month* survival advantage for the intervention group, his findings renewed interest in a role for psychological efforts in coping and living with cancer.

The *Lancet* report notwithstanding, the research literature on psychological therapies for cancer patients has had a relatively brief history, although the body of descriptive data documenting the psychologic–behavioral outcomes of cancer has grown rapidly (see Andersen, 1989, or *Cancer*, Vol. 67, No. 3 Supplement [whole issue], for reviews).[1] The dearth of intervention studies has occurred for a variety of research training and funding reasons (see Andersen, Beck, Ouelette-Kobasa, Revenson, & Temoshok, 1989, or Burish, 1991a, 1991b, for discussions); however, the dual expertise—cancer and psychotherapy outcome—required of investigators has been noted less often along with the scientific, ethical, and logistic difficulties surrounding research with ill, symptomatic individuals. Nevertheless, randomized dem-

Reprinted from *Journal of Consulting and Clinical Psychology, 60*(4), 552–568. (1992). Copyright © 1992 by the American Psychological Association. Used with permission of the author.

The author would like to thank individuals who provided constructive criticism on drafts of the article: Joan Bloom, John Cacioppo, Mark Elliot, Janice Kiecolt-Glaser, Michael Vasey, and two anonymous reviewers. Susan Doyle-Mirzadeh assisted with the literature search.

[1]The review of psychological efforts with cancer patients for the initial *Journal of Consulting and Clinical Psychology* behavioral medicine issue focused on behavioral treatments for aversive reactions to chemotherapy (Redd & Andrykowski, 1982). That literature has progressed in the decade with several cogent, recent reviews devoted to the topic (Andrykowski, 1990; Carey & Burish, 1988; Carnrike & Carey, 1990; Morrow & Dobkin, 1988) in addition to the rapidly progressing research on drug management and combination treatments of nausea and vomiting (Eyre & Ward, 1984; Morrow, 1989). Although psychologic efforts have been used to reduce these and other disruptive symptomatologies (e.g., anorexia, see Bernstein, 1986; pain, see Turk & Fernandez, 1990) and produce indirect improvement of adjustment, this article focuses on broad-based interventions to directly enhance general "adjustment" or improve "quality of life."

onstration projects, a major accomplishment in research development (Kazdin, 1986), have been conducted. I will begin with a critical review of the literature and conclude with two related discussions, (a) hypotheses of the components and mechanisms for intervention effectiveness and (b) future directions for research.

Review of Psychological Interventions With Cancer Patients

A classic question in psychotherapy outcome research has been, "What specific treatment, by whom, is most effective for this individual with that specific problem, and under which set of circumstances?" (Paul, 1969). Responding to this query is made difficult by the additional *circumstance* of cancer. That is, cancer is not one disease but several separate ones, each with multiple etiologies and disparate outcomes. In sum, there is not a prototypic "cancer patient." However, in this review I will highlight variables that may moderate overall risk and responses to psychological interventions. As a beginning point, Table 1 describes aspects of cancer that may affect an individual's risk for psychological and behavioral morbidity.

There is general support for the correlation between the "magnitude" of disease/ treatment and psychological and behavioral endpoints across sites of disease. For example, Cella et al. (1987) examined emotional distress in patients with lung cancer and found that a *composite* score for the extent of disease and physical impairment from treatment best predicted the magnitude of mood disturbance. Body satisfaction (Schain et al., 1983) and overall quality of life (de Haes, van Oostrom, & Welvaart, 1986) are correlated with extent of treatment for breast cancer. Among individuals

Table 1—*Cancer Characteristics That Contribute to the Individual's Risk for Psychological and Behavioral Morbidity*

Morbidity risk	Cancer characteristics		
	Extent of disease	Magnitude of treatment	Prognosis
Low	Localized/Stage I or II at diagnosis	Usually single modality (e.g., surgery or RT)	Favorable (e.g., 70–95% 5-year survival)
Moderate	Regional/Stage III at diagnosis; first recurrence for initially Stage I disease	Often combination therapy (e.g., surgery with RT for nodal disease; surgery with adjuvant chemotherapy)	Guarded (e.g., 40–60% 5-year survival)
High	Distant/Stage IV at diagnosis; first recurrence for regional disease or all stages of rapidly progressive disease (e.g., lung or pancreatic cancer)	Possibility of surgery or RT for debulking/ palliation. Systemic chemotherapy is likely; possibility of invasive treatments for pain/symptom control	Dismal (e.g., 15–40% 1-year survival; 4– 15% 5-year survival)

Note. RT = radiotherapy.

receiving surgical melanoma treatment, there is a positive correlation between the magnitude of distress and the depth of the indentation in the local scars (Cassileth, Lusk, & Tenaglia, 1983). In our research (Andersen, Anderson, & deProsse, 1989a), the magnitude of sexual morbidity was greatest among the patients treated with combined treatment (i.e., surgery plus radiotherapy), in comparison with either modality alone. Taken together, these data provide conceptual replications of specific cancer characteristics at risk factors for morbidity.

This conceptualization is used to organize the intervention studies into efforts for patients at low, moderate, or high risk. Within each category there are two sections. First, descriptive investigations are briefly summarized to highlight the general adjustment pattern(s) and provide a point of comparison for the findings for the no-treatment control groups. This discussion is limited to the methodologically strongest studies, longitudinal designs with and without comparison groups. Next for the review, studies using a quasi-experimental (e.g., the nonequivalent control group) or an experimental design are included. Studies using other designs (e.g., single-group pretest–posttest, the posttest only design, case reports) are omitted because of their limited scientific value.

To illustrate the concept of morbidity risk and its role in moderating outcome, I begin with the most comprehensive and well-documented outcome study conducted to date. (For this study, all patient and intervention details are included; however, these details for the remaining studies can be found in Table 2.) Published in the *Journal of Consulting and Clinical Psychology* in 1980, Wayne Gordon and his collaborators (Gordon et al., 1980) used a quasi-experimental design with repeated assessments for a psychosocial intervention for newly diagnosed melanoma, breast, and lung cancer patients. The intervention had three components: education (including teaching about the medical system, disease and treatment side effects, hypnosis and relaxation training to reduce emotional distress), counseling (including support and ventilation of feelings, issue clarification and problem solving and social support), and environmental change (referral for additional services and advocacy to health care personnel). The format was individual sessions with a "counselor" (a psychologist, social worker, or psychiatric nurse). The content and number of sessions were allowed to vary and were recorded as process variables. The research design involved a 6-month recruitment period for the first control group, followed by a 12-month recruitment for the intervention, and then a second 6-month control recruitment. There were differential rates of participation (15–16% of the control and 23% of the intervention recruitees declined), with refusers being significantly older. In total, 157 intervention (65 melanoma, 50 breast, and 42 lung cancer) and 151 control (62 melanoma, 48 breast, and 41 lung cancer) patients participated. Demographics indicated a mean age in years of 48 for the melanoma, 55 for the breast, and 59 for the lung samples. The entire sample was predominantly White (98%), married (79%), and high-school educated (96%) and had an occupation higher than skilled laborer (89%). Outcome was assessed pretreatment, posttreatment at hospital discharge, and at 3 and 6 months posttreatment using a structured interview. Measures included a problem-oriented survey of 13 life areas (e.g., physical discomfort, mobility, vocation, finances, social concerns, worry) and standardized questionnaires assessing emotional distress, recent life events, health locus of control, and activities of daily living. Preliminary analyses indicated similar rates of attrition (12–13% across conditions) but dissimilar sources. Control dropouts were more likely to

Table 2—*Summary of Patient and Intervention Characteristics Within Low-, Moderate-, and High-Risk Groups*

	Recruitment		Disease/treatment		Demographics				Intervention		
Study	Source	% refusal	Site/Stage	Time in illness	N	Age (years)	Gender	Race	Format	No. of sessions/ total treatment	Therapist(s)
Low risk											
Capone, Good, Westie, & Jacobsen (1980)	University medical center	13	Gynecol/ I: 51%; II: 22%; III: 15%; IV 12%	Diagnosis	56	50	Female	White: 79% Black: 21%	Individual	4+/—	N = 2; MA level psychologists
Houts, Whitney, Mortel, & Bartholomew (1986)	University medical center	22	Gynecol/ unknown	Diagnosis	32	50	Female	—	Individual: peer, phone contact, and bibliotherapy	3phonecalls/—	N = 2; MSW social workers
Davis (1986)	Regional cancer center	—	Breast/ I: 100%	6 weeks posttreatment	25	50	Female	—	Individual	13 sessions/ 9.75 hr	N = 1; BA level social worker
Christensen (1983)	Individual referral	—	Breast I/II: 100%	2–3 months posttreatment	20	40	Female	—	Conjoint with partner	4/—	PhD psychologist
Edgar, Rosberger, & Nowlis (1992)	University medical center	61	Breast (48%) I–II: 50% III: 43% IV: 7%	12 weeks postdiagnosis	205 35% loss by 12 months	56 years	75% female	—	Individual	5 sessions/5 hr	N = ? Nurses
Fawzy, Cousins, Fawzy, Kemeny, Elashoff, & Morton (1990)	University medical center	12	Melanoma/ I: 94% II: 6%	Immediate posttreatment	80; 25% dropout of controls	42 45 for I; 38 and C	53% female	White: 99%	Group	6 sessions/9 hr	N = 2; lay counselor and psychiatrist

Moderate risk

Study	Setting		Cancer/stage	Timing	N	Age	Gender	White	Format	Sessions/hr	Therapists
Heinrich & Coscarelli-Schag (1985)	VA medical center	13	Lung, colorectal, and prostate/—	Average 2 years postdiagnosis; 50% on chemotherapy	51; 27% dropout	56	32% female	White: 96%	Group ± spouse participation	6 sessions/12 hr	N = 2; MD psychiatrist and PhD psychologist
Jacobs, Ross, Walker, & Stockdale (1983)	University medical center	20	Hodgkin's disease/—	Average 1 year postdiagnosis; 31% on chemotherapy	105; 23% loss	20–40	34% female	—	Study I: bibliotherapy; Study II: group support	I: — II: 8 sessions/ 12 hr	I: — II: N = 3 MD oncologist, PhD psychologist and MSW social worker
Maguire, Brooke, Tait, Thomas, & Sellwood (1983)	UK university medical center	12	Breast/ I/II 100%	During and immediate posttreatment	152	—	Female	—	Individual	—	N = 1; nurse
Cain, Kohorn, Quinlan, Latimer, & Schwartz (1986)	University medical center	15	Gynecol/—	Diagnosis	80; 10% and 25% loss at follow-ups	59	Female	—	Individual versus group	8 sessions/—	N = 2; medical social workers
Forester, Kornfeld, & Fleiss (1985)	University medical center	—	Mixed: 36% lung, 30% gyn./—	Pretreatment (radiotherapy)	100	62	50% female	—	Individual	10 sessions/5 hr	N = 1; MD psychiatrist
Telch & Telch (1986)	University medical center	0—all referred and screened	Mixed: 36% breast, 29% Hodgkin's	On posttreatment follow-up	41	41	66% female	—	Group coping versus group support	6 sessions/9 hr	N = 2; MA psychologist and MSW social worker

(table continues)

Table 2—(Continued)

Study	Source	% refusal	Site/Stage	Time in illness	N	Age (years)	Gender	Race	Format	No. of sessions/ total treatment	Therapist(s)
	Recruitment		**Disease/treatment**			**Demographics**			**Intervention**		
					High risk						
Ferlic, Goldman, & Kennedy (1979)	University medical center	15	Mixed/ "advanced"	Diagnosis to 12 months post ($M = 7$ weeks postdiagnosis)	60	48	50% female	—	Group	6 sessions/9 hr	$N = 1+$; MSW social worker and occasional team member
Spiegel, Bloom, & Yalom (1981); Spiegel, Bloom, Kraemer, & Gottheil (1989)	Referral from community and university	17	Breast/ Metastatic, 5 years since diagnosis	During and posttreatment	86%; 33% loss to illness/ death at start; 48% loss by 12 months	54	Female	—	Group	52+ sessions/ 75+ hr	$N = 3$; MD psychiatrist or MSW social worker and peer counselor
Linn, Linn, & Harris (1982)	VA hospital	15	Mixed; 46% lung/Stage IV	Late/terminal stage	120; 58% death by 6 months	58	Male	White: 88%; Black: 12%	Individual but families occasionally included	"several/ weeks" until death/—	$N = 1$; hospice counselor
Yates, McKegney, & Kun (1981)	University affiliated hospital	10	Mixed: 40% lung, 14% breast/—	Late/terminal stage	199	58	48% female	—	Individual at home	1/month until death/—	$N = 1+$; nurse practitioners
McCorkle, Benoliel, Donaldson, Georgiadou, Moinpour, & Goodell (1989)	19 community hospitals	—	Lung/Stage II, III, or IV	Diagnosis	166; 66% death/ illness/lost by 6 months	Approx. 65	37% female	White: 89% Black: 7%; Other: 4%	Individual at home	1 week/mo, or as needed/—	$N = ?$; MA level nurses

Note. Gynecol = gynecological; VA = Veterans Administration; UK = United Kingdom; dash = data not available.

be male, older, less educated, receiving more treatment modalities, and reporting an external locus of control, whereas only intervention dropouts indicated more religious participation.

Cancer groups such as melanoma, breast, and lung patients would have cancer characteristics of low-, moderate-, and high-risk groups, respectively. Process data on the "magnitude" of the psychosocial intervention confirmed their differential outcomes. Whereas the mean intervention was 11 sessions of 20 min duration (a total of 3.7 hr), lung patients were seen for an average of 20 sessions, breast cancer patients for 13 sessions, and melanoma patients for 8 sessions. For emotional distress, the greatest improvement occurred for the lung cancer patients, moderate improvement for the breast, and no differences between the intervention and the control melanoma groups. These findings may have been due to the adjustment pattern for the no-treatment control subjects for each site. The highest levels of continuing distress were found for the lung patients, moderate levels for the breast group, and a rapid, stable decline in distress for the melanoma patients. Regarding outcome for other life areas, the intervention subjects as a group resumed daily activities significantly sooner (by 3 months) than the controls, and activities were more likely to be away from the home (e.g., grocery shopping) than at home (e.g., watching TV). Finally, there was a trend in more of the intervention subjects returning to work (74% vs. 59%), with the lowest rates for the lung cancer patients (49% vs. 73–79% for the melanoma and breast groups). In summary, this study is notable by its inclusion of a large sample and examination of disease site as a factor, a structured but individualized intervention, documentation of therapy content and process, and diverse outcome assessment. Finally, it provides evidence for the role of disease/treatment variables in moderating psychosocial outcomes.

Low Morbidity Risk

Overview of Descriptive Findings

Longitudinal data suggest that when localized disease is controlled and recovery proceeds unimpaired, the severe distress of diagnosis dissipates and emotions stabilize by 1 year posttreatment. In fact, the greatest improvement can be found as early as 3–4 months posttreatment. These were the outcomes of Stage I breast (Bloom, 1987; Vinokur, Threatt, Caplan, & Zimmerman, 1989) and Stage I and II gynecologic (Andersen, Anderson, & deProsse, 1989b) patients conducted in the United States and replicated with data from the Netherlands (de Haes et al., 1986) using controlled prospective longitudinal designs and comparisons with benign disease and healthy subjects. This consistency represents replications across site, treatment, and nationality for women with cancer. Unfortunately, comparable longitudinal studies, with or without comparison groups, have not been done with men.

Intervention Investigations

Two nonequivalent control group designs have provided brief interventions to gynecologic cancer patients. Capone, Good, Westie, and Jacobsen (1980) provided a crisis-oriented intervention to newly diagnosed women. The structured counseling

provided during hospitalization assisted women to express feelings and fears related
to their diagnosis or surgery, provided information about treatment sequelae, and
attempted to enhance self-esteem, feminity, and interpersonal relationships. For sexually active women, an additional component included sexual information and methods to cope and reduce anxiety when resuming intercourse. Fifty-six newly diagnosed
women participated, and a nonequivalent control group was obtained by recruiting
previously treated women on follow-up. Standardized outcome measures assessed
emotional distress (both by symptom ratings and the Profile of Mood States (POMS;
McNair, Lorr, & Droppleman, 1971) and self-concept and were supplemented with
self-reports of employment and frequency of intercourse. Data were gathered at pretreatment and 3-, 6-, and 12-month posttreatment. For the measures of emotional
distress, analyses indicated no differences between groups or within the intervention
group. A trend in the percentages of women returning to work favored the intervention participants (e.g., 50% vs. 25% at 3 months). In contrast, substantial differences
were found in the sexual outcomes across all posttreatment assessments (e.g., 16%
of the intervention vs. 57% of the control women reported less frequent or no sexual
activity at 12 months posttreatment).

The second quasi-experimental investigation was reported by Houts, Whitney,
Mortel, and Bartholomew (1986) and examined peer counseling. The structured intervention included encouragement to maintain interpersonal relationships; to make
positive plans for the future; to query the medical staff regarding treatments, side
effects, and sexual outcomes; and to maintain normal routines. These interventions
were delivered in three telephone contacts (one pretreatment and at 5 and 10 weeks
posttreatment) and with pretreatment provision of a booklet and coping audiotape.
Thirty-two women, 14 intervention and 18 control, newly diagnosed with gynecologic disease participated. The POMS assessed emotional distress, and an experimenter-derived measure assessed coping strategies at pretreatment and 6 and 12
weeks (3 months) posttreatment. Analyses indicated no differences between groups
at any point in time. In summary, both the quasi-experimental designs suggested that
interventions for gynecologic cancer patients produced limited gains, with the
greatest improvement in sexual functioning.

Edgar, Rosberger, and Nowlis (1992) used a repeated measures crossover design
to study the timing of intervention delivery. A coping skills intervention was used
and included instruction in problem solving, setting goals to increase feelings of
control, cognitive restructuring, relaxation training, and information about the hospital and health care system. Over 200 patients who had been diagnosed on average
11 weeks previously were randomized to receive the intervention *early* ($n = 103$) or
late ($n = 102$). Standardized outcome measures were used and assessed anxiety,
depression, perception of control, and distress from intrusive thoughts about the
illness. The individual difference variable of ego strength was studied as a moderator
of outcome. Measures were completed for both groups at baseline, and at 4, 8, and
12 months. Following the baseline assessment, the early group received the intervention and the late group received the intervention following the 4-month assessment. Analyses indicated that both groups improved with time, but there were greater
gains, albeit modest ones, for the late intervention group. The greater effectiveness
of the late delivery is puzzling, as there are no strong theoretical or empirical bases
for the effect. One confounding in the investigation is that the therapists may have
been more effective in the intervention delivery by the time they treated the second

group of subjects. Additional analyses suggested that the intervention effects were strongest for those with lower ego strength scores or more physical debilitation, perhaps because both variables are correlated with higher levels of distress.

There are only four experimental studies with low-morbidity-risk adult cancer patients, and two have small samples. Davis (1986) compared two behavior therapies with a no-treatment control. The first combined electromyography and temperature control biofeedback along with progressive relaxation training. The second treatment was cognitive–behavior therapy, including identifying current concerns, coping through positive problem-solving imagery and positive self-talk, and progressive relaxation training. Twenty-five women with breast cancer (10 biofeedback, 5 cognitive therapy, and 7 no-treatment) participated. Outcome measures were the Spielberger State Anxiety Inventory (STAI; Spielberger, Gorsuch, & Lushene, 1970) and urinary cortisol measured with a 24-hr sample, and data were collected pre- and posttreatment and at an 8-month follow-up. Analyses indicated a significant reduction with time in the state anxiety scores but no differential improvement. Cortisol levels for the intervention subjects were significantly lower at the 8-month follow-up only.

Christensen (1983) reported on a focused intervention for adjustment difficulties of mastectomy patients and their partners. The structured program included discussion of the history of the relationship, readings and discussions of the emotional and sexual aspects of mastectomy, disclosure of feelings and fantasies of the self and the spouse, and other exercises (communication training, role playing) to facilitate confronting and solving problems. Twenty women, 10 intervention and 10 no-treatment control, participated. Standardized outcome measures were used and assessed emotional distress (Beck Depression Inventory [BDI]; Beck, Ward, Mendelson, Mock, & Erbaugh, 1961; and Spielberger STAI), self-esteem, marital adjustment, sexual satisfaction, and personality (locus of control) and were administered pre- and posttreatment. Analyses indicated the intervention had modest effects in reducing distress for the breast cancer patients (i.e., significantly lower scores, 8 vs. 12, only on the BDI), but significant improvements in self-reported sexual satisfaction were found from both the woman and her partner. There were no significant differences on the remaining measures.

Finally, the largest investigation for low-risk patients was conducted by Fawzy, Cousins, Kemeny, and colleagues (Fawzy, Cousins, et al., 1990; Fawzy, Kemeny, et al., 1990) and attempted to reduce distress and enhance immune functioning in newly diagnosed and treated melanoma patients. A structured group support intervention included health education (e.g., reducing sun exposure), illness-related problem solving, stress management (relaxation training), and group support. Eighty patients, 40 intervention and 40 no-treatment control, were recruited. Outcome measures assessed emotional distress (POMS) and included an experimenter-derived coping styles inventory and an immunologic assessment (NK cells, T-cell subsets, CD8 and CD4 T cells, and activation markers on the major T-cell subsets) and were collected pretreatment, posttreatment, and at a 6-month follow-up. Despite randomization the control group was significantly younger, 38 versus 45 years, and there was greater distress (significantly higher anxiety, depression, and anger scores on the POMS) and more problematic coping strategies (higher avoidance and distraction) for the intervention subjects. There were no pretreatment immunologic differences. In analyzing the data, analysis of covariance was used. Regarding emotional distress, at posttreatment the intervention subjects reported significantly more vigor on the

POMS; there were no differences on the remaining scales. By 6 months, emotional distress had improved further for the intervention subjects with significantly lower total mood disturbance as a result of lower depression, confusion, and fatigue and higher vigor. Coping data indicated that the intervention subjects reported significantly more use of active-behavioral strategies by treatment's end, a pattern that continued with the addition of active-cognitive strategies by 6 months. Regarding the immunologic findings, there was a significant posttreatment difference between the groups in CD57 LGLs for the intervention subjects, and follow-up analyses suggested that these changes took place in the CD8 T-cell subpopulation and not in the NK cells. At 6 months, the difference in LGLs remained significant, but follow-up analyses indicated the increase was seen in CD16 NK cells but not in the CD8 cells, which had been the posttreatment pattern. Other significant changes were found for NK cells (as determined by markers, but not by cytotoxicity) and T cells (a small reduction in mean levels for CD4, whereas CD8 remained unchanged).

Methodology Summary

Drawing general conclusions is made difficult by the restricted study samples. Only three sites of disease have been studied (i.e., breast, gynecologic, and skin), which reflect 3% of the new cases in men and 47% of the new cases in women annually (Boring, Squires, & Tong, 1992). Related to this issue is the circumstance of gender, as only one study included any men (47% of the sample in Fawzy, Cousins, et al., 1990, and Fawzy, Kemeny, et al., 1990) whereas men represent 50% of all new cases (Boring et al., 1992). The samples were also not representative of national data on the sociodemographic characteristics of cancer patients. Non-Whites were poorly represented. The Capone et al. (1980) investigation was the only one to include significant numbers of Black women (21% of the sample). Study samples have been young, as the mean age for the breast sample in Christensen (1983) was 40 years, and the mean age for the melanoma sample in Fawzy, Cousins, et al. (1990) and Fawzy, Kemeny, et al. (1990) was 42 years, in comparison with mean ages of 55 years and 57 years, respectively, from national data (Axtell, Asire, & Meyers, 1976). These study group characteristics may be due in part to the research sites—university medical centers or a regional cancer center—for all of the investigations except one (Christensen, 1983).

The majority of the studies began during the diagnostic or immediate posttreatment period. Outcome was assessed by a variety of strategies; however, the domains that could be changed through the intervention included self-reports of emotional distress (e.g., POMS, BDI, STAI), coping, and target areas of vulnerability (e.g., sexuality or marital adjustment for women with breast or gynecologic cancer). Other life areas that might be less likely to be affected (e.g., employment status, self-esteem) yielded mixed results. The descriptive data and the quasi-experimental designs confirm the hypothesized profile of low psychosocial morbidity. The rapid emotional rebound that occurs without intervention may have contributed to the findings of no differential outcome (Capone, Good, Westie, & Jacobsen, 1980; Davis, 1986; Houts et al. 1986) or only modest improvement (Christensen, 1983; Edgar, Rosberger, & Nowlis, 1992; Fawzy, Cousins, et al., 1990) in emotional distress. Despite this, longer term follow-up data suggested some consolidation of intervention effects across time (upward of 6 months posttreatment), with lowered emotional distress or enhanced coping (Fawzy, Cousins, et al., 1990) coupled with confirming biologic outcomes (Davis, 1986; Fawzy, Kemeny, et al., 1990). Multiple posttreatment assessments (e.g., 3, 6, and 12 months posttreatment in Capone et al., 1980) provide an estimate of the reliability of these effects for a particular study. If long-term outcomes are replicable, they are made more impressive by their achievement with very brief therapy (e.g., 10 therapy hours). Unfortunately, no clear statements can be made regarding the types of therapists who can achieve these gains, as their training ranged from bachelors to doctoral level with several disciplines (e.g., psychology, psychiatry, nursing, social work) represented.

Moderate Morbidity Risk

Overview of Descriptive Findings

Psychosocial adjustment is variable for individuals with regional disease. Such were the outcomes in retrospective (Cella & Tross, 1986) and longitudinal (Devlen, Maguire, Phillips, Crowther, & Chambers, 1987) studies of Hodgkin's disease and non-Hodgkin's lymphoma patients. Studies of cancer patients receiving adjuvant therapy or single-, double-, or triple-agent chemotherapy report higher levels of affective distress while on therapy than those receiving no treatment or time-limited treatment such as radiotherapy (Hughson, Cooper, McArdle, & Smith, 1986; Meyerowitz, Watkins, & Sparks, 1983). Also, the extensive literature on aversive reactions to chemotherapy (see Carey & Burish, 1988, for a review) documents the difficult experience of those undergoing cancer treatment for regional disease.

Intervention Investigations

The single quasi-experimental design with moderate morbidity risk patients was conducted by Heinrich and Coscarelli-Schag (1985) using stress and activity management, cancer education, relaxation training, cognitive therapy and adaptive coping, and activity management. Fifty-one patients, 26 intervention and 25 control, completed several outcome measures, including ones for emotional distress (Symptom Checklist–90 [SCL-90]; Derogatis, 1977), cancer information, psychosocial adjustment to illness, the Karnofsky Performance Status Scale (Karnofsky & Burchenal, 1949), reports of daily activities, and self-report ratings of satisfaction with care and quality of life. Data were collected pre- and posttreatment and with a 2-month telephone follow-up. Concerning cancer information, all patients significantly improved with time, but the intervention subjects evidenced differential gains. Regarding emotional distress, psychosocial adjustment, and daily activities, all patients improved with time, but no differential improvement was found. There was no evidence for lowered levels of distress for the spouses across time or with the intervention.

Five diverse experimental investigations have been conducted. In the majority, patients continued in their treatment, chemo- or radiotherapy, during the psychological intervention. Jacobs, Ross, Walker, and Stockdale (1983) conducted two studies, one examining patient education and the other group support, for adults with Hodgkin's disease. One hundred five adults participated who were receiving or had recently completed chemotherapy. A single outcome, an experimenter-derived measure of distress, social adjustment, and life satisfaction, was administered pre- and posttreatment. A knowledge test of Hodgkin's disease was also used for the education study. Subjects were randomized to one of four groups: education intervention (n = 21), education control (n = 26), support intervention (n = 16), or support control (n = 18). In the education study, the intervention consisted of provision of a booklet about the disease/treatment and mailings of brief newspapers about advances in treatment. Analyses indicated that educational intervention subjects significantly improved on the measure of Hodgkin's disease knowledge. Significant improvement was also found on 2 (lower anxiety and fewer treatment problems) of the 14 adjustment scales. In the peer support study, analyses indicated positive psychosocial gains across time but no differential improvement for the intervention patients.

Several articles by Maguire and colleagues (Maguire, Brooke, Tait, Thomas, & Sellwood, 1983; Maguire, Hopwood, Tarrier, & Howell, 1985; Maguire, Tait, Brooke, Thomas, & Sellwood, 1980) have described the outcomes following individual counseling for women treated with mastectomy. A nurse specialist provided an intervention in the hospital presurgery and in the patient's home every 2 months until "it was clear that the patient had adapted well." The intent was to restore mobility to the affected arm through movement exercises, to facilitate adjustment to the scar and breast loss by disclosing feelings, and to encourage to return to social activities and employment. One hundred fifty-two women, 75 intervention and 77 no-treatment control, participated. Outcome measures were experimenter-derived and assessed physical rehabilitation outcomes (e.g., arm swelling, pain) and nurse judgments about social adjustment, return to work, marital adjustment, emotional distress, and sexual functioning, at 3 months and 12–18 months posttreatment. Physical outcomes appeared to be better for the counseled women, with fewer reporting problems with swelling or pain. Psychological responses to breast loss were judged to be better for the counseled women (68% vs. 52% had adapted "well"). Also, counseled women reported fewer difficulties with their social relationships and when returning to housework or employment. There were significantly more episodes and more severe episodes of anxiety or depression (e.g., 3% vs. 19% of the intervention and control groups, respectively, had "moderately severe" bouts of anxiety at 12–18 months). Finally, marital and sexual adjustment was also better for the counseled women. Only 7% of the experimental but 15% of the control marriages were "strained" by the illness and treatment, and by 12–18 months 8% of the experimental but 31% of the control women still reported sexual difficulties.

Cain, Kohorn, Quinlan, Latimer, and Schwartz (1986) compared individual and group therapy formats for a structured intervention for women with gynecologic cancer. The intervention had eight components including discussion of the causes of cancer at diagnosis, impact of the treatment(s) on body image and sexuality, relaxation training, emphasis on good dietary and exercise patterns, communication difficulties with medical staff and friends/family, and setting goals for the future to cope with uncertainty and fears of recurrence. Seventy-two women (21 individual intervention, 22 group intervention, and 29 no-treatment control) participated. Outcome measures were standardized and included depression and anxiety interviewer rating scales and a psychosocial adjustment to illness scale, which were administered pre- and posttreatment and at a 6-month follow-up. Posttreatment analyses indicated all groups improved with time; however, interviewer rated anxiety was significantly lower for the individual therapy subjects only. Gains were more impressive with the 6-month follow-up data. There were no differences between the intervention formats, but both groups reported less depression and anxiety and better psychosocial adjustment (including health perspectives, sexual functioning, and use of leisure time) than the no-treatment control group.

Forester, Kornfeld, and Fleiss (1985) provided individual psychotherapy to cancer patients during radiotherapy. Unlike many other structured interventions, individual psychotherapy sessions were offered to discuss "whatever the patient wished." Sessions included supportive therapy with "educational, interpretive, and cathartic components" (p. 23). One hundred patients (48 intervention and 52 no-treatment control) completed the study. A standardized interview (modified Schedule for Affective Disorders and Schizophrenia [SADS]; Endicott & Spitzer, 1978) was administered pretreatment, mid-radiotherapy (3 weeks), end of radiotherapy (6 weeks), postintervention, and at 1- and 2-month follow-ups. Using simple totals of SADS emotional distress symptoms, analyses indicated all groups improved with time, but the psychotherapy patients improved differentially through the 2-month follow-up. Simple totals of SADS physical symptom items—anorexia, fatigue, and nausea/vomiting—indicated significantly lower levels across all symptoms for the intervention group at the 1-month follow-up only.

Telch and Telch (1986) compared the effectiveness of coping skills instruction with supportive therapy offered in groups for cancer patients receiving routine follow-up care. A novel aspect is that potential participants were screened using an experimenter-derived structured interview, and only those with "clear evidence of psychological distress" (p. 803) were eligible. The intervention taught cognitive, behavioral, and affective coping strategies and included homework assignments, goal setting, self-monitoring, and role playing. Relaxation training and stress management skills were also included, and patients were asked to provide ratings of home practice. The group support intervention provided an environment for patients to discuss feelings, concerns, and problems, with no specific agenda or plan for at-home activities. Forty-one cancer patients (13 coping skills group, 14 group support, and 14 no-treatment control) completed the study. Posttreatment outcome measures were the POMS, the Cancer Inventory of Problem Situations (Heinrich, Coscarelli-Schag, & Ganz, 1984), and an experimenter-derived self-efficacy scale. Despite randomization, pretreatment analyses indicated that subjects in the coping skills intervention reported significantly more distress on the POMS and lower levels of coping efficacy, and analysis of covariance was used. Analyses for the POMS indicated that the coping skills group improved significantly across all scales, the group support group improved on the anxiety and depression scales only, but the no-treatment control worsened. The same pattern was found with the other measures. Also, the coping skills patients were rated as being significantly less distressed on both therapist and independent observer ratings than support group and no-treatment control patients, whose ratings did not differ. Despite the differential improvement of the intervention groups, patient ratings of treatment credibility indicated no difference between the groups in their satisfaction with therapy content or the therapists.

Methodology Summary

The elevated-risk profile for these patients is evident by the significant distress at study entry even though many had been diagnosed months previously. One source of distress is continued involvement in treatment, as subjects from half of the studies were still receiving radiotherapy or chemotherapy (Heinrich & Coscarelli-Schag, 1985; Jacobs et al., 1983; Forester, Kornfeld, & Fleiss, 1985). Participants were more representative on disease and sociodemographic variables. Three studies included a variety of cancer sites (Heinrich & Coscarelli-Schag, 1985; Forester et al., 1985; Telch & Telch, 1986) or a previously unstudied site (i.e., Hodgkins disease; Jacobs et al., 1983). Three studies included equal numbers or a predominance of men (Heinrich & Coscarelli-Schag, 1985; Jacobs et al., 1983; Forester et al., 1985), and the age means for some were more representative (e.g., 59 years for the gynecologic sample in Cain et al., 1986). However, it is likely that the study samples remained largely White, as all but one study (Heinrich & Coscarelli-Schag, 1985) failed to even report racial data. As for the studies with low-risk patients, all the investigations were conducted at university medical centers (or a Veterans Administration affiliate).

A wider variety of outcome measures detected improvement. Intervention effects were found reliably with self-reports of emotional distress and with modified versions of diagnostic interviews (SADS) or interviewer rated distress (Hamilton Rating for Depression). Unlike the weak effects at posttreatment for low-risk interventions subjects, more impressive posttreatment gains were found initially (excepting Heinrich and Coscarelli-Schag, 1985, and the group support intervention in Jacobs et al., 1983), and the effects appeared stronger with follow-up (Cain et al., 1986; Forester et al., 1985; Maguire et al., 1983), which extended as long as 12 months posttreatment. Interventions with an informational component improved patients' knowledge about their disease and treatment(s) and could be detected with experimenter-derived measures. Outcomes in other areas, such as listings of common concerns or activities of daily living, were more difficult to detect. Despite their relevance, there was only modest measurement of disease or treatment symptomatology, but some interventions did appear to lower symptom levels either directly (e.g., Maguire et al., 1983) or indirectly (e.g., Forester et al., 1985). As with the low-risk studies, brief interventions were offered by a diversity of professionals. Notably, two studies provided important data on treatment credibility and satisfaction with the therapists (Heinrich & Coscarelli-Schag, 1985; Telch & Telch, 1986).

High Morbidity Risk

Overview and Descriptive Findings

Individuals with systemic or rapidly progressing disease (e.g., pancreatic cancer) confront a life time line of months, as survival for the next year is possible but unlikely (e.g., 1-year rates for metastatic lung, breast, pancreatic, and liver cancers are 39%, 44%, 17%, and 32%, respectively; Axtell, Asire, & Meyers, 1976). This situation is devastating, and the magnitude of distress with recurrence eclipses that found with the initial diagnosis (Thompson, Andersen, & DePetrillo, 1992). Studies that have contrasted cancer patients showing no evidence of disease (i.e., low risk) and those receiving palliative treatment (i.e., moderate risk; Cassileth et al., 1985) have reported the greatest distress for those with disseminated disease (i.e., high risk; Bloom, 1987). In addition, there is often increasing physical debilitation or difficult-to-manage symptoms, such as pain.

Intervention Investigations

Despite the challenges in conducting research with this population, six experimental studies have been conducted. Ferlic, Goldman, and Kennedy (1979) published the first randomized intervention study, an interdisciplinary crisis intervention program that included patient education, presentations by medical team members, and supportive group therapy. Sixty adults, 30 intervention and 30 no-treatment control, with "advanced" cancer participated. Outcome measures were experimenter-derived and assessed hospital adjustment, communication with others, disease information, death perceptions, and self-concept. Analyses indicated the intervention group improved across all areas, whereas the controls improved in three—relationship strength, cancer information, and death perceptions—following the 2-week intervention. The self-concept score for the intervention group significantly increased, whereas that for the control group significantly decreased. A 6-month follow-up was attempted; however, there was significant mortality (18%) and insufficient questionnaire returns (55%).

As noted in the introduction, several papers have described the group support intervention of Spiegel, Bloom, and colleagues (Spiegel et al., 1981; Spiegel & Bloom, 1983) for women with breast cancer. Women were randomized to no treatment or a group treatment intervention that included discussion of death and dying, family problems, communication problems with physicians, and living fully in the context of a terminal illness. The intervention subjects were also randomized a second time to two conditions: (a) no additional treatment or (b) self-hypnosis for pain problems (Spiegel & Bloom, 1983), which was incorporated into the weekly intervention. At the end of the first year the groups formally ended, but members could continue to meet as they wished or were able; some groups lasted for an additional 2 years. Eighty-six women, 50 intervention and 36 no-treatment control, participated. Following random assignment, there was subject loss (e.g., refusal, too weak, death) with the study beginning with 34 intervention and 24 control participants; however, the survival data is reported for the original sample of 86. Outcome measures were the Health Locus of Control Scale, the POMS, a phobia checklist, a self-esteem measure, and experimenter-derived measures of maladaptive coping and denial, and they were administered pretreatment and at 4, 8, and 12 months during the intervention/control year. In analyzing the treatment outcome data, slopes analysis was used to maximize the use of the data collected, as only 52% of the subjects completed all assessments. Analyses indicated that the intervention group reported significantly fewer phobic responses and lower anxiety, fatigue, and confusion and higher vigor on the POMS than did the control subjects. These differences were evident at all assessments, but the magnitude increased from 4 to 12 months. There was also a significant decrease in the use of maladaptive coping responses by the intervention group. There were no significant differences on the remaining measures. Regarding the findings from the hypnosis substudy, women receiving hypnosis within the group support intervention reported no change in their pain sensations during the year, whereas pain sensations significantly increased for the other women in group support who did not receive hypnosis. Similar findings were reported for pain suffering—a slight decrease for the women who also received hypnosis and a significant increase in suffering for the remaining intervention women. It is important to note that pain sensation scores for both groups were, however, significantly lower than those for the no-intervention control subjects, suggesting that the hypnosis component provided an additive analgesic effect to other group treatment components. Using the Cox proportional hazards model (Spiegel et al., 1989), a striking difference of 18.9 months for the control subjects and 36.6 months for the intervention subjects was found from study entry until death. Follow-up analyses, controlling for initial disease stage, days of irradiation, or use of androgen or steroid treatments all indicated the same substantial survival differences.

The remaining four investigations included primarily lung cancer patients. The most psychological study was that of Linn, Linn, and Harris (1982). A supportive death-and-dying intervention program was offered to reduce denial but maintain hope, to increase environmental control, to continue meaningful activities, and to foster self-esteem and life satisfaction. In addition, the therapist was often with the intervention subject at death. One hundred twenty men were randomized to intervention ($n = 62$) or no-treatment control ($n = 58$) groups. Standardized outcome measures included emotional distress (depression scale from the POMS), self-esteem, life satisfaction, social isolation, and locus of control scale. Nurses rated functional status for daily activities, and a physician rated body system impairment. Measures were administered pretreatment and 1, 3, 6, 9, and 12 months later. There were no significant differences between the groups at the 1-month assessment, but significant differences in favor of the intervention emerged by 3 months and remained for the majority of the measures. Differences included lower POMS depression score at 3 months, higher life satisfaction, higher self-esteem, lower alienation from 3 to 12 months, and a more internal locus of control for the 9- and 12-month assessments. The results for the lung and other site samples were similar. Despite the more favorable psychological outcomes for the intervention subjects, there were no functional status, body system impairment, or treatment compliance (e.g., rehospitalization, complications) differences between the groups. By the 6-month assessment, 58% of the sample had died. Survival analyses showed no significant differences between groups.

Two investigations incorporating psychological techniques in the context of specialized nursing care for terminal patients provide relevant data. The no-treatment control condition for both investigations consisted of routine outpatient visits for monitoring medical and psychosocial difficulties. The first study was conducted by Yates, McKegney, and Kun (1981) and compared standard follow-up with monthly home visits by a nurse practitioner providing nursing, pain management, and nutritional services. One hundred ninety-nine patients were randomized to intervention ($n = 98$) or no-treatment control ($n = 101$) groups. Outcome measures were modest and included a visual analog pain rating, a self-report measure of life satisfaction, and the Karnofsky Performance Status Scale (Karnofsky & Burchenal, 1949). Measures were administered pretreatment and with monthly evaluations by a social worker or, during the latter years of the study, by independent evaluators because it appeared that the social workers began to provide psychosocial interventions despite prohibitions. Few significant differences between the groups were found, with the most notable finding being the stabilization of pain for the home care group with increasing pain for the routine care group. Although the economic costs of the intervention were demonstrated (i.e., more of the home care patients died at home, resulting in lower overall costs), there was no survival advantage for the home care group.

The second nursing intervention was conducted by McCorkle and colleagues (1989) and compared standard office care with two types of specialized home care: visits by a member of an interdisciplinary team and visits by an oncology nurse practitioner. One hundred sixty-six patients with lung cancer were randomized. Standardized outcome measures assessed mood (POMS), current adjustment concerns, need for assistance, and pain, other symptoms, and general health, and were administered pretreatment and every 6 weeks for 6 months. The majority of the subjects died before completion of the study; data analyses are reported only for the 78 subjects (47% of the total) with complete follow-up data. There were no significant pretreatment differences in the areas of mood, current concerns, or pain reports; but despite randomization, there were significant pretreatment differences between groups (better adjustment for the oncology home care group) for the remaining measures, and covariance analyses were used. Analyses indicated significant differences between the specialized home and standard office care models but no differences between the two home care variants. All patients became more debilitated with time, as indicated by increased distress with symptoms, increased dependency, and more negative health perceptions; however, these responses stabilized for the specialized home care groups before increasing to the range of those for the office care group at the final assessment. The only significant finding differentiating the two specialized programs was a trend for rehospitalization stays to be shorter (e.g., 50 vs. 76 days) for the patients visited by the oncology nurse.

Methodology Summary

Among the methodologic challenges, subject loss (usually from death) is salient, as it may even occur during the time from recruitment to study initiation. Researchers typically compare the initial participants and the "completers" (e.g., Spiegel et al., 1989), and no systematic bias is usually detected. However, if psychological variables are related to survival, then patients surviving longer may be "hardier" on some psychosocial dimension that may interact with treatment involvement. When conducting analyses across time, some investigators have chosen a slopes analysis to maximize the number of data points available for each subject (Spiegel et al., 1981). A less satisfactory solution is to eliminate subjects with incomplete data, as this results in a substantial reduction of statistical power (e.g., McCorkle et al., 1989) and increases the cost of already expensive studies.

Despite these problems with subject mortality, the study participants have been generally representative of adults with advanced or progressive cancer. The study that provided few sociodemographic data but described the patients as having "advanced" disease had the youngest study sample (mean age of 48 years; Ferlic et al., 1979), whereas the mean ages for the remaining studies ranged from 54 to 65 years. With the exception of the breast study by Spiegel and colleagues (1989), the remaining study samples were at least 50% male, with the Linn study including all men. Studies also included a variety of disease sites. Unfortunately, non-Whites remained underrepresented, with only 11–12% of the samples being Black in the two studies providing data (Linn et al., 1982; McCorkle et al., 1989). Like all other studies, patients were recruited from university or university-affiliated facilities, with the exception of the participants in the McCorkle et al. (1989) study, who came from several city hospitals.

The positive outcomes for high-risk cancer patients are notable considering their worsening pain and/or increasing debilitation as they approach death. Measures of emotional distress have been found to be sensitive to posttreatment improvements as well as gains with follow-up. In addition, change in other areas—self-esteem/concept, death perceptions, life satisfaction, and locus of control—were more often found (e.g., Ferlic et al., 1979; Linn et al., 1982); these effects were not detected in studies with low-risk patients. Important for quality of life, psychological interventions could also lower or stabilize pain reports (Spiegel & Bloom, 1983). Finally, it is important to note that the only study in this group that offered brief intervention (9 hr of total therapy time) was Ferlic et al. (1979), whereas the remainder were "several sessions," "until death," or at least 75 hr. Again, a diversity of professionals provided the interventions; however, the two studies with the weakest outcome had most psychological components provided by nurse specialists (McCorkle et al., 1989; Yates et al., 1981).

Intervention Effectiveness: Components and Mechanisms

Psychological interventions with cancer patients have addressed three phases in the disease time line: diagnosis/pretreatment, immediately posttreatment or during extended treatment (such as radiotherapy or chemotherapy), and disseminated disease or death. Typically, interventions were designed to address only the adjustment difficulties of a specific phase and were usually so time-limited that little overlap was possible. Although not a perfect correspondence, there has been a "matching" between the interventions for specific phases and the risk groups studied. That is, the majority of the study participants in the diagnostic/pretreatment studies included low-risk patients, studies of coping with treatment included moderate-risk, and, not surprising, studies of adjustment to disseminated disease or coping with death included high-risk patients. Although there appear to be unique intervention components for different phases, there are some commonalities.

Studies with newly diagnosed cancer patients have focused on the trauma of learning one has a potentially life-threatening illness. Despite some improvement in cancer prognoses in the last 30 years (e.g., there has been a 70% decline in cervix death rates and a 33% decline in liver death rates; American Cancer Society, 1992), Weisman and Worden's (1976–1977) label of *existential plight* remains descriptive of the emotional, cognitive, and behavioral turmoil. Both descriptive and intervention study data suggest a psychotherapeutic model of crisis intervention or brief therapy as the "best fit." Both are similar in terms of their rapid early assessment, present-day focus, limited goals, therapist direction, and prompt interventions (Kolotkin & Johnson, 1983). When applied in the context of cancer, therapy components have included an *emotionally supportive context* to address fears and anxieties about the disease (e.g., Cain et al., 1986; Capone et al., 1980; Forester et al., 1985; Maguire et al., 1983), *information about the disease and treatment* (e.g., Cain et al., 1986; Fawzy, Cousins, et al., 1990; Fawzy, Kemeny, et al., 1990; Houts et al., 1986; Jacobs et al., 1983; Maguire et al., 1983), *behavioral coping strategies* (e.g., role playing difficult discussions with family or the medical staff; Fawzy, Cousins, et al., 1990; Fawzy, Kemeny, et al., 1990; Houts, Whitney, Mortel, & Bartholomew, 1986), *cognitive coping strategies* (Cain, Kohorn, Quinlan, Latimer, & Schwartz, 1986; Davis, 1986; Houts et al., 1986; Telch & Telch, 1986), and *relaxation training* to lower "arousal" and/or enhance one's sense of control (Davis, 1986; Edgar, Rosberger, & Nowlis, 1992; Fawzy, Cousins, et al., 1990; Fawzy, Kemeny, et al., 1990). Also, *focused interventions* incorporating the above components for areas of increased morbidity for selected disease groups (e.g., sexual functioning for women treated for gynecologic or breast cancer; fertility loss for men treated for testicular cancer) have been included.

The multiple studies using some or all of these components have provided conceptual replications of their effectiveness. These positive outcomes can also be contrasted with null findings for (group) interventions that included *no structured content*. Reliance on group support alone may be insufficient to produce any measurable benefit (Jacobs et al., 1983; Telch & Telch, 1986).[2] Other data also provide clarifying information. The components appear to be more important than procedural variations. For example, therapy format appears to have a lesser impact, as these components have yielded favorable outcome whether delivered individually or in groups (e.g., Davis, 1986; Fawzy, Cousins et al., 1990; and Fawzy, Kemeny et al., 1990, for low risk; Maguire et al., 1980, and Forester et al., 1985, for moderate risk), and same-study contrasts of individual and group formats yielded equivalent improvement (Cain et al., 1986). Involvement of significant others may have some positive effects, but their participation appears to be unnecessary to achieve gains for the cancer patients. (As an aside, direct benefit for a spouse may be minimal [e.g., Heinrich & Coscarelli-Schag, 1985] unless the focus of treatment is on a mutually important issue, such as sexual problems [Christensen, 1983].) Finally, when distress is declining across time during recovery, as it does for low- and some moderate-risk individuals, it is unclear whether delivery of intervention "late" in the process rather than "early" is beneficial.

What are the mechanisms for intervention effectiveness when delivered during the diagnostic, treatment, or early recovery periods? In large measure, the psychologic mechanisms may not be significantly different from those for coping with other stressors. That is, learning more about a stressor, confronting it with positive cognitive states, active behavioral strategies, and, eventually, reduced emotional distress may provide realistic appraisals of current or impending stresses of the disease or treatment process and enhance one's sense of self-efficacy or feelings of control *early* in the adjustment process.

That the interventions produce more than situational improvement and may alter an individual's longer term psychologic/behavioral adjustment is suggested by the gains continuing (and often increasing) during the first posttreatment year (e.g., Cain et al., 1986; Forester et al., 1985), even when the therapy has been brief (e.g., 10 hr total). Also, long-term outcomes may be more easily achieved with the extended

---

[2]Some might consider the group-support-only condition in these studies as a conceptual approximation to a placebo condition. As such, the importance of the specific components is further highlighted.

interventions. Regardless of the length of the intervention, the continuation of active behavioral coping, positive cognitions, and so forth, may be the type of necessary conditions to enable *late* mechanisms, psychologic/behavioral, or biologic, to emerge. For example, a behavioral mechanism hypothesized for the Spiegel et al. (1989) results is that direct effects of the intervention (lower levels of emotional distress and maladaptive coping as well as containment of pain symptom levels) increase the likelihood and success of subsequent adaptive health behaviors (e.g., complying with medical therapy; improving diet, exercise), which may have, in turn, influenced the disease process.

The oft proposed biologic mechanism for findings such as Spiegel et al.'s (1989) is immune system enhancement. Evidence for its plausibility comes from two lines of data. First, some of the specific components highlighted above have been used singly with health subjects and positive immune system changes have been found. So it is not inconceivable that similar immune system enhancement might occur for cancer patients if the system is not overburdened/compromised from the disease or treatment. Specifically, relaxation with medical students before exams (Kiecolt-Glaser et al., 1984) and older adults in retirement facilities (Kiecolt-Glaser et al., 1985) has produced higher helper T-lymphocyte percentages and higher NK cell activity, respectively. Experimental study of self-disclosure of earlier traumatic experiences from healthy undergraduates found a higher mitogen response in disclosers and, furthermore, a better lymphocyte proliferative response for first-time disclosers (Pennebaker, Kiecolt-Glaser, & Glaser, 1988). Although there may be notable differences between disclosure of earlier traumas and active participation in a psychologic intervention, the magnitude of crisis reactions generated by a cancer diagnosis (or the circumstance of facing a rapidly approaching death) may increase their similarities. Second, the most relevant supporting data are those of Fawzy, Cousins, et al. (1990) and Fawzy, Kemeny, et al. (1990; see above), who used the intervention components with melanoma patients and found significant and positive immunologic changes. Also, the majority of these changes did not occur until 6 months, a time line consistent with the possibility that longer term behavioral/psychologic processes may be needed to effect immunologic change in a sample with disease.

In addition to the intervention components noted above, other ones (and, correspondingly, other mechanisms) may be operative for high-risk patients. Whereas many cancer patients at low or moderate risk for adjustment difficulties may improve without intervention, high-risk no-intervention patients worsen (McCorkle et al., 1989; Spiegel & Bloom, 1983). The reasons for this more difficult trajectory may include the existential distress that comes with cancer diagnosis in addition to the more difficult *confirmation* of a shortened life span, increased numbers and less controllable symptoms of disseminated disease or more toxic therapies, and a worsening of the latter difficulties with time.

Intervention for high-risk patients had many of the same components as those for low- or moderate-risk groups, but the more difficult circumstances appeared to shift content to specific death or quality of life issues. For example, coping with one's own (or a group member's) death or decisions of no treatment versus a toxic regimen became therapy tasks (Cassileth & Cassileth, 1983; Spiegel & Glafkedes, 1983). Other interventions focused on coping with debilitation or behavioral control of pain (Spiegel & Bloom, 1983). The psychologic mechanisms underlying the effectiveness of these therapy components may be as described above—enhanced self-efficacy, control, and realistic appraisals. However, additional ones may occur because one's worst fears of cancer (e.g., intolerable symptoms, physical debilitation and dependency, and dying) are often realized. Unavoidable circumstances of this sort may make the maintenance of self-efficacy or feelings of control fleeting. What other factors might then contribute to improved outcome for high-risk patients? One possibility is the benefit that accrues from the provision of social support by a therapist.

Interventions for high-risk patients were demanding. Studies noted that therapists needed to be comfortable with difficult topics and circumstances, such as bedside counseling (see Linn et al., 1982, or Spiegel & Yalom, 1978, for discussions). As patients must cope, these therapists do so as they maintain relationships with those about to die. Variables historically viewed as the critical ones for therapist effects in psychotherapy process and outcome research—empathy, warmth, and genuineness (Parloff, Waskow, & Wolfe, 1978)—may take on added significance in the context of cancer. Although there are many therapist variables that may be important, these have been universally accepted by all psychotherapy persuasions (Beutler, Crago, & Arizmendi, 1986). They may be pivotal for cancer patients who are confronting life and death issues when they feel least able or when significant others are unable to do so. When group therapies "work," the role of the therapist (and these qualities) shift to the group participants (Yalom, 1975). The hypothesis for the importance of therapeutic relationships is consistent with epidemiologic data suggesting that another significant other—a spouse—may provide social support for the survival advantage of marrieds with cancer (Goodwin, Hunt, Key, & Samet, 1987) or other illnesses (e.g., Berkman & Syme, 1979; House, Robbins, & Metzner, 1982).

It is unlikely that the qualities of therapeutic empathy, warmth, and genuineness evolve quickly when they are separate from an ongoing social relationship such as a marriage. The most demanding interventions were the individual support of Linn (Linn et al., 1982) and the group support of Spiegel, Bloom, and Yalom (1981); in fact, these interventions were so different (e.g., at least 75 *hours* in Spiegel) that they might best be considered in their own context. This magnitude of intervention is 6–7 times that of any other. Intervention for the Linn subjects may not have been as long, in part because the lung cancer participants died more rapidly. Despite potentially similar intensities of intervention, the remarkable survival advantage found by Spiegel was not replicated by Linn. Aside from the many methodology differences of the studies, one disease factor accounting for the discrepancy might be the shorter survival "window" for metastatic lung cancer patients in contrast to metastatic breast cancer patients. (Five-year survival rates are 14% and 72%, respectively, for initial Stage III disease and 2% and 19%, respectively, for initial Stage IV disease [Boring, Squires, & Tong, 1992].) That is, if "psychological factors" such as those accruing from long-term improvements in adjustment, continued gains from long-term therapy participation, or a significant therapeutic relationship influence survival through changes in health behaviors and/or immune system enhancement, the differences may be detected only when the "dose" of the factor is sufficient and when the disease provides a reasonable time interval for the factor to contribute.

Future Directions

Although intervention research with medically ill individuals is often not construed as psychotherapy outcome research, the same domains—patients; therapist and treatments; assessment strategy, outcome criteria, and tactical selection of research designs—are relevant. In addition, the important role of disease/treatment variables as moderators for outcome require description and control. All of these variables have been considered in the above review; I turn next to their consideration for future research directions.

Patient Variables

Attention to three classes of variables—sociodemographics, premorbid status, and individual differences—of study subjects is needed. For all, description is essential, and "manipulation" as factors in a design would move the field forward. First, we begin with sociodemographic variables—age, race, gender, education, and income —as their importance is usually ignored despite their *general role* as potential mediators for health-promoting or health-damaging behaviors (Matthews, 1989). Specifically for cancer, a clear relationship to disease risk has been found with *age*, with a consistent increase in the incidence rates across races, sexes,and cancer sites. Furthermore, there are disproportionate death rates for the elderly: the largest cancer burden is borne by those 55 years and older, and the increase is dramatic after age 65. Despite the latter, when emotional distress from cancer is considered, age is negatively correlated with distress such that "younger" patients are more distressed than "older." (Vinokur et al., 1989, contrasted women age 64 or less with those over 65 years who had been treated for breast cancer; Cassileth et al., 1984, found similar age-related adjustment patterns in six chronic illness groups.) Also, if individuals become physically impaired from the disease, younger patients experience significantly greater deterioration in their mental health and well-being than similarly impaired older patients (Vinokur, Threatt, Vinokur-Kaplan, & Satariano, in press). To summarize, although the majority of cancer patients will be "older," "younger" patients are at greater risk for adjustment difficulties. The studies reviewed seldom considered whether or not the sample was nationally representative, and, furthermore, "younger" cancer patients (who may be at "higher" risk for psychological distress) were disproportionately sampled.

There are epidemiologic data on cancer risk for the remaining sociodemographic factors, but there are few supporting psychologic data. Considering *race*, when Blacks and Whites are compared, Blacks have a greater incidence than Whites across the majority of cancer sites (exceptions include bladder cancer, breast cancer in women over 40 years, colon, lung, and ovary for women; Christensen & Baquet, in press). Current incidence rates for Hispanics are not representative (e.g., data from Hispanics in the Southwest are available, but they underestimate the rates for Puerto Ricans and Cubans); similar problems exist for the database on Native Americans, a situation compounded by their heterogeneity (tribal differences). Considering mortality, Blacks have the highest mortality rate (211.0) and lowest all-site survival rate (37.8) compared with Whites (166.2 and 50.3, respectively). In summary, Blacks have a disproportionate cancer burden, and that for Hispanics and Native Americans is negative but less clear. Despite this racial distribution of the disease, there are few descriptive data on the psychosocial responses of non-Whites; few non-Whites have participated in the intervention investigations, and efforts to remedy these situations are recent (e.g., Bal, 1992; Freeman, 1989). The psychosocial responses to cancer of Blacks or other minorities may not be identical to that of Whites; if they are dissimilar, their potential risk for adjustment difficulties may be increased because the health care system (including psychologists armed with interventions) may be less attuned to their needs.

For *socioeconomic status* (SES), the proxy measures of family income and educational level might be used. There is a relationship between both variables and age-adjusted cancer incidence and survival. The discouraging cancer results for some racial groups, Blacks in particular, appear to be due in large part to SES (Baquet, Horm, Gibbs, & Greenwald, 1991) and are likely to be the health consequences that befall the nations' poor (Freeman, 1989). Thus, examining the psychologic responses of various socioeconomic groups necessitates consideration of the circumstances that may arise from a lack of education, unemployment, substandard housing, poor nutrition, risk-promoting life-style and behavior, diminished access to health care, and others—all variables to consider in the context of one more stressor, cancer.

Within the rubric of *premorbid status, both physical and mental health* are considered. Existing health conditions (with their corresponding treatments) often limit the cancer treatments that can be offered as well as their efficacy. In addition, some chronic conditions serve as risk factors for cancer (e.g., obesity is a risk-factor for endometrial cancer; alcohol consumption is linked to cirrhosis, and cirrhosis is linked to liver cancer). Regardless of the linkage, comorbidity will result in greater decrements in social and role functioning, mental health, and health perceptions (Stewart et al., 1989). Psychiatric history, particularly depressive disorders, places an individual at increased risk for depression following cancer diagnosis (i.e., beyond the 6% base rate for depression in the healthy population). Thus, the presence of previous physical *or* mental health conditions may increase risk for adjustment difficulties following cancer and may interact with the efficacy of interventions. This conclusion is consistent with survey data indicating that the effects of depressive symptoms *and* chronic medical conditions (e.g., hypertension, diabetes, arthritis, gastrointestinal disorder) on functioning are additive, resulting in twice the reduction in social adjustment and physical functioning as either condition alone (Wells et al., 1989). Of all the studies reviewed, few noted any strategy for dealing with either of these issues in the context of subject recruitment. If these factors are allowed to vary and positive outcomes are found for an intervention, we have greater confidence in the robustness of the psychologic observations. However, variation rather than control may also make more difficult the clarification of biologic mechanisms.

This review serves as testimony for the generally positive effects of psychological interventions for cancer patients, and thus the literature would be moved forward with an examination of psychological/behavioral individual differences as a factor in research designs. Although there are potentially several relevant ones, three are highlighted.

1. Existing *social networks/support differences among patients* or *interventions that differ in the provision of social support* would provide important data. Future study will be assisted by the advances in the assessment of social support, but for adults a straightforward proxy variable may be marital status. Married persons live longer and have lower mortality for almost every major cause of death in comparison with single never married, separated, widowed, or divorced persons (Ortmeyer, 1974). More specifically, population-based studies of adults with cancer indicate that unmarrieds have a decreased overall survival because of initial presentations with

more advanced disease, a higher likelihood of being untreated for cancer, and, after adjustment for both factors, a poorer treatment response still remains for unmarrieds (Goodwin et al., 1987). Given the incidence rates for the disease, the unmarried group is also likely to be "older." What might be the mechanisms for such a risk status? The two most likely candidates are the benefits that accrue from the higher SES of marrieds (see discussion above) and social support. The importance of social support has been underscored in large community cohort studies that have controlled for income (e.g., Berkman & Syme, 1979; House et al., 1982). In addition to the role of social support as an individual difference variable, the discussion above and other authors (Broadhead & Kaplan, 1991; Taylor, Falke, Shoptaw, & Lichtman, 1986) have highlighted its potential contribution as a factor in moderating outcome along with other intervention components.

2. Consideration of the contribution of earlier (prediagnosis) or new *stresses* to intervention effectiveness would be important. Although there is no straightforward examination of this issue in the cancer literature, there is ample evidence for the moderating role of stress for both psychological and health outcomes. Convincing evidence for the importance of stress on an *illness endpoint* comes from Cohen, Tyrrell, and Smith (1991). Using a novel strategy to quantify "stress" (a composite index of negative life events, perceptions of one's coping capabilities, and negative affect), it related in a dose–response fashion to common cold infections, a pattern replicated across five cold viruses. Previous data have confirmed that acute (Kiecolt-Glaser et al., 1984) and chronic stressors (Kiecolt-Glaser et al., 1991) adversely affect health and immunity in otherwise healthy adults. Thus, we might hypothesize that the effects of ongoing or new stressors for cancer patients may adversely affect direct or indirect intervention outcomes or the psychological or biologic mechanisms.

3. Finally, study of psychological *individual differences* remains important. Although this suggestion is often made, it is more difficult to specify *which* differences, as both positive and negative findings exist for the majority of likely candidates. However, dimensions under current study with cancer groups that may hold promise include relatively stable coping processes (e.g., Charles Carver's study of optimism–pessimism; Scheier & Carver, in press) and positive affects (e.g., Levy, Lee, Bagley, & Lippman, 1988; but see Zonderman, Costa, & McCrae, 1989, for contrary data). Other studies that have highlighted adverse effects of negative emotions, specifically anger (either expression or control; e.g., Greer, Morris, & Pettingale, 1979; Derogatis, Abeloff, & Melisartos, 1979), might consider the broader construct of neuroticism as one possible basis for these findings.

Cancer Variables

This article begins by raising and attempting to dispel a "uniformity myth" in research with cancer patients and considers the "magnitude" of disease/treatment as an important factor in outcome. Although this view of the complexity of cancer and its treatment is not without problems (e.g., the direct effects of one aspect can be confounded by the other), the research summaries suggest the utility of such a classification at the present time. On the broadest levels, important medical decisions at diagnosis include the determination of site, stage of disease, and the histopathologic classification, including grading and cell type. Medical judgments about the disease and selection of treatment(s) consider these variables as well as many others, including the aggressiveness and predictability of the disease, the medical morbidity and mortality of the therapy, overall cure rate, and physician/institution experience in treating the disease (e.g., see Osteen, Steele, Menck, & Winchester, 1992, for an interesting example). Even when study samples having similar disease characteristics can be found, the subjects may still not receive similar therapies or may be more or less eligible for medical interventions to reduce psychological/behavioral risk. Obvious examples of the latter are the differential availability or selection of breast-preserving therapy or breast reconstruction and the control of disease or treatment symptomatology (e.g., control of nausea/vomiting from chemotherapy with antiemetic or behavioral pain control strategies.[3] Data have suggested that the availability of such interventions is risk reducing (e.g., examples of rehabilitative medical efforts include breast reconstruction, maxillofacial prosthetics for the head/neck patients, vaginal reconstruction for pelvic exenteration patients, or penile implants for men with prostate cancer), although they are not panaceas. Whereas some studies acknowledged the general importance of some of these variables in the form of stringent recruitment criteria (e.g., Fawzy, Cousins, et al., 1990; Fawzy, Kemeny, et al., 1990), the majority did not.

Future research must wrestle with this difficult issue. As a beginning, more comprehensive disease and treatment description of study participants is needed. Next, study of these variables as factors in a design using strategies such as those suggested here would provide data to identify risk groups at or shortly after the time of diagnosis, as even the most cost-effective interventions will not be available to or appropriate for all cancer patients.

Therapists and Therapeutic Techniques

Important for advancing the field is description, documentation, and testing mechanism(s) of the therapies studied. Few investigators publish supplementary clinical articles discussing aspects of the intervention (see Gordon et al., 1980, or Spiegel et al., 1981, for exceptions) or note that intervention manuals are available on request (see Fawzy, Cousins, et al., 1990, or Gordon et al., 1980, for exceptions). Only the Gordon study documented the content of the therapy sessions, total length per subject, and the interventions employed. With few exceptions, studies did not provide process measures of intervention components (see Telch and Telch, 1986, for their monitoring of homework assignments). Specification of the theoretical bases or the mechanisms by which interventions are to achieve their effectiveness would clarify the details of complex interventions, detail the conditions necessary for replication, and advance theory. Finally, it is suggested that "nonspecifics" require study as they may play an important role in moderating outcome in studies of high-risk patients.

---

[3]One group addressing this issue consists of investigators who are studying efforts to reduce symptoms of chemotherapy. Ratings of the emetogenic potential of the drugs have been used to predict outcome (Carey & Burish, 1988).

Assessment Strategies and Outcome Criteria

By definition, the intent of psychological intervention research is clinical improvement of distressing psychological states or behavior. Other intentions, such as making theoretical contributions or having indirect effects on other life areas, require additional outcome criteria and data collection. At a minimum, assessment for intervention studies in cancer may require familiarity with several nonoverlapping methodologies, including assessment of affective distress and psychopathology, "quality-of-life" measures, and relevant medical (i.e., biologic, disease, or treatment) endpoints, to note the obvious.

Considering the range of assessment measures, it appears that psychological interventions for cancer patients have been expected to provide "all things (outcomes) to all people." Beyond the direct impact on distressing states or behaviors, the outcome net has been cast widely (and perhaps wildly) to tap internal, stable patient characteristics (e.g., self-esteem), intimate relationships (e.g., marital adjustment), social relationships, major life areas (e.g., hours of employment), physical activity, disease and treatment-related symptoms, biologic responses (e.g., endocrine/immune variables), and finally disease endpoints. A number of perspectives have encouraged this diversity and complexity, including advocates of convergent operations, the advocates of divergent operations, the view that outcome research needs to document the mechanism (and more specifically, the biologic mechanism) of treatment efficacy, and the belief that casting a wide net is essential when knowledge is limited (e.g., see Ware, 1984, for an example). Whatever the rationale, this scenario might be balanced by other perspectives, such as the burden on patients, the economic cost of the research, and the appreciation that a single study need not address all issues.

The contributions of psychology to cancer research may be linked in part to the continued refinement of creative, feasible, and reliable/valid assessment methods. For example, this fact is made obvious by the accelerating attention to and press for quality-of-life assessment in clinical trials research (see Aaronson, 1989; Olschewski & Schumacher, 1990). It is important to note that significant progress has been made in the decade. Whereas early panels focused on assessment as the to-be-tackled problem (see American Cancer Society, 1984), recent panels have acknowledged the general success in the use of existing measures for many aspects of adjustment (e.g., see Burish, 1991a, 1991b; American Cancer Society, 1992).

A Final Comment on Impediments: Funding for Psychological Intervention Research With Cancer Patients

Complexities confronting the researcher studying psychological interventions for cancer patients were detailed. Other articles can provide discussions of many impediments, such as the training circumstances, for example, that have resulted in relatively few psychologists' having a primary focus on cancer (see Andersen et al., 1989, or Burish, 1991b). However, it is clear that the magnitude of clinical psychology's (or behavioral science's) contribution to addressing the cancer problem has been constricted by the lack of attention to and funding of this research by federal agencies. Even "modest" interventions are time- and labor-intensive undertakings made possible only with external funding. This reality, coupled with cancer as the number two cause of death of Americans, makes the level of previous research support disheartening. In addition, the data suggest that the funding for cancer rehabilitation research has worsened in the decade. For example, Ferlic et al. (1979) reported the first randomized psychological intervention study with cancer patients in 1979. Counting the 18 major investigations since then, only 16% of the studies were reported in the last 5 years. Although what is studied is driven by the quality of grant applications submitted, it is difficult to conceive that the *disciplines* of psychology, psychiatry, and nursing, for example, could not (or did not) submit more than 18 fundable intervention studies in the last 13 years. The thrust of this article is to underscore the meaningful differences psychological interventions can make for cancer patients, but I will end with the concern that their impact will be negligible without psychology also *advocating* for their importance to policy makers and funding agencies.

References

Aaronson, N. K. (1989). Quality of life assessment in clinical trials: Methodologic issues. *Controlled Clinical Trials, 10*, 195s–208s.

American Cancer Society. (1984). Proceedings of the working conference on methodology in behavioral and psychosocial cancer research—1983. *Cancer, 53*(Suppl. 10), 2217–2384.

American Cancer Society. (1992). *Cancer facts & figures: 1992.* Atlanta, GA: Author.

Andersen, B. L. (1989). Health psychology's contribution to addressing the cancer problem: Update on accomplishments. *Health Psychology, 8*, 683–703.

Andersen, B. L., Anderson, B., & deProsse, C. (1989a). Controlled prospective longitudinal study of women with cancer: I. Sexual functioning outcomes. *Journal of Consulting and Clinical Psychology, 57*, 683–691.

Andersen, B. L., Anderson, B., & deProsse, C. (1989b). Controlled prospective longitudinal study of women with cancer: II. Psychological outcomes. *Journal of Consulting and Clinical Psychology, 57*, 692–697.

Andersen, B. L., Beck, G., Ouelette-Kobasa, S., Revenson, T. A., & Temoshok, L. (1989). Directions for a psychology research agenda in cancer. *Health Psychology, 8*, 753–760.

Andrykowski, M. A. (1990). The role of anxiety in the development of anticipatory nausea in cancer chemotherapy: A review and synthesis. *Psychosomatic Medicine, 52*, 458–475.

Axtell, L. M., Asire, A. J., & Meyers, M. H. (Eds.). (1976). *Cancer patient survival* (Report No. 5, NCI Pub. No. NIH 771-992). Washington, DC: U.S. Government Printing Office.

Bal, D. G. (1992). Cancer in African Americans. *Ca-A Cancer Journal for Clinicians, 42*, 5–6.

Baquet, C. R., Horm, J. W., Gibbs, T., & Greenwald, P. (1991). Socioeconomic factors and cancer incidence among Blacks and Whites. *Journal of the National Cancer Institute, 83*, 551–557.

Beck, A., Ward, C., Mendelson, M., Mock, J., & Erbaugh, J. (1961). An inventory for measuring depression. *Archives of General Psychiatry, 4*, 561–571.

Berkman, L. F., & Syme, S. L. (1979). Social networks, host resistance, and mortality: A 9-year follow-up study of Alameda County residents. *American Journal of Epidemiology, 109*, 186–204.

Bernstein, I. L. (1986). Etiology of anorexia in cancer. *Cancer, 58*, 1881–1886.

Beutler, L. E., Crago, M., & Arizmendi, T. G. (1986). Therapist variables in psychotherapy process and outcome. In S. L. Garfield & A. E. Bergin (Eds.), *Handbook of psychotherapy and behavior change* (3rd ed., pp. 257–311). New York: Wiley.

Bloom, J. R. (1987). Psychological response to mastectomy. *Cancer, 59*, 189–196.

Boring, C. C., Squires, T. S., & Tong, T. (1992). Cancer statistics, 1992. *Ca-A Cancer Journal for Clinicians, 42*(1), 19–38.

Broadhead, W. E., & Kaplan, B. H. (1991). Social support and the cancer patient: Implications for future research and clinical care. *Cancer, 67*, 794–799.

Burish, T. G. (1991a). Behavioral and psychosocial research in cancer: Building on the past, preparing for the future. *Cancer, 67*, 865–867.

Burish, T. G. (1991b). Progress in psychosocial and behavioral cancer research: The need for enabling strategies. *Cancer, 67*, 860–864.

Cain, E. N., Kohorn, E. I., Quinlan, D. M., Latimer, K., & Schwartz, P. E. (1986). Psychosocial benefits of a cancer support group. *Cancer, 57*, 183–189.

Capone, M. A., Good, R. S., Westie, K. S., & Jacobsen, A. F. (1980). Psychosocial rehabilitation of gynecologic oncology patients. *Archives of Physical Medicine and Rehabilitation, 61*, 128–132.

Carey, M. P., & Burish, T. G. (1988). Etiology and treatment of the psychological side effects associated with cancer chemotherapy. *Psychological Bulletin, 104*, 307–325.

Carnrike, C. L. M., & Carey, M. P. (1990). Assessing nausea and vomiting in adult chemotherapy patients: Review and recommendations. *Annals of Behavioral Medicine, 12*, 79–85.

Cassileth, B. R., Lusk, E. J., Strouse, T. B., Miller, D. S., Brown, L. L., & Cross, P. A. (1985). A psychological analysis of cancer patients and their next-of-kin. *Cancer, 55*, 72–76.

Cassileth, B. R., Lusk, E. J., Strouse, T. B., Miller, D. S., Brown, L. L., Cross, P. A., & Tenaglia, A. N. (1984). Psychosocial status in chronic illness: A comparative analysis of six diagnostic groups. *New England Journal of Medicine, 311*, 506–511.

Cassileth, B. R., Lusk, E. J., & Tenaglia, A. N. (1983). Patients' perceptions of the cosmetic impact of melanoma resection. *Plastic and Reconstructive Surgery, 71*, 73–75.

Cassileth, P. A., & Cassileth, B. R. (1983, March). Clinical care of the terminal cancer patient: Part 1. *Medical Times*, pp. 57s–66s.

Cella, D. F., Orofiamma, B., Holland, J. C., Silberfarb, P. M., Tross, S., Feldstein, M., Perry, M., Maurer, L. H., Comis, R., & Oraz, E. J. (1987). The relationship of psychological distress, extent of disease, and performance status in patients with lung cancer. *Cancer, 60*, 1661–1667.

Cella, D. F., & Tross, S. (1986). Psychological adjustment to survival from Hodgkin's disease. *Journal of Consulting and Clinical Psychology, 54*, 616–622.

Christensen, D. N. (1983). Postmastectomy couple counseling: An outcome study of a structured treatment protocol. *Journal of Sex & Marital Therapy, 9*, 266–274.

Christenson, G. M., & Baquet, C. (in press). What is known about the conditions and behavior of those people disproportionately affected by cancer? *Cancer Prevention*.

Cohen, S., Tyrrell, D. A., & Smith, A. P. (1991). Psychological stress in humans and susceptibility to the common cold. *New England Journal of Medicine, 325*, 606–612.

Davis, H. (1986). Effects of biofeedback and cognitive therapy on stress in patients with breast cancer. *Psychological Reports, 59*, 967–974.

de Haes, J. C. J. M., van Oostrom, M. A., & Welvaart, K. (1986). The effect of radical and conserving surgery on quality of life of early breast cancer patients. *European Journal of Surgical Oncology, 12*, 337–342.

Derogatis, L. R. (1977). *SCL-90: Administration, scoring, and procedures manual–I for the (R)evised Version*. Baltimore: Johns Hopkins University School of Medicine.

Derogatis, L. R., Abeloff, M. D., & Melisartos, N. (1979). Psychological coping mechanisms and survival time in metastatic breast cancer. *Journal of the American Medical Association, 242*, 1504–1508.

Devlen, J., Maguire, P., Phillips, P., Crowther, D., & Chambers, H. (1987). Psychological problems associated with diagnosis and treatment of lymphomas: 1. Retrospective study and 2. Prospective study. *British Medical Journal, 295*, 953–957.

Edgar, L., Rosberger, Z., & Nowlis, D. (1992). Coping with cancer during the first year after diagnosis: Assessment and intervention. *Cancer, 69*, 817–828.

Endicott, J., & Spitzer, R. L. (1978). A diagnostic interview: The Schedule for Affective Disorders and Schizophrenia. *Archives of General Psychiatry, 35*, 837–844.

Eyre, H. J., & Ward, J. H. (1984). Control of cancer chemotherapy-induced nausea and vomiting. *Cancer, 54*, 2642–2648.

Fawzy, F. I., Cousins, N., Fawzy, N., Kemeny, M. E., Elashoff, R., & Morton, D. (1990). A structured psychiatric intervention for cancer patients: I. Changes over time in methods of coping and affective disturbance. *Archives of General Psychiatry, 47*, 720–725.

Fawzy, F. I., Kemeny, M. E., Fawzy, N., Elashoff, R., Morton, D., Cousins, N., & Fahey, J. L. (1990). A structured psychiatric intervention for cancer patients: I. Changes over time in immunological measures. *Archives of General Psychiatry, 47*, 729–735.

Ferlic, M., Goldman, A., & Kennedy, B. J. (1979). Group counseling in adult patients with advanced cancer. *Cancer, 43*, 760–766.

Forester, B., Kornfeld, D. S., & Fleiss, J. L. (1985). Psychotherapy during radiotherapy: Effects on emotional and physical distress. *American Journal of Psychiatry, 142*, 22–27.

Freeman, H. P. (1989). Cancer in the socioeconomically disadvantaged. *Ca-A Cancer Journal for Clinicians, 39*(5), 266–288.

Goodwin, J. S., Hunt, W. C., Key, C. R., & Samet, J. M. (1987). The effect of marital status on stage, treatment, and survival of cancer patients. *Journal of the American Medical Association, 258*, 3125–3130.

Gordon, W. A., Freidenbergs, I., Diller, L., Hibberd, M., Wold, C., Levine, L., Lipkins, R., Ezrachi, O., & Lucido, D. (1980). Efficacy of psychosocial intervention with cancer patients. *Journal of Consulting and Clinical Psychology, 48*, 743–759.

Greer, S., Morris, T., & Pettingale, K. W. (1979). Psychological response to breast cancer: Effect on outcome. *Lancet, 2*, 785–787.

Heinrich, R. L., & Coscarelli-Schag, C. (1985). Stress and activity management: Group treatment for cancer patients and their spouses. *Journal of Consulting and Clinical Psychology, 53*, 439–446.

Heinrich, R. L., Coscarelli-Schag, C., & Ganz, P. A. (1984). Living with cancer: The Cancer Inventory of Problem Situations. *Journal of Clinical Psychology, 40*, 972–980.

House, J. S., Robbins, C., & Metzner, H. L. (1982). The association of social relationships and activities with mortality: prospective evidence from the Tecumseh community health study. *American Journal of Epidemiology, 116*, 123–140.

Houts, P. S., Whitney, C. W., Mortel, R., & Bartholomew, M. J. (1986). Former cancer patients as counselors of newly diagnosed cancer patients. *Journal of the National Cancer Institute, 76*, 793–796.

Hughson, A. V., Cooper, A. F., McArdle, C. S., & Smith, D. C. (1986). Psychological impact of adjuvant chemotherapy in the first two years after mastectomy. *British Medical Journal of Clinical Research, 293*, 1268–1271.

Jacobs, C., Ross, R. D., Walker, I. M., & Stockdale, F. E. (1983). Behavior of cancer patients: A randomized study of the effects of education and peer support groups. *American Journal of Clinical Oncology, 6*, 347–353.

Karnofsky, D. A., & Burchenal, J. H. (1949). The clinical evaluation of chemotherapeutic agents in cancer. In C. M. Macleod (Ed.), *Evaluation of chemotherapeutic agents* (pp. 191–205). New York: Columbia University Press.

Kazdin, A. (1986). The evaluation of psychotherapy: Research design and methodology. In S. L. Garfield & A. E. Bergin (Eds.), *Handbook of psychotherapy and behavior change* (3rd ed., pp. 23–68). New York: Wiley.

Kiecolt-Glaser, J. K., Dura, J., Speicher, C., Trask, B., & Glaser, R. (1991). Spousal caregivers of dementia victims: Longitudinal changes in immunity and health. *Psychosomatic Medicine, 53*, 345–362.

Kiecolt-Glaser, J. K., Garner, W. K., Speicher, C., Penn, G. M., Holliday, J., & Glaser, R. (1984). Psychosocial modifiers of immunocompetence in medical students. *Psychosomatic Medicine, 46*, 7–14.

Kiecolt-Glaser, J. K., Glaser, R., Williger, D., Stout, J., Messick, G., Sheppard, S., Richer, D., Romisher, S. C., Briner, W., Bonnell, G., & Donnerberg, R. (1985). Psychosocial enhancement of immunocompetence in a geriatric population. *Health Psychology, 4*, 25–41.

Kolotkin, R. L., & Johnson, M. (1983). Crisis intervention and measurement of treatment outcome. In M. J. Lambert, E. R. Christensen, & S. S. DeJulio (Eds.), *The assessment of psychotherapy outcome* (pp. 132–159). New York: Wiley.

Levy, S. M., Lee, J., Bagley, C., & Lippman, M. (1988). Survival hazards analysis in first recurrent breast cancer patients: Seven-year follow-up. *Psychosomatic Medicine, 50*, 520–528.

Linn, M. W., Linn, B. S., & Harris, R. (1982). Effects of counseling for late stage cancer patients. *Cancer, 49*, 1048–1055.

Maguire, P., Brooke, M., Tait, A., Thomas, C., & Sellwood, R. (1983). The effect of counselling on physical disability and social recovery after mastectomy. *Clinical Oncology, 9*, 319–324.

Maguire, P., Hopwood, P., Tarrier, N., & Howell, T. (1985). Treatment of depression in cancer patients. *Acta Psychiatric Scandia, 72*(Suppl. 320), 81–84.

Maguire, P., Tait, A., Brooke, M., Thomas, C., & Sellwood, R. (1980). Effect of counselling on the psychiatric morbidity associated with mastectomy. *British Medical Journal, 281*, 1454–1456.

Matthews, K. A. (1989). Are sociodemographic variables markers for psychological determinants of health? *Health Psychology, 8*, 641–648.

McCorkle, R., Benoliel, J. Q., Donaldson, G., Georgiadou, F., Moinpour, C., & Goodell, B. (1989). A randomized clinical trial of home nursing care for lung cancer patients. *Cancer, 64*, 1375–1382.

McNair, D. M., Lorr, M., & Droppleman, L. F. (1971). *Profile of Mood States*. San Diego, CA: Educational and Industrial Testing Service.

Meyerowitz, B. E., Watkins, I. K., & Sparks, F. C. (1983). Psychosocial implications of adjuvant chemotherapy: A two-year follow-up. *Cancer, 52*, 1541–1545.

Morrow, G. R. (1989). Chemotherapy-related nausea and vomiting: Etiology and management. *Ca-A Cancer Journal for Clinicians, 39*, 89–104.

Morrow, G. R., & Dobkin, P. L. (1988). Anticipatory nausea and vomiting in cancer patients undergoing chemotherapy treatment: Prevalence, etiology, and behavioral interventions. *Clinical Psychology Review, 8*, 517–556.

Olschewski, M., & Schumacher, M. (1990). Statistical analysis of quality of life data in cancer clinical trials. *Statistics in Medicine, 9*, 749–763.

Ortmeyer, C. F. (1974). Variations in mortality, morbidity, and health care by marital status. In L. L. Erhardt & J. E. Berlin (Eds.), *Mortality and morbidity in the United States* (pp. 159–184). Cambridge, MA: Harvard University Press.

Osteen, R. T., Steele, G. D., Menck, H. R., & Winchester, D. P. (1992). Regional differences in surgical management of breast cancer. *Ca-A Cancer Journal for Clinicians, 42*, 39–43.

Parloff, M. B., Waskow, I. E., & Wolfe, B. E. (1978). Research on therapist variables in relation to process and outcome. In S. L. Garfield & A. E. Bergin (Eds.), *Handbook of psychotherapy and behavior change* (2nd ed., pp. 233–282). New York: Wiley.

Paul, G. L. (1969). Behavior modification research: Design and tactics. In C. M. Franks (Ed.), *Behavior therapy: Appraisal and status* (pp. 29–62). New York: McGraw-Hill.

Pennebaker, J. W., Kiecolt-Glaser, J. K., & Glaser, R. (1988). Disclosure of traumas and immune function: Health implications for psychotherapy. *Journal of Consulting and Clinical Psychology, 56*, 239–245.

Redd, W. H., & Andrykowski, M. (1982). Behavioral intervention in cancer treatment: Controlling aversive reactions to chemotherapy. *Journal of Clinical and Consulting Psychology, 50*, 1018–1029.

Schain, W., Edwards, B. K., Gorrell, C. R., deMoss, E. V., Lippman, M. E., Gerber, L. H., & Lichter, A. S. (1983). Psychosocial and physical outcomes of primary breast cancer therapy: Mastectomy vs. excisional biopsy and irradiation. *Breast Cancer Research and Treatment, 3*, 377–382.

Scheier, M. F., & Carver, C. S. (in press). Effects of optimism on psychological and physical well-being: Theoretical overview and empirical update. *Cognitive Therapy and Research.*

Silberberg, E., & Lubera, J. A. (1989). Cancer statistics, 1989. *Ca-A Cancer Journal for Clinicians, 39*, 3–20.

Spiegel, D., & Bloom, J. R. (1983). Group therapy and hypnosis reduce metastatic breast carcinoma pain. *Psychosomatic Medicine, 45*, 333–339.

Spiegel, D., Bloom, J. R., Kraemer, H. C., & Gottheil, E. (1989, October 14). Effect of psychosocial treatment on survival of patients with metastatic breast cancer. *Lancet*, pp. 888–891.

Spiegel, D., Bloom, J. R., & Yalom, I. (1981). Group support for patients with metastatic cancer: A randomized outcome study. *Archives of General Psychiatry, 38*, 527–533.

Spiegel, D., & Glafkedes, M. C. (1983). Effects of group confrontation with death and dying. *International Journal of Group Psychotherapy, 33*, 433–447.

Spiegel, D., & Yalom, I. D. (1978). A support group for dying patients. *International Journal of Group Psychotherapy, 28*, 233–245.

Spielberger, C. D., Gorsuch, R. L., & Lushene, R. E. (1970). *Manual for the State–Trait Anxiety Inventory*. Palo Alto, CA: Consulting Psychologists Press.

Stewart, A. L., Greenfield, S., Hays, R. D., Wells, K., Rogers, W. H., Berry, S. D., McGlynn, E. A., & Ware, J. E. (1989). Functional status and well-being of patients with chronic conditions: Results from the Medical Outcomes Study. *Journal of the American Medical Association, 262*, 907–913.

Taylor, S. E., Falke, R. L., Shoptaw, S. J., & Lichtman, R. R. (1986). Social support, support groups, and the cancer patient. *Journal of Consulting and Clinical Psychology, 54*, 608–615.

Telch, C. F., & Telch, M. J. (1986). Group coping skills instruction and supportive group therapy for cancer patients: A comparison of strategies. *Journal of Consulting and Clinical Psychology, 54*, 802–808.

Thompson, L., Andersen, B. L., & DePetrillo, D. (1992). The psychological processes of recovery from gynecologic cancer. In M. Coppleson, P. Morrow, & M. Tattersall (Eds.), *Gynecologic oncology* (2nd ed., pp. 1499–1505). Edinburgh, England: Churchill Livingstone.

Turk, D. C., & Fernandez, E. (1990). On the putative uniqueness of cancer pain: Do psychological principles apply? *Behavior Research and Therapy, 28*, 1–13.

Vinokur, A. D., Threatt, B. A., Caplan, R. D., & Zimmerman, B. L. (1989). Physical and psychosocial functioning and adjustment to breast cancer: Long-term follow-up of a screening population. *Cancer, 63*, 394–405.

Vinokur, A. D., Threatt, B. A., Vinokur-Kaplan, D., & Satariano, W. A. (in press). The process of recovery from breast cancer for younger and older patients: Changes during the first year. *Cancer.*

Ware, J. E., Jr. (1984). Methodological considerations in the selection of health status procedures. In N. K. Wenger, M. E. Mattson, C. D. Furberg, & J. Elinson (Eds.), *Assessment of quality of life in clinical trials of cardiovascular therapies* (pp. 84–95). New York: Le Jacq.

Weisman, A. D., & Worden, J. W. (1976–1977). The existential plight in cancer: Significance of the first 100 days. *International Journal of Psychiatry in Medicine, 7*, 1–15.

Wells, K. B., Stewart, A., Hays, R. D., Burnam, A., Rogers, W., Daniels, M., Berry, S., Greenfield, S., & Ware, J. (1989). The functioning and well-being of depressed patients: Results from the Medical Outcomes Study. *Journal of the American Medical Association, 262,* 914–919.

Yalom, I. D. (1975). *The theory and practice of group psychotherapy* (2nd ed.). New York: Basic Books.

Yates, J. W., McKegney, F. P., & Kun, L. E. (1981). A comparative study of home nursing care of patients with advanced cancer. *Proceedings of the National Conference on Human Values and Cancer* (pp. 207–218). New York: American Cancer Society.

Zonderman, A. B., Costa, P., & McCrae, R. R. (1989). Depression as a risk for cancer morbidity and mortality in a nationally representative sample. *Journal of the American Medical Association, 262,* 1191–1195.

Chapter 7
EFFECTS OF PSYCHOSOCIAL INTERVENTIONS WITH ADULT CANCER PATIENTS:
A Meta-Analysis of Randomized Experiments

Thomas J. Meyer and Melvin M. Mark

Though the field of psychosocial oncology is relatively young, intervention studies and indeed even narrative reviews of those studies are no longer rare. Meta-analytic investigations, however, are conspicuously absent from the literature. In the present article, the results of treatment–control studies of psychosocial interventions with adult cancer patients are assessed meta-analytically. The focus is on the effects of nonpharmacological interventions intended to improve the quality of life of adults who have already been diagnosed with one of the neoplastic diseases. Outcomes of interest are measures of emotional adjustment, functional adjustment, treatment- or disease-related symptoms, medical status, or some combination of these categories.

Some previous narrative reviewers have addressed psychosocial interventions broadly, whereas others have focused on specific types of interventions; in both cases, past reviews have tended to conclude cautiously that controlled studies show the interventions to be at least promising and probably beneficial to cancer patients (e.g., Andersen, 1992; Trijsburg, van Knippenberg, & Rijpma, 1992; Watson & Marvell, 1992). A mixture of significant and nonsignificant results in controlled studies has led traditional reviewers to be cautious in their conclusions. As many meta-analysts (e.g., Hedges & Olkin, 1985; Hunter & Schmidt, 1990) have noted, such a pattern of significant and nonsignificant outcomes will arise if the underlying effect size is positive but moderate and study samples are small. By combining results across studies, a meta-analysis can more powerfully address the question: Is there an overall benefit to psychosocial interventions with cancer patients, and if so, how large is it?

In addition to the question of overall effectiveness of psychosocial interventions, we examine a set of more specific questions. First, because many researchers have suggested that certain types of interventions are preferable to others, we assess whether different classes of interventions are equally effective. Second, we investigate whether treatment effectiveness varies as a function of the severity of disease and treatment, factors that Andersen (1992) focused on in a recent review (also see

Reprinted from *Health Psychology*, *14*(2), 101–108. (1995). Copyright © 1995 by the American Psychological Association. Used with permission of the author.

A portion of this article was reported at the 98th Annual Convention of the American Psychological Association, Boston, August 1990, and in Thomas J. Meyer's doctoral dissertation at Pennsylvania State University. This research was supported in part by a dissertation research award from the American Psychological Association and by a National Institute of Mental Health fellowship in Mental Health Statistics at the Division of Biostatistics, Columbia University School of Public Health.

We thank the Interlibrary loan staffs at Pennsylvania State University and Columbia University's Health Science Campus for their assistance; Laurie Cohen for reliability coding; Juris Draguns for German translation; and Janet Swim, Barbara A. Meyer, Elizabeth J. Susman, William J. Ray, Juris Draguns, William Redd, and three anonymous reviewers for their comments on earlier versions of this article. We also thank the many researchers who sent additional information regarding their work.

Ahles, Cohen, & Blanchard, 1984; Watson, 1986). Third, we consider whether effect size differs for studies that screen potential participants and include only those with clear difficulties relative to studies without such screening. Several researchers have suggested that scarce services need only be offered to (e.g., Greer, 1987; Worden & Weisman, 1980), or are more effective for (e.g., Watson, 1983, 1986; Watson & Marvell, 1992), those at risk or in need (though Greer also noted that studies have shown that medical staff underestimate need). Finally, we attempt to determine if effect size depends on whether the intervention is focused specifically on coping with chemotherapy, pain, or radiation treatment.

Method

Search Strategy

Following common practice in many behavioral medicine meta-analyses (e.g., Fredrikson & Matthews, 1990), only published randomized experiments were included in the analyses reported here. Appropriate studies were defined as published randomized trials in which (a) a group of adult cancer patients receiving a psychosocial, behavioral, or psychoeducational intervention was compared with another group of cancer patients receiving either no psychosocial intervention or an extremely minimal sham procedure, and (b) the outcome variables included the patients' behavioral, emotional, physiological, or medical state. Hospice and terminal home care studies were excluded because there were few randomized studies and because preliminary work had indicated that they were quite distinct from other psychosocial interventions (Meyer, 1991). Studies were located from *Psychological Abstracts*, *Medline*, the reference sections of located studies and review articles, by writing to researchers in the field and through informal inquiries (see Meyer, 1991, for details).

Results of the Search

Forty-five studies, reporting 62 treatment–control comparisons[1] relevant to the meta-analysis, were retrieved.[2] Five studies were from Great Britain, 2 from Canada, 1 each from Colombia and Egypt, and the remaining 36 from the United States. The primary source articles are listed in the Reference section. Supplementary information was sometimes obtained directly from the authors, from a dissertation report on which the study was based, or from an additional published report.

Table 1 presents information about patient age, diagnosis, and sex. For those studies in which the mean age was reported, samples clustered around the 50s.

[1] The results for the two biofeedback treatment groups in Shartner, Burish, and Carey (1985) have been combined and analyzed as a single treatment–control comparison because of the small numbers involved (8 intervention patients and 4 controls). Because this review does not focus on different types of control groups, results for multiple control groups were combined for the two studies with two control groups.

[2] Two psychotherapy studies reported by Grossarth-Maticek (Grossarth-Maticek & Eysenck, 1989; Grossarth-Maticek, Schmidt, Vetter, & Arndt, 1984) are excluded from all results in this article. The integrity of some of Grossarth-Maticek's other data has been challenged by researchers (van der Ploeg, 1991) including one of his coauthors (Vetter, 1991).

Table 1—*Age, Type of Cancer, and Sex*

Group	No. studies	% of studies reported
Mean age of sample		
49 or below	10	28.6
50–59	18	51.4
60 and over	7	20.0
Not reported	10	—
Single type or location of cancer		
Yes	14	31.1
Breast	4	8.9
Hodgkins	2	4.4
Lung	2	4.4
Skin	2	4.4
Bladder	1	2.2
Female reproductive	1	2.2
Male reproductive	1	2.2
Hematological	1	2.2
No	31	69.9
Proportion (in percentages) of study sample that is female		
0	2	5.0
1–20	0	0.0
21–40	3	7.5
41–59	13	32.5
60–79	14	35.0
80–99	2	5.0
100	6	15.0
Not reported	5	—

Fourteen of the studies were limited to a single type of cancer, including four with only breast cancer patients. There was a tendency for studies to have a preponderance of women such that in 55% of the studies reporting gender more than 60% of the patients were female, whereas in only 12.5% of the studies 60% of the patients were male.

Only eight of the studies from the United States reported quantitative information about race or ethnicity. Three of those reported samples in which at least 10% of participants were African American; no North American studies reported as many Latino/Hispanic, Asian American, or Native American Indian patients.

Variables

Dependent Measures

Five higher order categories of dependent measures were developed. Emotional adjustment involved measures of such constructs as mood state, fear and anxiety, depression, denial or repression, self-esteem, locus of control, satisfaction with medical care, other attitudes, personality traits, and any other type of emotional adjustment or distress. Functional adjustment consisted of indicators of behavioral functioning in normal life settings (e.g., socializing and going back to work). Illustrative measures included the Karnofsky Performance Status, self-report measures of social behaviors, and other life indicators of adjustment and functioning. The category treatment- or disease-related symptoms related to chemotherapy-related nausea and vomiting, pain, coughing, nutritional measures, including body weight, and similar symptoms related to cancer and its treatment. The medical measures category included such indicators as leukocyte activity, tumor response to chemotherapy, and physician rating of disease progression. The category compound or global measures included measures combining clear, core aspects of more than one of the preceding categories. An example would be the Cancer Inventory of Problem Situations (Schag, Heinrich, & Ganz, 1983), which explicitly addresses emotional adjustment, functional adjustment, and treatment- and disease-related symptoms. This category of measures also included global measures for which overall ratings implicitly cut across the preceding categories (despite potential interpretive problems, this compound category was included for completeness).

Treatment Style Categories

The five categories of interventions were defined as follows. Cognitive–behavioral interventions include cognitive, cognitive–behavioral, and behavioral methods focused on changing specific thoughts or behaviors or on learning specific coping skills. Procedures coded here included progressive muscle relaxation training, meditation, hypnotherapy, systematic desensitization, biofeedback, and behavior modification or reinforcement. If a treatment had a substantial behavioral component, it was placed in this cognitive–behavioral category even if it also had considerable emphasis on information and education (cf. Mazzuca, 1982). This category is similar to the behavioral supercategory developed by Smith and Glass (1977) in their pioneering meta-analysis of the psychotherapy outcome studies except that cognitive interventions have been transferred into it, to some extent dealing with Presby's (1978) objections to Smith and Glass's category.

Informational and educational treatments included interventions primarily providing sensory, procedural, or medical information; coping information, if provided, did not include active rehearsal of new behaviors. An example is the booklet Goodwin (1979) provided to patients before lung surgery that described normal breathing, symptoms to expect after the surgery, and self-care measures to promote optimum recovery and cope with symptoms.

Nonbehavioral counseling or psychotherapy interventions referred to noncognitive and nonbehavioral verbal psychotherapy and counseling, including psychodynamic, existential, supportive or general counseling, and crisis intervention. This category is similar to Smith and Glass's (1977) verbal psychotherapy supercategory except that it does not include cognitive interventions. This category included social support by professionals.

Social support (by nonprofessionals) referred to cases in which fellow patients or family members provide the intervention by being supportive (e.g., in a support group run by fellow patients rather than professionals). Structured social support interventions by nonprofessionals (other patients or family members) are important in the cancer literature (Lieberman, 1988) and made a natural category.

Another category included unusual treatments (e.g., music therapy) and cases in which clearly dissimilar or incongruous approaches were combined, especially when the different aspects of the intervention were given by different practitioners. For instance, this label was given to Spiegel and Bloom's (1983) well-known study because it combined hypnosis, classified here as a behavioral method, with a psychodynamic process group. The category 'other' was not used for the many interventions with some aspects of education and behavioral coping skills. In such cases, we determined whether the content of the intervention was nearly exclusively educational or whether there was a substantial behavioral component, and the intervention was assigned accordingly.

Moderator Variables

Three potential moderator variables were examined: Andersen's (1992) categories of risk for psychological distress, whether the intervention was focused on a particular symptom or treatment side effect, and whether patients were screened. Following Andersen, we categorized studies as having patients low, medium, or high in risk for psychological distress by weighing three dimensions. Low risk was defined as corresponding with local disease, low intensity of treatment, and favorable prognosis. High risk was defined as corresponding with disseminated disease, high intensity of treatment, and bleak prognosis. For the intervention-focus variable, studies were classified as being focused on treating chemotherapy-related symptoms, radiation-related symptoms, and pain or as not being so focused. For the patient-screening variable, studies with screening of patients were defined as those in which only patients with clear signs of distress (emotional distress, particular chemotherapy side effects, or pain) were treated, as contrasted with studies that included cancer patients regardless of distress level.

Method of Coding and Analysis

Coding Strategy

We attempted to calculate the effect size for every measure in an article. Following Matt (1989), if a measure was discussed in the Method section but no detailed results were reported, the effect size was assumed to be zero. However, if most effect sizes reported only as nonsignificant were in fact nonzero in the same direction as the average effect size, then treating these unreported effect sizes as zero provides a conservative estimate. To find an upper bound estimate so as to bracket effect sizes, calculations were also conducted with such results (i.e., those reported only as nonsignificant or not explicitly reported) completely omitted from the analysis.

To avoid overrepresenting studies with multiple measures, when a treatment–control comparison provided more than one effect size for a dependent measure category (e.g., several different emotional adjustment measures) the results were averaged (weighted by sample sizes if the different measures or sampling occasions had different Ns).

Multiple Treatment–Control Comparisons

So that overall significance levels would not be based on subjects counted twice or even three times, the number of subjects in the control group was divided by the number of treatment groups compared with it.

Reliability Coding

All of the studies on which the present meta-analysis is based were coded by the first author. Reliability coding conducted in preliminary analyses (Meyer, 1991) indicated that it was reasonable to accept the primary coder's judgments for this work. For example in a broader set of studies, for frequently encountered classifications, kappas ranged from .81 to .88 (Meyer & Mark, 1994).

Data Analysis

Hedges and Olkin's (1985) methods were used to conduct separate meta-analyses of effect sizes for each of the five types of dependent measures. A unit-free effect size *g* was obtained from outcome measure scores by obtaining the difference between the control group mean and the treatment group mean and dividing the result by the pooled standard deviation. For certain complex designs, Shadish and Montgomery's (1986) methods were used to determine *g*. The effect size *g* was then multiplied by a small sample size correction factor to obtain an unbiased value of *d*, the effect size used in the rest of the analysis (Hedges & Olkin, 1985).

Homogeneity tests were also conducted to test whether a set of effect sizes could be considered as a sample from a single underlying effect size. The different treatment categories were compared in terms of the magnitude of effect size associated with each. Similar analyses were conducted for the moderator variables. Johnson's (1989) software for meta-analyses was used.

Results

Homogeneity

For four of the five categories of dependent measure categories, the set of effect sizes was homogenous. The exception was for measures of emotional adjustment; when one outlier was removed, however, the remaining studies had homogenous effect sizes. The discrepant study (Ali & Khalil, 1989) was the only one from a country (Egypt) in which patients were not notified of their cancer diagnosis. Following the method of Hedges and Olkin (1985), that study has been deleted from all the results.

Average Effect Sizes

Overall average effect sizes are presented in Table 2. Significant beneficial effects ranging from .19 to .28 were found for the four dependent measure categories for

Table 2—*Weighted Effect Sizes for Dependent Measure Categories*

Measure	Studies	Comparisons	Total N	d	d 95% CI
Emotional adjustment	41	56	2,840	.24	.17/.32
Functional adjustment	16	21	940	.19	.06/.32
Treatment- and disease-related symptoms	28	39	1,606	.26	.16/.37
Medical	5	7	232	.17	−.10/.44
Compound and global	5	7	373	.28	.08/.49

Note. CI = confidence interval.

which the most patients were studied. For the fifth category, medical measures, the slightly smaller effect size of .17 was not statistically significant.

For the analyses summarized in Table 2, effect sizes reported as nonsignificant are assumed to be zero. To establish an upper bound, weighted average effect sizes were also calculated excluding these effect sizes. The resulting average effect sizes were .31 for emotional adjustment, .32 for functional adjustment, .41 for treatment- and disease-related symptoms, .39 for medical measures, and .28 (unchanged) for compound and global measures.

Treatment Style and Potential Moderator Variables

For all five outcome variables, there were no significant differences on post hoc comparisons among any of the treatment categories. Table 3 presents the effect sizes, by dependent measure category, for each intervention type.

There was no significant effect of Andersen's (1992) risk categories; for emotional adjustment, $QB(2) = 3.13$, $p = .21$; for functional adjustment, $QB(1) = 2.50$, $p = .11$, with high risk tending to be associated with larger effects than moderate risk; and for symptoms, $QB(2) = 0.14$, $p = .93$. There was no significant effect of study focus (e.g., pain-focused and radiation-focused; all $ps > .15$) or screening for distress on effect sizes (all $ps > .20$) for any of the dependent measure categories. As with the nonsignificant differences among treatment style categories, these results must be interpreted with caution. Type II errors are possible because the effect sizes and the number of treatment–control comparisons are relatively small.[3]

[3] The present article is adapted from a longer manuscript by Meyer and Mark (1994), available from Melvin M. Mark, which presents a meta-analysis including both nonrandomized and unpublished studies. No significant differences were observed between published and unpublished studies or between random and nonrandom studies. Nevertheless, in the large set of studies, effect sizes were generally larger, with d = .29 for emotional adjustment, .26 for functional adjustment, .27 for treatment- and disease-related symptoms, .21 for medical measures, and .13 for compound and global measures. In addition, screening was a significant moderator, with studies that included only patients in distress having higher effect sizes on measures of emotional adjustment and treatment- and disease-related symptoms. The Meyer and Mark (1994) manuscript also includes a discussion of the file drawer problem and analyses of fail-safe N.

Table 3—*Weighted Effect Size (ES), N, and 95% Confidence Interval (CI) for Treatments by Dependent Measure*

Treatment	Emotional adjustment	Functional adjustment	Symptoms	Medical	Compound and global
Behavioral					
ES	.19, $n = 1{,}323$	.10, $n = 194$	.32, $n = 727$	.13, $n = 184$	.20, $n = 203$
CI	+0.08/+0.30	−0.20/+0.40	+0.16/+0.48	−0.17/+0.43	−0.07/+0.49
Informational and educational					
ES	.25, $n = 988$	.27, $n = 465$	.21, $n = 416$	.80, $n = 26$	.35, $n = 118$
CI	+0.12/+0.37	+0.08/+0.46	+0.01/+0.40	+0.00/+1.60	−0.02/+0.72
Nonbehavior counseling/ therapy					
ES	.39, $n = 422$	.12, $n = 263$	.17, $n = 339$	−.20, $n = 22$	.45, $n = 52$
CI	+0.19/+0.58	−0.12/+0.37	−0.05/+0.39	−1.04/+0.64	−0.12/+1.02
Social support					
ES	−.23, $n = 19$	−.08, $n = 18$	—	—	—
CI	−1.14/+0.67	−1.02/+0.85			
Other					
ES	.33, $n = 88$	—	.45, $n = 124$	—	—
CI	−0.10/+0.76		+0.09/+0.82		

Discussion

We consider first the overall average effect size for the interventions. The results clearly indicate that psychosocial interventions have positive effects on emotional adjustment, functional adjustment, and treatment- and disease-related symptoms in adult cancer patients. Previous reviewers (e.g., Greer, 1987; Trijsburg et al., 1992) have been concerned that studies have not consistently shown statistically significant results. However, such a pattern of results could be expected because of the small sample size and consequent low statistical power of the average study in this area (Hedges & Olkin, 1985; Hunter, Schmidt, & Jackson, 1982). In the few studies (5 of 45) that included medical outcome measures, there was no statistically significant effect of psychosocial interventions on those variables. However, these studies represented far fewer patients than the other outcome categories (232, as contrasted with 2,840 for emotional adjustment, the most-reported category).

Interpretation of Effect Sizes

Are the statistically significant effect sizes clinically significant? Depending on one's perspective, it is possible to interpret the effect sizes found as very important or as relatively small. First, consider the effect sizes in relation to other psychological interventions. The magnitude of the present effects is somewhat smaller than that found by Matt (1989) for psychotherapy outcome studies. Matt found a *d* of .35

when he replicated Smith and Glass's (1977) meta-analysis using methods similar to those used here (though Matt did not exclude unpublished and nonrandom studies). Thus, the present effects represent a range somewhat smaller in clinical significance than those of psychotherapy in general. Note, however, that Hunter and Schmidt (1990) considered effect sizes in the range of .20 to .40 as fairly typical of psychological interventions that work, and the effects observed here generally fall within that range.

It is nevertheless possible to view the observed effects simply as small. Cohen (1977) has called effect sizes of .2, .5, and .8 "small," "medium," and "large," respectively. From this perspective, the observed effect sizes tend to be fairly small.

On the other hand, Rosenthal (1984) has pointed out that in the medical field even tiny effects may be of crucial importance. An effect size d of .08, which raises success rates from 48% to 52%, can be of considerable importance to the individuals affected. Using the methods of Rosenthal and Rubin (1982), differential success rates of intervention versus control subjects were 56% versus 44% for measures of emotional adjustment, 55% versus 45% for functional adjustment, 57% versus 43% for treatment- and disease-related symptoms, 54% versus 46% for medical measures, and 57% versus 43% for compound and global measures.

Even if one views the effect sizes as relatively small, it is still possible to find reasons to be impressed that any positive effect has occurred. It is also possible that cancer patients will benefit in ways that are not reflected in the dependent measures used in outcome studies. For example, Cella et al. (1989) have documented that cancer patients score significantly lower on Total Mood Disturbance on the Profile of Mood States than the published normative groups. Thus, cancer patients may not be able to improve much from better than average. Phrased differently, it may be that cancer patients who are fairly well-adjusted before diagnosis show no improvement because of ceiling effects. Those who are not well-adjusted may require extensive intervention for obvious benefits (Watson, 1983); their illness is an ongoing objective stressor complicating the resolution of premorbid issues. Vachon (1988) has suggested another possibility: "[by intervening] we may risk having . . . patients, family members and survivors appear to be doing worse because they have learned to identify and express their emotions and emotional needs, rather than repressing them" (p. 48). In sum, we believe the positive effects are noteworthy.

Substantive Implications of Meta-Analytic Methodology

There were a number of methodological choices that may result in conservative effect size estimates. First, we assumed nonsignificant results were zero in the primary analyses. Second, we took a comprehensive approach to including dependent measures (following Matt, 1989). As we reported, excluding nonsignificant results, rather than assuming them to be zero, caused effect size estimates to increase from a range of .17–.28 to .28–.41. Similarly, Matt (1989) obtained effect size estimates for psychotherapy interventions half the size of those reported by Smith, Glass, and Miller (1980). A third possible source of conservative bias is that all interventions were included from multiple treatment studies even though some were studies in which components of complex treatments were examined both separately and in combination and in which not all interventions were expected to be equally effective.

Fourth, multiple measures were weighted equally even though some researchers included measures on which they expected little or no change. Fifth, measures were not corrected for unreliability even though many studies used instruments with as few as one item (see Hunter & Schmidt, 1990, for a discussion). In addition, larger effect sizes are obtained if nonrandom and unpublished studies are included (see Footnote 3).

Impact of Treatment Styles and Moderator Variables

The failure to reject the null hypothesis of no differences between categories in all subset analyses raises two possibilities: There really may not be differences between the effect sizes of different categories, or there may have been insufficient statistical power to find true differences. Given that the main effects were not large, the power to find interaction effects in this sample of studies was small. To move beyond our general finding that psychosocial interventions have a beneficial effect on most outcome measures, reporting of interaction effects needs to be improved and cumulated across studies.

Note that questions about the relative efficacy of treatment styles or the impact of the moderator variables can only be partially illuminated by study-level analyses such as those undertaken here. A relationship based on the average values for variables across studies can conceal a different relationship between the variables within studies (Light & Pillemer, 1984). For instance, individual studies that included a range of risk among the patients served might have found a consistent relationship between risk and treatment effect if this had been investigated. In addition, within-study comparisons avoid problems of confounding between studies, as Shapiro and Shapiro (1982) have noted. Future attention to potential moderators in primary research seems desirable.

Questions of External Validity

The studies included in the meta-analysis predominantly included White women from the United States.[4] The search strategy uncovered only two studies from nonindustrialized countries. Some caution is indicated in assuming that the results apply equally to men, to ethnic minorities in the United States, and to other nations. Future studies focusing on these populations would be desirable to assess the extent to which the present results can be extended (cf. Burish, 1991, regarding the need for research on ethnic minorities).

Many researchers have noted that substantial numbers of patients refuse the opportunity to receive psychosocial interventions. The results reported here represent only those who agreed to participate in studies and who completed outcome measures. The beneficial results found should therefore be considered to apply only to those patients interested in participating in psychosocial interventions.

---

[4] Although there was no direct evidence to this effect, the underrepresentation of men might indicate some subtle biases about the appropriateness of psychosocial interventions for men versus women.

Future Research

We believe that the cumulative evidence is sufficiently strong that it would be an inefficient use of research resources to conduct more studies in the United States to ask the simple question: Is there an effect of behavioral, educational, social support, and nonbehavioral counseling and therapy interventions on the emotional adjustment, functional adjustment, and treatment- and disease-related symptoms of cancer patients? These interventions have a consistent beneficial effect on all three areas.

On the other hand, several other directions for future research seem important and should replace simple tests of the efficacy of psychosocial interventions on emotional and functional adjustment and on treatment- and disease-related symptoms. First, more direct comparisons of different treatments should be made. We believe it would be premature to conclude that there is no difference between treatment categories on the basis of the present meta-analysis, given possible confounds.

Another productive direction involves focusing on medical outcomes and survival, especially in longitudinal studies that simultaneously measure emotional adjustment, treatment compliance, treatment- and disease-related symptoms, and social support. Few long-term controlled studies of survival time have been reported, ironically in some cases with results opposite the predictions of the authors: Morgenstern, Gellert, Walter, Ostfeld, and Siegel (1984, with additional follow-up by Gellert, Maxwell, & Siegel, 1993) found no evidence that their intervention increased survival time, whereas Spiegel, Bloom, Kraemer, and Gottheil (1989) unexpectedly did. One desirable strategy would be to integrate such research on psychosocial interventions into new or existing studies of medical interventions. The increased monitoring of patients' treatment in cancer medical treatment could promote psychosocial research (W. H. Redd, personal communication, August 31, 1994). In addition, as Greer suggested in 1987, increased attention to studying the mechanisms of beneficial outcomes would be useful. This approach has proved helpful in the behavioral treatment of chemotherapy side effects (Watson & Marvell, 1992) and merits more study. In other words, mediational processes should be studied.

Finally, there is a need to investigate ways of increasing the impact of interventions and of decreasing their cost (Rimer, Keintz, & Glassman, 1985). Some research on replacing expensive professionals with audiotapes in relaxation training has had disappointing results (Carey & Burish, 1988), but it seems worthwhile to consider other methods to increase cost-effectiveness, including alternative approaches to treatment delivery and implementation. In a related vein, improving the acceptability of psychosocial interventions for both medical personnel and patients, as well as ensuring easy accessibility, would be worthwhile. Additional research, designed with attention to statistical power, might also fruitfully address whether psychosocial interventions are less effective for low-distress and for low-risk patients.

References

References marked with an asterisk indicate studies included in the meta-analysis.

Ahles, T. A., Cohen, R. E., & Blanchard, E. B. (1984). Difficulties inherent in conducting behavioral research with cancer patients. *Behavior Therapist, 7*(4), 69–70.

*Ali, N. S., & Khalil, H. Z. (1989). Effect of psychoeducational intervention on anxiety among Egyptian bladder cancer patients. *Cancer Nursing, 12,* 236–242.

Andersen, B. L. (1992). Psychological interventions for cancer patients to enhance the quality of life. *Journal of Consulting and Clinical Psychology, 60,* 552–568.

*Bindemann, S., Soukop, M., & Kaye, S. B. (1991). Randomised controlled study of relaxation training. *European Journal of Cancer, 27,* 170–174.

*Bridge, L. R., Benson, P., Pietroni, P. C., & Priest, R. G. (1988). Relaxation and imagery in the treatment of breast cancer. *British Medical Journal, 297,* 1169–1172.

Burish, T. G. (1991). Behavioral and psychosocial cancer research: Building on the past, preparing for the future. *Cancer, 67,* 865–867.

*Burish, T. G., Carey, M. P., Krozely, M. G., & Greco, F. A. (1987). Conditioned side effects induced by cancer chemotherapy: Prevention through behavioral treatment. *Journal of Consulting and Clinical Psychology, 55,* 42–48.

*Burish, T. G., & Jenkins, R. A. (1992). Effectiveness of biofeedback and relaxation training in reducing the side effects of cancer chemotherapy. *Health Psychology, 11,* 17–23.

*Burish, T. G., & Lyles, J. N. (1981). Effectiveness of relaxation training in reducing adverse reactions to cancer chemotherapy. *Journal of Behavioral Medicine, 4,* 65–78.

*Burish, T. G., Snyder, S. L., & Jenkins, R. A. (1991). Preparing patients for cancer chemotherapy: Effect of coping preparation and relaxation interventions. *Journal of Consulting and Clinical Psychology, 59,* 518–525.

*Cain, E. N., Kohorn, E. I., Quinlan, D. M., Latimer, K., & Schwartz, P. E. (1986). Psychosocial benefits of a cancer support group. *Cancer, 57,* 183–189.

*Cannici, J., Malcolm, R., & Peek, L. A. (1983). Treatment of insomnia in cancer patients using muscle relaxation training. *Journal of Behavior Therapy and Experimental Psychiatry, 14,* 251–256.

*Carey, M. P., & Burish, T. G. (1987). Providing relaxation training to cancer chemotherapy patients: A comparison of three delivery techniques. *Journal of Consulting and Clinical Psychology, 55,* 732–737.

Carey, M. P., & Burish, T. G. (1988). Etiology and treatment of the psychological side effects associated with cancer chemotherapy: A critical review and discussion. *Psychological Bulletin, 104,* 307–325.

Cella, D. F., Tross, S., Orav, E. J., Holland, J. C., Silberfarb, P. M., & Rafla, S. (1989). Mood states of patients after the diagnosis of cancer. *Journal of Psychosocial Oncology, 7*(1–2), 45–54.

Cohen, J. (1977). *Statistical power analysis for the behavioral sciences* (Rev. ed.). New York: Academic Press.

*Cotanch, P. H., & Strum, S. (1987). Progressive muscle relaxation as antiemetic therapy for cancer patients. *Oncology Nursing Forum, 14*(1), 33–37.

*Dalton, J. A. (1987). Education for pain management: A pilot study. *Patient Education and Counseling, 9,* 155–165.

*Davis, H., IV. (1986). Effects of biofeedback and cognitive therapy on stress in patients with breast cancer. *Psychological Reports, 59,* 967–974.

*Decker, T. W., Cline-Elsen, J., & Gallagher, M. (1992). Relaxation therapy as an adjunct in radiation oncology. *Journal of Clinical Oncology, 48,* 388–393.

*Dixon, J. (1984). Effect of nursing interventions on nutritional and performance status in cancer patients. *Nursing Research, 33,* 330–335.

*Dodd, M. J. (1984). Measuring informational intervention for chemotherapy knowledge and self-care behavior. *Research in Nursing and Health, 7*(1), 43–50.

*Dodd, M. J. (1987). Efficacy of proactive information on self-care in radiation therapy patients. *Heart and Lung, 16,* 538–544.

*Dodd, M. J. (1988). Efficacy of proactive information on self-care in chemotherapy patients. *Patient Education and Counseling, 11,* 215–225.

*Domar, A. D., Noe, J. M., & Benson, H. (1987). The preoperative use of the relaxation response with ambulatory surgery patients. *Journal of Human Stress*, *13*(3), 101–107.

*Eardley, A. (1988). Patients' worries about radiotherapy: Evaluation of a preparatory booklet. *Psychology and Health*, *2*, 79–89.

*Edgar, L., Rosberger, Z., & Nowlis, D. (1992). Coping with cancer during the first year after diagnosis: Assessment and intervention. *Cancer*, *69*, 817–828.

*Fawzy, F. I., Kemeny, M. E., Fawzy N. W., Elashoff, R., Morton, D., Cousins, N., & Fahey, J. L. (1990). A structured psychiatric intervention for cancer patients: II. Changes over time in immunological measures. *Archives in General Psychiatry*, *47*, 729–735.

*Flórez-B. H. (1979). Psicoterapia de grupo en pacientes de cáncer [Group psychotherapy in cancer patients]. *Rivista Latinoamericana de Psicología*, *11*(1), 47–63.

*Forester, B., Kornfeld, D. S., & Fleiss, J. L. (1985). Psychotherapy during radiotherapy: Effects on emotional and physical distress. *American Journal of Psychiatry*, *142*, 22–27.

Fredrikson, M., & Matthews, K. A. (1990). Cardiovascular responses to behavioral stress and hypertension: A meta-analytic review. *Annals of Behavioral Medicine*, *12*, 30–39.

Gellert, G. A., Maxwell, R. M., & Siegel, B. S. (1993). Survival of breast cancer patients receiving adjunctive psychosocial support therapy: A 10-year follow-up study. *Journal of Clinical Oncology*, *11*, 66–69.

*Goldberg, R. J., & Wool, M. S. (1985). Psychotherapy for the spouses of lung cancer patients: Assessment of an intervention. *Psychotherapy and Psychosomatics*, *43*(3), 141–150.

*Goodwin, J. O. (1979). Programed instruction for self-care following pulmonary surgery. *International Journal of Nursing Studies*, *16*, 29–40.

Greer, S. (1987). Psychotherapy for the cancer patient. *Psychiatric Medicine*, *5*, 267–279.

*Greer, S., Moorey, S., Baruch, J. D. R., Watson, M., Robertson, B. M., Mason, A., Rowden, L., Law, M. G., & Bliss, J. M. (1992). Adjuvant psychological therapy for patients with cancer: A prospective randomised trial. *BMJ: British Medical Journal*, *304*, 675–680.

Grossarth-Maticek, R., & Eysenck, H. J. (1989). Length of survival and lymphocyte percentage in women with mammary cancer as a function of psychotherapy. *Psychological Reports*, *65*, 315–321.

Grossarth-Maticek, R., Schmidt, P., Vetter, H., & Arndt, S. (1984). Psychotherapy research in oncology. In A. Steptoe & A. Mathews (Eds.), *Health care and human behaviour* (pp. 325–341). New York: Academic Press.

Hedges, L. V., & Olkin, I. (1985). *Statistical methods for meta-analysis*. Orlando, FL: Academic Press.

Hunter, J. E., & Schmidt, F. L. (1990). *Methods of meta-analysis: Correcting error and bias in research findings*. Newbury Park, CA: Sage.

Hunter, J. E., Schmidt, F. L., & Jackson, G. B. (1982). *Meta-analysis: Cumulating research findings across studies*. Beverly Hills, CA: Sage.

*Jacobs, C., Ross, R. D., Walker, I. M., & Stockdale, F. E. (1983). Behavior of cancer patients: A randomized study of the effects of education and peer support groups. *American Journal of Clinical Oncology*, *6*, 347–353.

Johnson, B. T. (1989). *DSTAT: Software for the meta-analysis review of research literatures*. Hillsdale, NJ: Erlbaum.

*Johnson, J. (1982). The effects of a patient education course on persons with a chronic illness. *Cancer Nursing*, *5*(2), 117–123.

*Johnson, J. E., Nail, L. M., Lauver, D., King, K. B., & Keys, H. (1988). Reducing the negative impact of radiation therapy on functional status. *Cancer*, *61*, 46–51.

Lieberman, M. A. (1988). The role of self-help groups in helping patients and families cope with cancer. *CA: A Cancer Journal for Clinicians*, *38*(3), 162–168.

Light, R. J., & Pillemer, D. B. (1984). *Summing up: The science of reviewing research*. Cambridge, MA: Harvard University Press.

*Linn, M. W., Linn, B. S., & Harris, R. (1982). Effects of counseling for late stage cancer patients. *Cancer*, *49*, 1048–1055.

*Lyles, J. N., Burish, T. G., Krozely, M. G., & Oldham, R. K. (1982). Efficacy of relaxation training and guided imagery in reducing the aversiveness of cancer chemotherapy. *Journal of Consulting and Clinical Psychology, 50*, 509–524.

*Maguire, P., Brooke, M., Tait, A., Thomas, C., & Sellwood, R. (1983). The effect of counseling on physical disability and social recovery after mastectomy. *Clinical Oncology, 9*, 319–324.

Matt, G. E. (1989). Decision rules for selecting effect sizes in meta-analysis: A review and reanalysis of psychotherapy outcome studies. *Psychological Bulletin, 105*, 106–115.

Mazzuca, S. A. (1982). Does patient education in chronic disease have therapeutic value? *Journal of Chronic Diseases, 35*, 521–529.

Meyer, T. J. (1991). Meta-analysis of controlled studies of psychosocial interventions with adult cancer patients (Doctoral dissertation, Pennsylvania State University). *Dissertation Abstracts International, 52*, 4475B–4476B.

Meyer, T. J., & Mark, M. M. (1994). *The effects of psychosocial interventions with adult cancer patients: A meta-analysis of controlled studies.* Unpublished manuscript.

Morgenstern, H., Gellert, G. A., Walter, S. D., Ostfeld, A. M., & Siegel, B. S. (1984). The impact of a psychosocial support program on survival with breast cancer: The importance of selection bias in program evaluation. *Journal of Chronic Diseases, 37*, 273–282.

*Morrow, G. R., Asbury, R., Hammon, S., Dobkin, P., Caruso, L., Pandya, K., & Rosenthal, S. (1992). Comparing the effectiveness of behavioral treatment for chemotherapy-induced nausea and vomiting when administered by oncologists. oncology nurses, and clinical psychologists. *Health Psychology, 11*, 250–256.

*Morrow, G. R., & Morrell, C. (1982). Behavioral treatment for the anticipatory nausea and vomiting induced by cancer chemotherapy. *New England Journal of Medicine, 307*, 1476–1480.

Presby, S. (1978). Overly broad categories obscure important differences between therapies. *American Psychologist, 33*, 514–515.

Rimer, B., Keintz, M. K., & Glassman, B. (1985). Cancer patient education: Reality and potential. *Preventive Medicine, 14*, 801–818.

*Rimer, B., Levy, M. H., Keintz, M. K., Fox, L., Engstrom, P. F., & MacElwee, N. (1987). Enhancing cancer pain control regimens through patient education. *Patient Education and Counseling, 10*, 267–277.

*Roffman, R. A. (1986). Stress inoculation training in the control of THC toxicities. *International Journal of the Addictions, 21*, 883–896.

Rosenthal, R. (1984). *Meta-analytic procedures for social research.* Newbury Park, CA: Sage.

Rosenthal, R., & Rubin, D. B. (1982). A simple, general purpose display of magnitude of experimental effect. *Journal of Educational Psychology, 74*, 166–169.

Schag, C. C., Heinrich, R. L., & Ganz, P. A. (1983). Cancer Inventory of Problem Situations: An instrument for assessing cancer patients' rehabilitation needs. *Journal of Psychosocial Oncology, 1*, 11–24.

Shadish, W. R., & Montgomery, L. M. (1986). *Marital/family therapy meta-analysis coding manual* (Version 4.1). Unpublished manual.

Shapiro, D. A., & Shapiro, D. (1982). Meta-analysis of comparative therapy outcome studies: A replication and refinement. *Psychological Bulletin, 92*, 581–604.

*Shartner, C. D., Burish, T. G., & Carey, M. P. (1985). Effectiveness of biofeedback with progressive muscle relaxation training in reducing the aversiveness of cancer chemotherapy: A preliminary report. *Japanese Journal of Biofeedback Research, 12*, 33–40.

Smith, M. L., & Glass, G. V. (1977). Meta-analysis of psychotherapy outcome studies. *American Psychologist, 32*, 752–760.

Smith, M. L., Glass, G. V., & Miller, T. I. (1980). *The benefits of psychotherapy.* Baltimore: Johns Hopkins University Press.

*Spiegel, D., & Bloom, J. R. (1983). Group therapy and hypnosis reduce metastatic breast carcinoma pain. *Psychosomatic Medicine, 45*, 333–339.

Spiegel, D., Bloom, J. R., Kraemer, H. C., & Gottheil, E. (1989). Effect of psychosocial treatment on survival of patients with metastatic breast cancer. *Lancet*, 888–891.

*Syrjala, K. L., Cummings, C., & Donaldson, G. W. (1992). Hypnosis or cognitive behavioral training for the reduction of pain and nausea during cancer treatment: A controlled clinical trial. *Pain*, *48*, 137–146.

*Telch, C. F., & Telch, M. J. (1986). Group coping skills instruction and supportive group therapy for cancer patients: A comparison of strategies. *Journal of Consulting and Clinical Psychology*, *54*, 802–808.

Trijsburg, R. W., van Knippenberg, F. C. E., & Rijpma, S. E. (1992). Effects of psychological treatment on cancer patients: A critical review. *Psychosomatic Medicine*, *54*, 489–517.

Vachon, M. L. S. (1988). Counseling and psychotherapy in palliative/hospice care: A review. *Palliative Medicine*, *2*, 36–50.

Van der Ploeg, H. M. (1991). What a wonderful world it would be: A reanalysis of some of the work of Grossarth-Maticek. *Psychological Inquiry*, *2*, 280–285.

*Vasterling, J., Jenkins, R. A., Tope, D. M., & Burish, T. G. (1993). Cognitive distraction and relaxation training for the control of side effects due to cancer chemotherapy. *Journal of Behavioral Medicine*, *16*, 65–80.

Vetter, H. (1991). Some observations on Grossarth-Maticek's database. *Psychological Inquiry*, *2*, 286–287.

Watson, M. (1983). Psychosocial intervention with cancer patients: A review. *Psychological Medicine*, *13*, 839–846.

Watson, M. (1986). Results of supportive therapy, In B. A. Stoll (Ed.), *Coping with cancer stress* (pp. 123–129). Dordrecht, The Netherlands: Martinus Nijhoff.

Watson, M., & Marvell, C. (1992). Anticipatory nausea and vomiting among cancer patients: A review. *Psychology and Health*, *6*, 97–106.

*Weintraub, F. N., & Hagopian, G. A. (1990). The effect of nursing consultation on anxiety, side effects, and self-care of patients receiving radiation therapy. *Oncology Nursing Forum*, *17*(3, Suppl.), 31–38.

Worden, J. W., & Weisman, A. D. (1980). Do cancer patients really want counseling? *General Hospital Psychiatry*, *2*, 100–103.

*Zimmerman, L., Pozehl, B., Duncan, K., & Schmitz, R. (1989). Effects of music in patients who had chronic cancer pain. *Western Journal of Nursing Research*, *11*, 298–309.

Chapter 8
ETHNICITY AND CANCER OUTCOMES:
Behavioral and Psychosocial Considerations

Beth E. Meyerowitz, Jean Richardson, Sharon Hudson, and Beth Leedham

Cancer is the second leading cause of death in the United States (National Center for Health Statistics, 1993). The American Cancer Society estimates that one in three Americans alive today will be diagnosed with cancer at some point during their lives. With over 8 million Americans currently living with or surviving cancer (American Cancer Society, 1995), it clearly is a major public health concern.

Although many studies examine behavioral and psychosocial factors relevant to how people survive cancer and the quality of that survival (e.g., see Holland & Rowland, 1989), the focus of this literature has been almost entirely on non-Hispanic Whites. The extent to which findings can be generalized beyond the majority population is unknown. This lack of information is particularly unfortunate in light of rapidly increasing ethnic diversity within the United States and the high cancer rates within some ethnic groups.

Our goal in this review is threefold. First, we propose a framework to organize and summarize what is known about the links between ethnicity and two general cancer-related outcomes—adherence behaviors and responses to cancer and its treatments, including both survival and quality of life. Second, we consider socioeconomic, knowledge–attitudinal, and medical system–patient interaction variables that might mediate the relation between ethnicity and these outcomes. Finally, we identify gaps in the literature that may be especially useful to explore in future research. In each of these areas—outcomes, mediators, and recommendations—we draw on three distinct literatures from public health and psychology. Despite apparent connections, the literatures on screening–follow-up behaviors, survival, and quality of life–coping are not well integrated and are inconsistent in their coverage of issues related to ethnicity. Before presenting the framework, we discuss difficulties inherent in studying ethnicity in these literatures.

Studying Ethnic Diversity and Cancer

The 1990 U.S. Census describes the United States population of 249 million, using their labels, as 71.3% non-Hispanic White, 9.0% Hispanic, 12.1% Black, 2.9% Asian/Pacific Islander, 0.8% Native American, and 4.0% "other race." Between 1980 and 1990, the Asian/Pacific Islander population increased by 108%, the Hispanic population by 53%, the Native American population by 38%, the Black population by 13%, and the non-Hispanic White population by only about 7% (U.S. Bureau of the Census, 1990a). Notwithstanding that there may have been an undercount of various

Reprinted from *Psychological Bulletin, 123*(1), 47–70. (1998). Copyright © 1998 by the American Psychological Association. Used with permission of the author.

The writing of this article was supported, in part, by American Cancer Society Grant SIG20.

immigrant and other groups, the growth in ethnic minority populations is remarkable. Clearly, information relevant to these populations is essential. Yet, understanding the role that ethnicity and race play in the behavioral and psychosocial aspects of cancer is complex and difficult for at least three reasons, which we discuss below.

The Complexity of Ethnic Diversity

Ethnicity is a complex and imprecise term that is difficult to operationalize. General ethnic groupings belie the diversity that exists within these groups; many countries of origin and languages are represented within each. Approximately 30 countries of origin for Latinos and 43 for Asian/Pacific Islanders were identified in the 1990 U.S. Census. Over 100 different languages and dialects have been identified for Asian/ Pacific Islanders, and over 200 distinct languages have been identified for Native Americans (Scott & Suagee, 1992). Most of the African American population has been in the United States for generations, but there are several recent immigrant groups from the Caribbean who speak English, Spanish, or French. The White population is also far from homogeneous, with new arrivals coming primarily from Eastern Europe and the Middle East. There are many Americans who are of mixed race or ethnicity but who are categorized into one ethnic group based on surname, self-identification, or other characteristics.

In addition to country of origin and language, generation of immigration may convey information about religion, health care practices, food consumption, and other beliefs and behaviors that may have significant implications for health. The historical conditions of immigration—slave, political refugee, opportunity seeker—may also have importance.

This within-group heterogeneity makes it very difficult to form ethnic categorizations that identify distinct, homogeneous groupings.[1] For example, a recent refugee from El Salvador may share little in common with a third-generation Spanish American, both of whom are likely to be categorized as Latino/Hispanic on the basis of Spanish surnames. Furthermore, ethnic populations are not uniformly distributed within the United States. California's Latinos are primarily of Mexican origin (79.6%), Florida's are largely Cuban (49.1%), and New York's are largely Puerto Rican (49.1%; U.S. Bureau of the Census, 1990b). Thus, studies of Latinos in different parts of the country may be describing individuals with different national and

[1]In addition to the problems with identifying homogeneous ethnic groupings, it is difficult to settle on appropriate labels. Name designation is inherently political and carries with it implications far beyond simple identification. In this article, we have attempted to use the terminology that currently appears to be preferred by a majority of individuals for self-identification. We recognize that these terms are flawed and will likely evolve to new labels in time. When precise information about national origin or immigrant status was not provided, we used the following terms. (a) *African American* refers to Blacks living in the United States, regardless of whether they hold American citizenship. To our knowledge, the vast majority of such participants in these studies have been African Americans rather than Caribbean Islanders, for example. (b) *Latino* refers to persons of Mexican, Central American, and South American heritage, including descendants of both Spanish and indigenous peoples in these countries. This term also refers to individuals from Spanish-speaking Caribbean islands, such as Cuba and Puerto Rico. (c) *Asian American* refers to individuals who immigrated from, or whose ancestors immigrated from, Asia, Southeast Asia, or the Pacific Island countries. (d) *White* refers to non-Hispanic Whites. This term is rarely defined in the literature but appears to include a variety of ethnicities, except those listed above.

cultural origins. Similarly, ethnic designations give little attention to the fact that the socioeconomic status (SES) within ethnic groups is not homogeneous. Wilson (1987) carefully described the deep divisions between the life experiences and expectations of a large African American upper and middle class that has professional education and access to services and societal institutions and a smaller but substantial African American population that has been trapped in inner cities. This latter group, which Wilson termed *the truly disadvantaged*, has high unemployment rates, poor education, little opportunity, and disrupted family composition.

The Heterogeneity of Cancers Across Ethnic and Racial Groups

Appendixes A and B provide information from the National Cancer Institute's (NCI) Surveillance, Epidemiology, and End Results (SEER; Miller et al., 1996) Program concerning differences between non-Hispanic Whites, Latinos, African Americans, Asian Americans, and Native Americans in the incidence and mortality rates of common cancers (for a description of the NCI SEER national cancer registry, see Miller et al., 1993). Several important differences emerge. For example, African Americans have the highest incidence rates for cancer overall, accounted for largely by high rates of lung and prostate cancer among men. The mortality rates for African Americans also are higher than for Whites. For example, despite the lower breast cancer incidence rates for African American versus White women, the breast cancer mortality rates are nearly equivalent due to lower 5-year survival rates among African Americans (Miller et al., 1993). Latinos have a relatively low rate of cancer in general, with the exception of high rates of cervical cancer. Asian groups have low incidence rates of all cancers except stomach cancer. The 5-year survival rates are highest among Japanese with cancer. Native Hawaiians have very high rates of cancer, while Native Americans have low rates. Thus, consideration of ethnicity and cancer may differ by the anatomical site of the disease, the prognosis for the disease, and the treatments received. This situation makes it difficult to study ethnicity and cancer without introducing confounds.

Further problems in understanding cancer incidence and survival rates arise when measurement issues, such as those described earlier, are considered. Federal directives stipulate that federal agencies must collect and present data on at least four racial groups (American Indian or Alaska Native, Asian/Pacific Islander, Black, and White) and one ethnic group (Hispanic). On the 1990 U.S. Census, respondents were asked to report the one race with which they most closely identified and all persons were asked whether they identified as Hispanic (McKenney & Bennett, 1994). These census data provide the denominator for cancer incidence and mortality rates. Unfortunately, the validity of health statistics derived from these racial–ethnic groups is based on several faulty assumptions, including (a) the categories of race and ethnicity are consistently defined and ascertained and (b) the categories are understood by the populations questioned. Two examples of the problems with the assumptions of consistency and understanding are noteworthy. First, of the 10 million people who self-reported as "other race," 98% identified themselves as "Hispanic," indicating that they misinterpreted the subtle distinction intended between race and ethnicity. Second, the assignment of race–ethnicity at time of death was misclassified for 0.5% of Whites and 1.0% of African Americans. However, 21.0% of Asians and

23.7% of Native Americans were misclassified, most often as White. In the event of missing reports of race from next of kin, the mortician or a computer algorithm assigned race (i.e., not a person who knew the deceased or his or her appearance before the ravages of cancer; Hahn, 1992). Thus, the cancer mortality statistics on which researchers rely include cases misclassified on race–ethnicity.

The assignment to one of four racial groups in obtaining cancer statistics rests on the assumption that the four categories are naturally occurring, mutually exclusive, and not arbitrary. However, the study of human genetics does not provide evidence that there are four distinct racial groups. In fact, the differences within racial groups can be larger than the differences between groups (Yu, 1993). What is measured as "race" in public health surveillance is not a biological characteristic but rather a self-perception for which phenotypic characteristics may be one among many criteria (Hahn & Stroup, 1994). Skin color, in particular, commonly serves as a surrogate for race in this country, excluding consideration of culture, biology, values, or behavior (LaVeist, 1994). Biological notions of race may be confused with cultural and behavioral notions of "ethnicity" (Hahn, 1992). We suggest that culture and behavior may have greater explanatory value and greater construct validity than potentially unreliable measures of racial or ethnic categorization.[2]

The Atheoretical Basis of Ethnicity

Ethnicity is an atheoretical construct that provides little information to help us understand and explain phenomena. Even if individuals could be categorized into appropriate and homogeneous ethnic groupings, this is insufficient to develop useful predictive models. The role of ethnicity may be best understood by considering the mediating variables through which it has its impact—such as socioeconomic indicators that may influence access to care and attitudinal indicators that may influence access to care and attitudinal indicators that may influence willingness to obtain care —which may have more direct relations to cancer-related outcomes. Exploring possible explanatory variables allows for consideration of areas of intragroup differences and intergroup similarities, thereby decreasing the risk of overgeneralization and stereotyping.

Reliance on ethnicity as an analytic tool often leads to simplistic, misleading, or inappropriate conclusions unless the broader social and political implications of intergroup relations are considered (Wilkinson & King, 1987). Within health services research, the classification of people into racial or ethnic groups becomes meaningful only when the classification leads to a better understanding of the factors that have lead to disparity in disease treatment and health outcome (Schulman, Rubenstein, Chesley, & Eisenberg, 1995). Thus, it is not possible to examine the issues of ethnic influence on health without examining such issues as culture, economics, and racism.

---

[2]We do not argue that race is irrelevant to cancer outcomes. Scientists do not know yet how genetics relate to differences in cancer incidence between ethnic groups, but we suspect that important differences may emerge. For example, recent articles show a higher prevalence of the BRCA1 gene among Ashkenazi Jewish women (Struewing et al., 1995), suggesting that at least the prevalence of certain markers for breast cancer may differ among ethnic groups. Thus, we do not claim that there is no relationship between racial–ethnic categories and genetic characteristics of importance to understanding cancer. Rather, we suggest that these differences have little relevance or usefulness as psychosocial constructs.

Ethnicity as a Psychological Construct

Unfortunately, the health psychology literature, similar to the public health literature, tends to use ethnicity as a biological category or as a proxy for other variables, such as poverty. Reference to the multicultural mental health literature, which is rarely consulted in the literature on cancer and ethnicity, provides a more meaningful conceptualization. Phinney (1996) suggested ethnicity is composed of three components, culture, ethnic identity, and minority status. These aspects of ethnicity, which are overlapping and multidimensional, allow for the measurement of ethnicity along psychologically meaningful continua. Many of the difficulties associated with studying ethnicity can be avoided when it is conceptualized as a multidimensional, psychological construct rather than as a set of discrete categories. Such a conceptualization allows for full inclusion of people who are of mixed race or ethnicity. It also provides far more promise for understanding cancer outcomes than when ethnicity is viewed as a demographic category.

Culture

Phinney (1996) defined culture as "the norms, values, attitudes, and behaviors that are typical of an ethnic group and that stem from a common culture of origin transmitted through generations" (p. 920). It is likely that these cultural influences have an impact on thoughts and feelings about health care, illness, and cancer. Therefore, it is important to identify relevant and measurable components of culture while avoiding common pitfalls. First, researchers must avoid simply replacing ethnic labels with overgeneralized and oversimplified cultural labels (i.e., people from Group x believe y). As with ethnic labels, such an approach blurs important within-group differences and between-group similarities and risks reducing meaningful cultural attributes to stereotypes. Second, identifying components of ethnic cultures is useful only insofar as cultural attributes can be associated in a conceptually meaningful way to cancer outcomes. Meeting this goal requires recognizing that the nature of the relations between cultural variables and cancer outcomes may differ by ethnicity and within ethnicity by nationality (Vega, 1992), raising the further question of what mediates these relations. Vega (1992) suggested that

> the notion that psychological traits have identical cognitive presentation and behavioral sequelae in all cultural groups is more an article of faith than demonstrated fact .... Perhaps it is more precise to declare constructs to be culture specific or at least to have culture specific expressions since they involve belief systems, culturally sanctioned behavior and culturally conditioned cognitive processes. (p. 380)

Finally, any model of cultural influences on cancer outcomes will need to be flexible and developmental. Culture is not static at either the group or the individual level (Vega, 1992). Native-born Americans are constantly exposed to new cultural influences, and immigrants face the potential burdens of social incorporation and cultural adaptation.

Ethnic Identity

Ethnic identity refers to the extent to which an individual experiences a sense of belongingness and commitment in relation to a culture (or cultures) that he or she views as salient and important in daily life. Ethnic identity is rarely studied directly in health psychology research. However, a few studies do assess acculturation, which is sometimes operationalized to include aspects of both culture and ethnic identity. Most current conceptualizations of acculturation do not describe it as unidimensional or linear but rather allow for the possibility of biculturalism (LaFromboise, Coleman, & Gerton, 1993). Thus, individuals can operate effectively in a new culture without relinquishing their native ethnic identity (Szapocznik & Kurtines, 1993). La-Fromboise et al. described an "alternation model" of acculturation, whereby individuals can move back and forth from their native culture to the majority culture. They proposed that bicultural competence leads to better psychological outcomes by allowing individuals to maintain multiple ethnic identities and, thus, to adapt their responses to the demands of specific situations.

Research on the impact of acculturation and of maintaining ethnic identity has yielded inconsistent findings (Rogler, Cortes, & Malgady, 1991). Berry and Kim (1988) suggested that acculturation can have both positive and negative effects on health and mental health outcomes through physical, biological, cultural, and psychological changes. The process of acculturation is unlikely to proceed in a uniform manner. Specific values, beliefs, and attitudes will change at different times and rates, and some will not change at all. Moreover, the impact of changes is impossible to understand without considering the economic and psychosocial context in which changes occur. Adopting a mainstream ethnic identity, for example, may be problematic if it conflicts with the values of other family members (Szapocznik & Kurtines, 1993) or if it serves to highlight barriers to meeting important expectations for acculturation, such as economic advancement (Rogler et al., 1991). The discrepancy between expected and actual outcomes may become increasingly apparent, and increasingly disturbing, with greater acculturation, perhaps especially when departure status from the country of origin is higher than entry status in the United States. Additionally, accurate measurement of the impact of changes on mental health outcomes resulting from acculturation is difficult because with acculturation individuals change the way that they express psychological distress (Rogler et al., 1991).

When studying the specific relation of acculturation and ethnic identity to cancer outcomes, two questions merit consideration. First, To what extent has the individual and his or her family acculturated to Western medical culture? Even patients who identify fully with mainstream, White, American culture may feel that they are in a foreign environment when they are forced to enter the medical system. Second, To what extent have the medical caregivers developed bicultural competence? Successful acculturation to the medical system does not require giving up one's ethnic identity, but ethnicity can only be fully integrated into ongoing care with a sensitive and culturally aware medical team.

Minority Status

Minority status involves two components: (a) that one's culture and ethnic identity may be unfamiliar to many people and (b) the discrimination and prejudice that can accompany ethnic minority status for people of color in the United States. Although researchers do not know the specific mechanisms by which discrimination and prejudice affect health (Williams, Lavizzo-Mourey, & Warren, 1994), a full understanding of the relation between ethnicity and cancer outcomes requires their consideration. Minority status could influence cancer outcomes at many levels, including access to educational and economic resources, availability of care, quality of care, attitudes toward doctors and treatment, and physician and patient behavior. Cancer is primarily a disease of aging; therefore, most minority cancer patients have had a lifetime of exposure to these influences.

Moreover, because scientists are not immune from prejudice, research itself may be biased. For example, Osborne and Feit (1992) concluded that "a review of the English-language medical literature reveals that there is a predilection for making comparisons between black and white patients, particularly with diseases associated with promiscuity, underachievement, and antisocial behavior" (p. 275). They suggested that racism and an emphasis on racial categorization may promote these biases and, thus, restrict the focus and content of research.

Ethnicity and Cancer Outcomes: An Organizational Framework

In Figure 1, we propose a simple framework for structuring the literature on psychosocial and behavioral aspects of cancer and ethnicity and for identifying areas in need of further study. The framework pertains only to variables that may be relevant

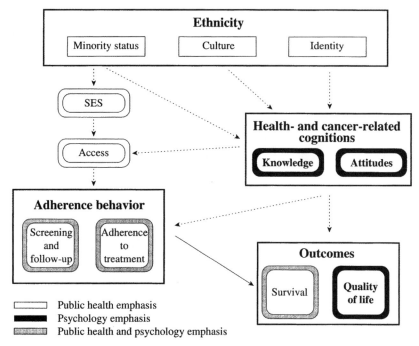

Figure 1. Proposed mediational framework linking ethnicity to cancer outcomes. SES = socioeconomic status.

to cancer outcomes after an individual has developed the disease; we make no attempt to include factors related to cancer onset. Primary outcomes of interest for patients with cancer are length of survival and quality of life. Behaviors that minimize the time between the appearance of cancer and the start of treatment, specifically, obtaining cancer-related screening and following up on suspicious symptoms, are important intermediate outcomes because they can improve survival and quality of life. Similarly, adherence to cancer treatment can influence cancer outcomes. The framework is designed to illuminate the relation between ethnicity and these three outcomes—adherence behaviors, survival, and quality of life.

Information about differences among ethnic groups in cancer outcomes alone is not sufficient to understand how or why these differences exist or to develop appropriate interventions. We present two general categories of variables that may mediate differences in cancer outcomes among ethnic groups, SES and knowledge of and attitudes toward cancer detection, and treatment. These mediating variables, in turn, may influence the extent to which the patient has access to adequate medical care. In this framework, adequate medical care refers both to treatment per se and to the nature of the relationship between physicians and patients. Finally, access to care may contribute to the patient's ability and willingness to adhere to medical recommendations for the diagnosis and treatment of cancer.

This framework is not meant to be a comprehensive predictive model. The arrows in Figure 1 denote relations that might be of primary interest to psychologists studying psychosocial and behavioral aspects of cancer outcomes. Other relations, although important in understanding cancer outcomes, have not been included. For example, an arrow from SES to survival would be necessary to take into account the general effects of poverty on health, and an arrow directly from minority status to access could indicate racist reactions of doctors to middle-class patients of color. We focus on patient behaviors and cognitions, not because all predictors of survival and quality of life are mediated through patient responses but because the current focus of the psychosocial oncology literature is on these variables as proximal concerns. Moreover, the entire framework must be considered in the context of other individual difference variables, such as personality, biology, and social functioning, and of larger sociological and economic issues, such as class and the politics of health care delivery.

We have not attempted to provide an exhaustive review of all of the literature relevant to the outcomes of interest. We focus on key studies that deal directly with ethnicity and cancer among adults in the United States. This research is contained in three distinct and virtually unrelated literatures, each of which deals with one of the cancer outcomes. Although the outcomes are studied in both the psychology and public health literatures, the focus of the research tends to differ by discipline, as depicted in Figure 1. Unfortunately, it is not common for studies in either discipline to move beyond using ethnicity as a demographic category. We suggest that an interdisciplinary approach in which ethnicity is viewed as a multidimensional, psychological construct is more likely to yield meaningful results.

Cancer Screening and Follow-Up

Cancer screening is intended to detect cancers at the earliest stage possible when the chances for successful treatment are greatest. Although screening tests are available to identify several different types of cancer, including breast, cervix, lung, colon, prostate, and testicular, the screening literature focuses primarily on screening for breast and cervical cancers. Our discussion of screening also considers follow-up because screening tests are only useful if patients seek treatment for positive or suspicious findings.

Ethnic Differences in Screening Behavior

Much of the research on cancer screening has focused on non-Hispanic White populations. There is a growing literature on African Americans and Latinos, and almost no published research on screening in Asian Americans or Native Americans. The most comprehensive source of data on rates of cancer screening among White, African American, and Latina women is through several large, national studies. National Health Interview Surveys (NHIS), conducted in 1987 and 1990, used personal household interviews with nationwide samples of the civilian population of the United States. These surveys included tens of thousands of respondents and had response rates exceeding 76%. The 1986 Access to Care Study used a nationwide telephone survey of over 4,500 people to assess rates of cervical and breast cancer screening.

The nature of the relation between ethnicity and screening for cervical and breast cancers appears to depend on the screening technique in question. Only in the case of Pap screening for cervical cancer does there seem to be a consistent relation between screening and ethnicity. For breast cancer screening—mammography, clinical breast examinations, and breast self-examination (BSE)—the results are mixed.

Three national studies have demonstrated that even after controlling for such factors as martial status, income, education, and age, African American women were significantly more likely to report having had a Pap smear in the past year than White women (Calle, Flanders, Thun, & Martin, 1993; Duelberg, 1992; Hayward, Shapiro, Freeman, & Corey, 1988). One of these studies also found that Latina women were significantly less likely than African Americans or Whites to report ever having had a Pap smear (Calle et al., 1993). A fourth study found that in bivariate analyses, African Americans were significantly more likely than Whites to have had a Pap smear within the past 3 years, and both groups were significantly more likely to have been screened than Latinas (Harlan, Bernstein, & Kessler, 1991). Multivariate analyses did not include ethnicity. Rather, researchers included a variable identifying the primary language spoken, which makes it impossible to distinguish ethnicity from acculturation fully. After controlling for age and two variables that may be associated with ethnicity, education and usual source of care, women who spoke Spanish as their primary language were significantly less likely to have received a Pap smear within the past 3 years than English-speaking women.

In general, these studies suggest that the direct, independent effect of race is small to moderate in size. For example, in the Calle et al. (1993) report, the adjusted odds ratio for never having had a Pap smear was 1.0 for Whites, 0.8 for African Americans (95% confidence interval [CI] = 0.6–1.0), and 3.2 for Latinas (95% CI = 2.3–4.5). Hayward et al. (1988) demonstrated a stronger effect for race in their comparison of African American and White women. After controlling for age, health insurance, income, education, and whether women were in the labor force, these investigators found that African Americans were 1.5 times as likely as Whites to have received a Pap smear within the recommended 3–5-year period. Race accounted for 2.7% of the variance in the model.

Three studies of national data also have been used to examine the relation between race–ethnicity and breast cancer screening. Hayward et al. (1988) analyzed data from the 1986 Access to Care Survey and found that urban residence, younger age, more education, poorer health status, and health insurance membership were significant multivariate predictors of mammography whereas neither ethnicity nor income was significant. Calle et al. (1993) focused on data collected in the 1987 NHIS. Their results showed that after adjusting for age, income, education, and other factors, there were no significant differences between African Americans and Whites on mammography use in the past year. Latinas were significantly less likely than the other two groups to report ever having had a mammogram; a greater percentage of Latinas also reported not having had a mammogram in the past year, although this difference did not reach significance. In the multivariate models, income remained a strong predictor of mammography, except at the lowest income levels. Although initial reports from the 1987 NHIS appeared to show differences in screening by ethnicity, this finding did not persist in 1990 nor did it hold up under further analysis (Rakowski, Rimer, & Bryant, 1993). Furthermore, the effect size of the significant relationship was small. After adjusting for several factors, including age, income, and education, the odds of never having had a mammogram were 1.0 for Whites, 1.0 for African Americans (95% CI = 0.8–1.2) and 1.4 for Latinas (95% CI = 1.1–1.9). Breen and Kessler (1994) compared data from the 1987 NHIS and the 1990 NHIS. After controlling for income and education, there were no significant differences by race–ethnicity at either time point.

These national data confirm the results of some smaller studies that also failed to demonstrate a significant relation between race–ethnicity and participation in mammography screening (Douglas, Bartolucci, Waterbor, & Sirles, 1995; Fink & Shapiro, 1990; Perez-Stable, Sabogal, & Otero-Sabogal, 1995; Vogel, Graves, Coody, Winn, & Peters, 1990). A number of other studies, however, have shown Whites to be significantly more likely to be screened (Kaplan, Weinberg, Small, & Herndon, 1991; Lackland, Dunbar, Keil, Knapp, & O'Brien, 1991; Rimer, Keintz, Kessler, Engstrom, & Rosan, 1989; Vernon et al., 1992). Most studies suggest that other variables, such as income and education, mediate the bivariate relation found between race–ethnicity and mammography. A few studies suggest direct, independent associations with both ethnicity and income, particularly among older women (Burns et al., 1996; Calle et al., 1993; Rimer et al., 1989; Stein, Fox, & Murata, 1991).

The three national studies examining the relation between ethnicity and clinical breast exams produced conflicting results. Duelberg's (1992) analysis of the 1985 NHIS data found race to be a significant bivariate predictor of having had a breast exam: African American women were more likely to report having had an exam than were White women. When the researcher controlled for urban residence, age, martial status, education, and income, race remained significant and even had a stronger relationship. Breen and Kessler's (1994) report of the 1987 and 1990 NHIS results showed that in both years, larger percentages of African Americans than Whites or Latinas reported having had a clinical breast exam. They did not state whether these analyses included such variables as income or education or whether the results were statistically significant. The 1986 Access to Care Survey data indicated that those with lower incomes and no health insurance were less likely to get physician breast exams. Ethnicity was not a significant predictor in the multivariate model (Hayward et al., 1988).

At least one study failed to support an independent relation between ethnicity and BSE (Fletcher, Morgan, O'Malley, Earp, & Degnan, 1989). A second study (Kaplan et al., 1991) found that Whites reported doing BSE more frequently than non-Whites but failed to report if this result was statistically significant.

The results of these studies are difficult to reconcile entirely with differences in cancer diagnosis and survival data. The less frequent Pap screening reported by Latina women is consistent with their higher rates of cervical cancer. However, although the SEER data clearly show a later stage of disease diagnosis among African American women with breast cancer, there is little evidence to suggest that they are screened less often. These reports are from large national studies and are difficult to dismiss. Several possibilities may help to explain these seemingly conflicting findings. It may be that many of the public programs designed to increase access to screening among low-income and minority populations had indeed been successful, but consequent differences in stage of diagnosis and survival were yet to emerge. It may also be that minority or low-income women interviewed in these national studies are a biased sample of women who were more interested in cancer screening, had homes and telephones to allow researchers to solicit their participation, and were willing to be interviewed. Women residing in dangerous neighborhoods, such as those whom Wilson (1987) described as truly disadvantaged, may have been less likely to have been interviewed. Assuming that questions were asked in a way that was clear to participants and that they answered accurately, we suggest that some of the problem of late stage diagnosis may be related to lack of response to warning signs of cancer, delay in responding to positive test results, or system overload resulting in delay of work up or treatment.

Ethnic Differences in Follow-Up of Abnormal Findings

Research has documented the relation between delay in seeking treatment after symptoms appear and later stage at diagnosis (Richardson et al., 1992). However, little is known about ethnic differences in delay. Some data suggest that after symptoms are identified, African Americans (Weissman, Stern, Fielding, & Epstein, 1991) and Latinos may be at risk for delaying medical care, even controlling for SES (Richardson et al., 1987), comorbidity, social support, other health practices, and access to care (Coates et al., 1992). For example, Mandelblatt et al. (1993) found that in a sample of older African American women in New York City (New York), 27% of women who were referred for further evaluation following an abnormal mammogram or clinical breast exam declined to follow-up. However, in interviews with African American and White women diagnosed with invasive breast cancer, Coates et al. found that African American women were far more likely to have advanced disease at diagnosis, but the median time between symptom recognition and medical consultation was only slightly longer for African American women (16 days) than for White women (14 days). Adjustment for other characteristics predictive of the length of this interval had little effect on racial differences. Similarly, Lauver (1994) found no differences between White and African American women on the number of days between detecting breast cancer symptoms and seeking care.

Little is known about ethnic differences in time to follow up in response to abnormal findings on cancer screening tests. There are a few studies that have focused on follow-up after abnormal Pap smears, but little research exists on other tests. Reports of adherence to abnormal Pap screening follow-up range from as low as 43% (Lerman et al., 1992) to 85% (Lauver, Barsevick, & Rubin, 1990). The majority of follow-up studies have found that adherence does not differ significantly by race (Laedtke & Dignan, 1992; Lerman et al., 1992; Michielutte, Diseker, Young, & May, 1985; Paskett, Carter, Chu, & White, 1990). Marcus et al. (1992) found that in bivariate analyses, African Americans and Latinos were less likely to comply with follow-up than were Whites; however, no significant differences were found after controlling for age, type of treatment facility (county vs. noncounty clinic), and severity of Pap results.

As was the case with screening, these data indicate no direct path from ethnicity to follow-up. In both cases, patterns may vary somewhat across screening behaviors. However, even when significant relations between ethnicity and behavior are found, they are rarely maintained when other variables are controlled in multivariate analyses. The results of these multivariate analyses indicate, as suggested earlier, that mediating variables may prove to be more useful predictors than ethnicity, per se.

Possible Mediating Variables

Socioeconomic status.   In most studies, SES is defined narrowly, often as income level. Income differs among ethnic groups in the United states, with 7.0% of Whites falling below the poverty level, 26.3% of African Americans, 22.3% of Latinos, 11.6% of Asian/Pacific Islanders, and 27.0% of Native Americans (U.S. Bureau of the Census, 1990a). In addition to the link with ethnicity, there appears to be an association between SES and cancer screening. Most studies of the association between income and mammography have shown a significant positive relationship (Bloom, Hayes, Saunders, & Flatt, 1987; Calle et al., 1993; Fox, Murata, & Stein, 1991; Kaplan et al., 1991; Lackland et al., 1991; Stein et al., 1991; Suarez, 1994; Vernon et al., 1992). Investigation of income and Pap screening has produced less consistent results. Hayward et al. (1988) and Suarez found income related positively to Pap smears; Spurlock, Nadel, and McMannon (1992), in contrast, found a negative association for women over age 60, and Peters, Bear, and Thomas (1989) and Sawyer, Earp, Fletcher, Daye, and Wynn (1990) found no association. Because ethnicity and income covary, the inclusion of both in a multivariate model may contribute to the lack of significance of one or the other.

A potential explanation for the relation between income and screening behavior may lie in the costs of the tests. Cost is frequently examined as a potential structural barrier in studies of mammography usage and to a lesser degree in studies of Pap screening. The cost of mammography is often cited as one of the most important barriers to screening for women of all ethnicities (Bastani, Marcus, & Hollatz-Brown, 1991; Frazier & Cummings, 1990; Vernon et al., 1992). At least one study of Pap screening behavior also asked participants about cost. Of those who had not been screened, cost was the most frequently cited barrier (Dietrich et al., 1989).

In addition to the direct costs of the screening tests, other associated costs may play a role. For example, a study of a large, multi-ethnic sample in Los Angeles (California) demonstrated that transportation incentives were the only intervention that significantly increased follow-up for abnormal Pap results among low SES women (Marcus et al., 1992). Similarly, among Mexican Americans, one third encountered significant income-related instrumental barriers (e.g., transportation, child care) the last time they sought medical care (Estrada, Treviño, & Ray, 1990).

Costs alone, however, may not fully explain the income–screening behavior relation. Engaging in BSE incurs no direct costs, but it also has been shown to be positively associated with income in some studies (Hayward et al., 1988; Jacob, Penn, & Brown, 1989; Nemcek, 1989), although others have not confirmed this finding (Fletcher et al., 1989; Kaplan et al., 1991; Lackland et al., 1991).

Knowledge and attitudes. Knowledge of screening procedures typically precedes screening, and knowledge of disease warning signs or symptoms is a necessary cue to seeking health care for those symptoms. Descriptive studies document a discouraging lack of accurate information about cancer among Latinos (Garcia & Lee, 1988; Perez-Stable, Sabogal, Otero-Sabogal, Hiatt, & McPhee, 1992), Asians (Garcia & Lee, 1988; Jenkins, McPhee, Bird, & Bonilla, 1990; Pham & McPhee, 1992), and African Americans (Manfredi, Warnecke, Graham, & Rosenthal, 1977; Price, Colvin, & Smith, 1993; Price, Desmond, Wallace, Smith, & Stewart, 1988a). The knowledge deficits appear to be greater among non-Whites than Whites across content areas, from general knowledge about cancer risk and symptoms (Coreil, 1984; Cotugna, Subar, Heimendinger, & Kahle, 1992; Price, Desmond, Wallace, Smith, & Stewart, 1988b) to specific knowledge about breast cancer (Caplan, Wells, & Haynes, 1992; Pham & McPhee, 1992), prostate cancer (Demark-Wahnefried et al., 1995), and testicular self-exams (Vaz, Best, & Davis, 1988). Although measures and data analysis procedures vary, existing data reliably demonstrate moderate-sized differences in knowledge, with the likelihood of accurate knowledge being up to 20% higher for Whites than African Americans, for example (e.g., Michielutte & Diseker, 1982).

Multivariate studies have yielded similar results. Two small studies have shown that Whites had higher levels of knowledge with regard to cancer (Robinson, Kessler, & Naughton, 1991) and could name more warning signs and types of cancer treatments than African Americans (Michielutte & Diseker, 1982). In a larger study, African Americans and Latinos scored lower on knowledge than Whites and Asians (Stone & Siegel, 1986). In a large sample of Latino and White health maintenance organization (HMO) subscribers, Latino ethnicity and low acculturation were significantly associated with more misinformation about cancer (Perez-Stable et al., 1992). All four of these studies controlled for potential confounds, such as education, gender, and age.

Research rarely connects knowledge to other variables of more urgent interest, such as health behavior, early diagnosis, or care received. In the studies that do, familiarity with Pap screening and belief in the value of early detection have been found to relate positively to adherence to screening and follow-up recommendations (Harlan et al., 1991; Mamon et al., 1990; Mandelblatt, Traxler, Lakin, Kanetsky, & Kao, 1992; Paskett et al., 1990; Peters et al., 1989). Knowledge of Pap smears has been shown to differ significantly by ethnicity. More Latinas than African Americans or Whites have never heard of Pap smears, and fewer African Americans and Latinas than Whites know how often Pap smears should be obtained (Harlan et al., 1991). Knowledge also has been demonstrated to have significant associations with performance of BSEs (Fletcher et al., 1989; Nemcek, 1989). Similarly, knowledge of breast cancer and mammography has consistently been associated with screening for all ethnicities (Bastani et al., 1991; Champion, 1992; Fox et al., 1991; Mandelblatt et al., 1992). However, the link between ethnic differences in knowledge and screening behavior has not been as convincingly made. In one study, White women were found to be more aware of mammography or other general information about radiologic screening than African Americans or Latinas (Fox et al., 1990). However, SES and educational differences were found among ethnic groups as well and were not controlled. Moreover, all women in that study, regardless of level of knowledge, received mammography due to physician recommendation—the importance of which is discussed in the next section.

Education is a possible explanation for differences in knowledge. In the United States, educational levels for individuals over age 25 do differ by ethnicity, with 79.8% of Whites having a high school education or better, 65.2% of African Americans, 50.2% of Latinos, 77.6% of Asian/Pacific Islanders, and 70.6% of Native Americans (U.S. Bureau of the Census, 1990a). The association between education and screening, however, is not clear cut. For mammography, this relation is difficult to assess because results are divided. Three studies have found that education relates significantly and positively to mammographic screening (Fink & Shapiro, 1990; Hayward et al., 1988; Suarez, 1994), while three have found no relation (Bloom et al., 1987; Kaplan et al., 1991; Vogel et al., 1990). Studies of Pap screening have almost universally found significant positive associations between Pap screening frequency and education among ethnically diverse samples (Cockburn, White, Hirst, & Hill, 1992; Harlan et al., 1991; Hayward et al., 1988; Mandelblatt et al., 1992; Michielutte et al., 1985; Suarez, 1994). However, education has not been associated with performance of BSE (Hayward et al., 1988; Kaplan et al., 1991). In addition to formal schooling, specific exposure to information about cancer may vary by ethnicity. For example, in a study of older Latina women, exposure to media-based health information predicted both symptom knowledge and screening (Ruiz, Marks, & Richardson, 1992). Language acculturation, in turn, predicted media exposure but did not predict screening and knowledge after controlling for exposure. These data suggest one route through which acculturation may have an impact on cancer outcomes.

In studies on follow-up, education has usually failed to relate significantly to adherence (Lerman et al., 1992; Marcus et al., 1992; Stewart, Buchegger, Lickrish, & Sierra, 1994). Only two of the studies reviewed found a significant relation for education. One found this relation to be inverse but did not include any covariates (Paskett et al., 1990). The other found a significant, positive relation between education and follow-up (Michielutte et al., 1985).

In addition to general knowledge, specific beliefs about cancer, whether accurate or inaccurate, may influence willingness to obtain screening. The cultural component of ethnicity as well as access to information may help to form these beliefs. Rubel and Garro (1992) suggested that individuals may make health decisions on the basis of their health culture, which is defined as

> the information and understanding that people have learned from family, friends, and neighbors as to the nature of a health problem, its cause, and its implications. Sick people use their health culture to interpret their symptoms, give them meaning, assign them severity, organize them into a named syndrome, decide with whom to consult, and for how long to remain in treatment. (p. 627)

It does appear that beliefs about cancer may vary somewhat by ethnicity. Chavez and colleagues (Chavez, Hubbell, McMullin, Martinez, & Mishra, 1995; Hubbell,

Chavez, Mishra, Magana, & Valdez, 1995) indicated that for breast cancer, while physicians ranked family history as the highest risk factor, Mexican immigrants ranked injuries to the breast, never breast feeding, excessive fondling, taking drugs or smoking, and using birth control pills as more important; family history ranked 12th. For cervical cancer, Latina women ranked behaviors that are morally questionable to some as most important, such as having abortions, getting sexually transmitted diseases, having multiple sexual partners, and using birth control pills. Similarly, over one third of Vietnamese women surveyed in San Francisco (California) reported that breast or cervical cancer could be caused by poor hygiene (Pham & McPhee, 1992). Although behaviors such as multiple sex partners have been shown to increase risk of cervical cancer, beliefs that are based on sexual morality and punishment are inaccurate, in general. With regard to attitudes toward breast screening, Fulton, Rakowski, and Jones (1995) found that Latinas were more likely than Whites or African Americans to agree with the statements "If your doctor gives you a breast exam, then you do not need to have a mammogram" and "Once you have a couple of mammograms in a row that show no problems, you don't need any more mammograms."

Other beliefs, such as perceived susceptibility to cancer, perceived efficacy of screening and treatment, and perceived severity of cancer, have been examined frequently as predictors of screening in the health psychology literature. Although model building investigations have rarely considered ethnic status, there are some data to support the link between these beliefs and screening. Perceived susceptibility to breast cancer has been associated with obtaining mammography among African American women (Bloom et al., 1987; Price, Desmond, Slenker, Smith, & Stewart, 1992), and perceived susceptibility to cervical cancer has been associated with obtaining Pap smears (Mandelblatt et al., 1992). There are also positive correlations among African American women between perceived benefits and obtaining Pap smears (Mandelblatt et al., 1992), being receptive to mammograms (Price et al., 1992), and obtaining mammograms (Burack & Liang, 1989). Perceived severity has been shown to be associated with receiving a mammogram in the past year among Latina women (Zapka, Stoddard, Barth, Costanza, & Mas, 1989). However, in a study of approximately 600 older Latina women, Richardson et al. (1987) found that neither perceived susceptibility nor perceived benefits were associated with screening. Instead, emotional reactions, such as nervousness and embarrassment, were strong negative predictors of BSE.

These latter findings suggest that the affective component of attitudes may play a role in predicting screening behavior. In one study, Latina and African American women were significantly more likely than White women to report that fear of radiation is an important barrier to mammography for them (Fox & Stein, 1991). Latina women were also more likely to describe fear of cancer and anxiety about the procedure to be strong barriers. In another study, Latinos were more likely than Whites to view cancer as a "death sentence" (Perez-Stable et al., 1992). There is some evidence to suggest that the strength of these views may be moderated by acculturation. For example, Balcazar, Castro, and Krull (1995) found that Mexican American women who were low (vs. high) in acculturation to the majority culture were more likely to endorse the statement "I am so afraid of being told I have cancer that I avoid going to the doctor" (p. 71).

In addition to any direct impact on avoiding treatment that these feelings might have, cancer-related anxieties and fears may also impede cancer-related information processing. Jepson and Chaiken (1990) found that fear about cancer inhibited systematic processing of information about the disease. Thus, having less knowledge about cancer may result partially from increased anxiety when cancer information is presented. However, this possibility needs to be tested directly with a multi-ethnic sample because there is some evidence to suggest that the relation of anxiety to cognitive performance may vary by ethnicity (Payne, Smith, & Payne, 1983).

Access to care and interactions with health care providers. The differences in SES and knowledge documented above may influence patients' interactions with health care providers and the health care system overall. There have been striking inequities between the health care received by Whites and non-Whites in the United States. Despite recent improvements, African Americans and Latinos see health care providers less frequently than non-Hispanic Whites (Blendon, Aiken, Freeman, & Corey, 1989; Hubbell, Waitzkin, Mishra, Dombrink, & Chavez, 1991; Wells, Golding, Hough, Burnam, & Karno, 1988).

Even within ethnic groupings, there are discrepancies in the availability of regular sources of health care. Both Mexican and Puerto Rican Americans are less likely to have a regular source of health care than Whites or African Americans (Lewin-Epstein, 1991). Among Latino subgroups, Mexican Americans tend to average fewer medical visits than Cuban or Puerto Rican Americans (Solis, Marks, Garcia, & Shelton, 1990). In addition to country of origin, acculturation levels and immigration status appear to predict health care use among Mexican Americans (Chesney, Chavira, Hall, & Gary, 1982; Wells, Hough, Golding, Burnam, & Karno, 1987). Immigrants, especially those who are undocumented, and Spanish-speaking people are least likely both to have health insurance and to use nonemergency health care (Chavez, Cornelius, & Jones, 1985; Stein & Fox, 1990).

Not surprisingly, these differences in access to health care are associated with screening behaviors. Having health insurance and a regular source of health care have been consistently associated with mammography use, Pap screening, and BSE practice (Fink & Shapiro, 1990; Fox et al., 1991; Harlan et al., 1991; Hayward et al., 1988; Jacob et al., 1989; Kang & Bloom, 1993; Longman, Saint-Germain, & Modiano, 1992; Mamon et al., 1990; Mickey, Durski, Worden, & Danigelis, 1995; Sawyer et al., 1990; Spurlock et al., 1992; Suarez, 1994). Acculturation also appears to be positively correlated with ever having had a mammogram among Latina women (Stein & Fox, 1990; Suarez & Pulley, 1995).

Even after a patient has made contact with a physician, appropriate screening and follow-up are not assured. Data document that medical caregivers miss key opportunities to increase care provided to underserved populations by failing to make appropriate referrals for further care (e.g., mammography; Caplan et al., 1992; Fox & Stein, 1991; Mandelblatt et al., 1992). In fact, some researchers have found that lack of physician recommendation, not patient behavior, is the most common reason for not having a mammogram (Bastani et al., 1991; Fox et al., 1991; Harper, 1993; Howe, 1992; Lackland et al., 1991; Mah & Bryant, 1992; Rimer, Ross, Cristinzio, & King, 1992; Skinner, Strecher, & Hospers, 1994; Stein, Fox, Murata, & Morisky, 1992; Vernon et al., 1992). For example, Fox and Stein reported that a physician recommendation increased the likelihood of mammography approximately sevenfold for African Americans, Latinas, and Whites. Physicians are less likely to provide screening mammography to older women, regardless of their risk category (Weinberger et al., 1991). They also perceive cost to be one of the greatest barriers to mammography for their patients, and those who see more Medicaid (a proxy for income) patients are less likely to refer for such a screening (Gemson, Elinson, & Messeri, 1988; Weinberger et al., 1991). Language is also related because doctors are less likely to discuss mammography with patients who speak only Spanish (Stein & Fox, 1990), suggesting another route through which acculturation may influence screening. Special efforts on the part of physicians to encourage mammography seem to be especially helpful for some low-income patients of color (Skinner et al., 1994).

Having a medical provider recommend Pap screening also relates positively to compliance with screening (Harlan et al., 1991; Mamon et al., 1990; McCurtis, 1979; Spurlock et al., 1992). In contrast to the mammography literature, however, these studies have not included attempts to identify specific factors associated with providers' recommendations.

Conclusion

The preceding findings suggest that the relation between ethnicity and screening and follow-up is complex. The results differ by screening test and by ethnicity. In no case, however, is there strong evidence for a direct link between ethnicity and behavior. Ethnicity appears to be an inexact proxy for other variables that hold greater promise for predicting and explaining screening and follow-up behavior. Indeed, in those cases in which positive bivariate associations between behavior and ethnicity are found, multivariate analyses indicate that these associations are typically the result of the relation between ethnicity and other variables. The correlates with the strongest empirical support are income, knowledge, access to health care, and physician recommendation.

There are serious limitations to this body of research. First, many studies fall prey to common methodological problems, including operationalizing variables inexactly, relying on samples of convenience, using assessment strategies of undetermined reliability and ecological validity, drawing causal conclusions from correlational data, and so on.[3] Furthermore, the vast majority of studies categorize individuals into ethnic groups, often without explaining how ethnicity is defined. Rarely is the multidimensional nature of ethnicity as a psychological construct considered. Nonetheless, that some findings are consistent despite these problems suggests that they may be robust. Perhaps more troubling is the narrow focus of much of the research. The research is limited to only a few screening behaviors and ignores some ethnic groups, such as Asian and Native Americans, almost completely. Because of the screening behaviors on which researchers have focused, studies also

---

[3]Some researchers also have described the reliance on self-report for data on participation in screening as a methodological drawback. Recent studies that have attempted to validate self-reported mammography data with institutional records have obtained confirmation rates ranging from approximately 66% to 99% (Bowman, Redman, Dickinson, Gibberd, & Sanson-Fisher, 1991; Degnan et al., 1992; Etzi, Lane, & Grimson, 1994; King, Rimer, Trock, Balshem, & Engstrom, 1990). However, while women have been shown to report accurately whether they have had a particular screening test, they are less able to remember precisely when they had it (Etzi et al., 1994; King et al., 1990). Thus, actual use may be overreported due to a tendency to recall incorrectly the lapse of time between each screen (Sawyer, Earp, Fletcher, Daye, & Wynn, 1989; Walter, Clarke, Hatcher, & Stitt, 1988).

have excluded men. With few exceptions, intra-ethnic differences, for example, variation associated with country of origin, immigration status, level of acculturation to the majority culture, and primary language, have not been adequately explored.

The variables that have been found to have predictive value are correlated with ethnicity. Thus, to understand the specific relation between ethnicity and screening and follow-up fully, researchers must adopt a coherent, multivariate approach that does not rely on ethnicity alone. A focus on possible mediating variables is more likely to lead to the development of useful conceptual models and successful intervention programs. Unfortunately, most of the research reviewed here fails to draw on psychological theory. One goal of this review is to point out the need for greater integration of public health and psychological approaches to these issues.

Treatment Outcomes: Survival and Quality of Life

The primary reason for interest in screening and follow-up is their association with treatment outcomes. It is well established that an earlier diagnosis of cancer is associated with better survival outcome (Baquet et al., 1986). In addition, to the extent that cancer can be treated successfully and with less invasive or toxic treatments, quality of life is likely to benefit. In this section, we consider ethnic differences in treatment outcomes and, then, describe variables that might mediate relations between ethnicity and cancer survival and quality of life.

Ethnic Differences in Length of Survival

As indicated in Appendix B, there are ethnic differences in cancer mortality rates associated with specific disease sites. Five-year survival rates also differ by ethnicity (Miller et al., 1993). Young, Ries, and Pollack (1984), for example, published a comparison of survival rates among 462,613 cancer cases from eight racial–ethnic groups in the United States using SEER data. They found that survival rates were comparable for Latinos, Chinese Americans, Hawaiians, and Whites. Japanese Americans experienced the highest survival rates. African Americans and Filipinos had lower survival rates, while Native Americans had the lowest rates. In addition to these overall survival rates, poorer survival of African Americans, as compared with Whites, is well documented for specific cancers, such as prostate, lung, and breast (e.g., Austin et al., 1990; Axtell & Meyers, 1978; Baquet et al., 1986; Dansey et al., 1988; Vernon, Tilley, Neale, & Steinfeldt, 1985); whereas for other specific cancer sites, there may be no differences (e.g., see Graham et al., 1992, for non-small-cell lung cancer). In contrast, better survival among Japanese is found consistently across most cancer sites (LeMarchand, Kolonel, & Nomura, 1984).

Some of this disparity in survival rates among ethnic groups is due to the stage of cancer at the time of diagnosis (Dayal, Power, & Chiu, 1982; Mandelblatt, Andrews, Kerner, Zauber, & Burnett, 1991; Miller et al., 1993; Richardson et al., 1992). Austin et al. (1990), for example, found that young African American men with prostate cancer were diagnosed at a later stage and had a shorter survival time than young White men. Several studies suggest that Latinos are also affected by late-stage diagnosis (Daly, Clark, & McGuire, 1985; Horm, 1987; Villar & Menck, 1994).

Villar and Menck showed that for seven of eight types of cancer studied, Latinos had a less favorable stage of disease at diagnosis than non-Hispanic Whites.

When researchers have controlled for stage or other indicators of disease progression, however, ethnic differences in survival sometimes remain. Most clearly, studies indicate that with few exceptions (e.g., Optenberg et al., 1995; Sutherland & Mather, 1986), the poor survival of African Americans persists within stage of disease (Baquet et al., 1986; Dayal et al., 1982; Fisher, Redmond, Fisher, & Bass, 1990; Kimmick, Muss, Case, & Stanley, 1991; Miller et al., 1993; Ragland, Selvin, & Merrill, 1991). Research also indicates that the survival advantage of Japanese is often maintained when stage of disease at diagnosis and other prognostic factors are held constant (LeMarchand, 1991).

In an effort to explain these survival differences, researchers have posited several biological factors that covary with ethnicity. For example, several studies have suggested that African American women have a greater proportion of estrogen receptor-negative breast tumors, which are associated with poor survival, than White women (Natarajan, Nemoto, Mettlin, & Murphy, 1985; Stanford & Greenberg, 1989). Similarly, levels of androgen metabolites differ among Japanese, White, and African American men. These metabolites may be key indicators of biological processes important in the development of prostate cancer and may underlie the very different incidence rates in these three groups (R. K. Ross et al., 1992). It is clearly beyond the scope of this article to review all of the medical literature on cancer prognosis. The previous examples notwithstanding, it is important to note that these medical models have not succeeded in fully explaining racial–ethnic differences in cancer survival rates. Thus, it is especially important to consider psychosocial factors, such as differences in SES, attitudes toward cancer detection and treatment, and access to care, that may help to explain survival patterns.

Ethnic Differences in Quality of Life

The past 2 decades have brought an increasing awareness of the importance of considering quality of life as well as survival following the diagnosis of cancer. Nonetheless, there is remarkably little research on quality of life following cancer among persons of color. Although there is a large literature on quality of life among non-Hispanic White Americans and Europeans, these studies almost never include sufficient diversity to report findings separately by ethnicity.

With few exceptions, the available data describing quality of life in non-Whites come from studies conducted in other countries. These findings are consistent with descriptions of quality of life following cancer for patients in the United States with similar diagnoses and treatments. For example, the concerns of Chinese breast cancer survivors, the reactions of Japanese patients to breast reconstruction, and the sexual difficulties of Chinese patients with cervical cancer are all similar to findings obtained from primarily White patients with breast and gynecological cancer in the United States (Alagaratnam & Kung, 1986; Bando, 1990; Ngan & Tang, 1988; O'Hoy & Tang, 1985).

While these studies provide useful information, they do not help us to understand the role that minority status, immigration or refugee status, language differences, ethnic identity, acculturation, and so forth may play in adjusting to cancer in the

United States. The few studies conducted with ethnic minorities in the United States tend to report more difficulties than are typically reported by non-Hispanic Whites or by Asians in their native countries. O'Hare, Malone, Lusk, and McCorkle (1993), for example, assessed symptom distress and unmet needs in a group of recently discharged, low-income, urban African American patients. They compared their results with previously collected data from middle-class White patients and found that the African American sample reported greater distress and more unmet needs. In another study, in-depth qualitative interviews with 26 African American patients with breast cancer from the rural South yielded similar information about the difficulties patients faced in dealing with medical institutions (Mathews, Lannin, & Mitchell, 1994). Low-income, Latino chemotherapy inpatients also reported a number of unmet needs in ethnographic interviews designed to tap the meanings of comfort from a cultural perspective (Neves-Arruda, Larson, & Meleis, 1992). For example, patients described discomfort with the unfamiliarity of the food and other aspects of the hospital environment.

Several case studies also suggest areas in which quality of life may be disrupted if the culture of the medical establishment conflicts with the patient's native culture (e.g., Brotzman & Butler, 1991; Eisenbruch & Handelman, 1990; Lima & Cohen, 1991; Mo, 1992; Sawyers & Eaton, 1992). For example, Eisenbruch and Handelman pointed out how it was necessary to consider a Cambodian family's belief that their son's advanced brain tumor was due to bad karma, dangerous house spirits, and neglect of an ancestral spirit. Only by respecting and encouraging, rather than attempting to discredit, the family's health beliefs was the medical staff able to support the ceremonial cures that the family required in order to come to terms with their son's illness. In contrast, Lima and Cohen described the case of a Latina women who was cajoled through a bilingual case conference into accepting palliative radiation and chemotherapy, despite her strong desire to avoid further treatment for terminal cancer.

Ethnic Differences in Adherence to Treatment

Ethnic differences in survival and, to a lesser extent, in quality of life may be associated with the extent to which patients adhere to treatment recommendations. Poor adherence has been shown to be the cause of poor disease control among patients with numerous chronic diseases, including cancer (Bonadonna & Valagussa, 1981; Coronary Drug Project Research Group, 1980; Lipid Research Clinics Program, 1984; Pizzo et al., 1983; Richardson et al., 1990; Sackett, Haynes, Gibson, & Johnson, 1976; Stanway, Lambie, & Johnson, 1985; Wagner, Truesdale, & Warner, 1981). Although the impact on quality of life may be less direct, better disease control is likely to lead to better quality of life. Conversely, adherence to aversive treatments has been found to disrupt quality of life temporarily, although the impact of treatments on patients of color has not been studied directly.

Numerous studies have indicated that approximately 50% of all patients across a wide range of diseases, therapies, and individual patient characteristics are non-compliant with prescribed medical regimens (Morrow, Leirer, & Sheikh, 1988; Sackett & Snow, 1979; Shope, 1981). Some researchers have examined the level of compliance with cancer chemotherapy and have found that compliance is low, in general (Feld, Rubinstein, & Thomas, 1993; Lebovits et al., 1990; Levine et al., 1987; Smith, Rosen, Trueworthy, & Lowman, 1979). Low-income and private, community-based care are associated with still lower compliance (Lebovits et al., 1990).

The extent to which nonadherence to treatment mirrors ethnic differences in survival outcomes is unclear. There is very little research assessing adherence across ethnicities and its impact on survival. A study of patients with hematologic cancers showed a clear and definite relation between compliance and survival (Richardson, Shelton, Krailo, & Levine, 1990). All patients were of low SES, and approximately half were Latino; however, no differences in compliance by ethnicity were noted (Levine et al., 1987; Richardson et al., 1990). Formenti et al. (1995) found that compliance to radiation treatment among indigent Latina patients with cervical cancer was extremely low—far lower than rates for middle-class White populations reported in other studies. Survival was not assessed in the study, although adherence to that radiation protocol has a strong positive correlation with local disease control and survival. In both of these studies, income rather than ethnicity may have been the more important predictor of adherence.

Possible Mediating Variables

Socioeconomic status. Cancer patients with lower income survive for shorter periods of time than patients with greater financial resources (Berg, Ross, & Latourette, 1977; Farley & Flannery, 1989; Karjalainen & Pukkala, 1990; LeMarchand, 1991; Lipworth & Parker, 1972). For example, Berg et al. analyzed 20,000 cases of 39 types of cancer and found the 5-year survival rates for indigent patients were lower than those for nonindigent patients. The patients in the study received health care from the same staff, leading to the assumption that host factors, such as immune competence, nutrition, and concurrent disease, may have accounted for the difference. It is also possible that different care was provided or adhered to by the indigent patient. Greenwald and Henke (1991), for example, showed that there was a substantial survival advantage for patients with prostate cancer seen in an HMO, where access to and quality of care are standardized, versus patients seen in a fee-for-service setting. This difference was especially marked for those with incomes under $20,000.

Ethnic differences in SES appear to account for at least some of the variance in survival rates across ethnicities. Most studies indicate that after SES is controlled, the effect of ethnicity on survival is reduced (Bassett & Krieger, 1986; Dayal et al., 1982; McWhorter, Schatzkin, Horm, & Brown, 1989; also see Coates et al., 1990, for an exception). Cella et al. (1991) assessed survival in a cooperative protocol research group studying lung, multiple myeloma, gastric, pancreatic, and breast cancer and Hodgkin's disease. There was no significant difference in survival related to ethnicity after adjusting for age, all clinical variables, and initial physical impairment. Education and income, however, continued to be significant predictors of survival. Similarly, Gordon, Crowe, Brumberg, and Berger (1992) found that for 1,392 patients with breast cancer, race was a significant predictor of survival after adjustment for key prognostic factors; but after adjustment for SES, it ceased to be significant. When analyses were stratified by race, SES was a significant predictor of survival in White but not African American patients, perhaps due to the small number of higher SES

African Americans in their study. Other research has found SES to be predictive of survival among African American patients as well. Freeman and Wasfie (1989) showed lower survival rates for breast cancer among poor African American women in Harlem (New York) than among African American women nationally, for example.

Latino health statistics raise questions about the extent to which poverty determines cancer survival outcomes, however. The overall health status and cancer survival rates of Latinos are similar to those of non-Hispanic Whites and better than those of African Americans and Native Americans. SES for Latinos, however, is similar to that of African Americans and Native Americans. Nickens (1995) suggested that groups that have remained poor in the United States for several generations may suffer ongoing psychological and physical damage as compared with new immigrant groups. Thus, comprehensive consideration of SES must go beyond simple reliance on measures of income to include a broader conceptualization of the social and historical context in which income differences occur.

It is highly likely that SES is associated with quality of life. Golding and Burnam (1990) found that a community sample of Mexican Americans had higher depression scores than non-Hispanic Whites, accounted for by their greater exposure to stress. In a study of indigent Latina patients with cervical cancer, the general stress associated with poverty and immigration status was a strong predictor of psychosocial difficulties, separate from cancer-related stressors (Meyerowitz, Formenti, Ell, & Leedham, 1997).

Knowledge and attitudes.   Lack of knowledge about cancer and its treatment is likely to contribute to nonadherence (Loehrer et al., 1991). As we described in our discussion on knowledge related to screening behaviors, members of ethnic minority groups in the United States report less cancer-related knowledge on a range of topics. Loehrer et al. demonstrated, however, that misinformation is common among low SES patients with cancer, regardless of ethnicity. As with screening behaviors, inaccurate knowledge about cancer was inversely related to level of education.

The attitudes and beliefs that individuals hold may influence their willingness to adhere to treatment and their quality of life following diagnosis and treatment as well (Hartog & Hartog, 1983; Trill & Holland, 1993). Although the literature on attitudes and beliefs tends to focus on ethnic or racial groups individually—typically African American, Asian American–Asian, or Latino—it appears that there is considerable similarity across these cultures as well as considerable variance within cultures. It seems that there is a fairly consistent set of beliefs on which persons of color may agree and with which non-Hispanic Whites—and therefore the medical system in the United States—seem to disagree. One set of beliefs is not necessarily superior to the other, but the mismatch may lead to distress and difficulty for patients whose values are not consistent with the values of the people treating them. Much of this literature is speculative and, with few studies providing strong empirical support, risks promoting stereotypes. Nonetheless, the consistency with which these belief patterns are described in the literature suggests that they may be a fruitful area for research that could link ethnic culture and identity with cancer-related attitudes. The many descriptions of potentially important culture-specific beliefs that may be associated with adherence and reactions to the diagnosis and treatment of cancer can be condensed into four general categories: acceptance of death and suffering and "fatalism," familism, beliefs in folk medicine, and attitudes toward coping.

Acceptance of death and suffering and fatalism. Several writers have suggested that African Americans, Latinos, and Asians–Asian Americans tend to view death and suffering as integral parts of life and, therefore, may be less likely than physicians to place emphasis on "fighting" the cancer (Kagawa-Singer, 1987; Mathews et al., 1994; Uba, 1992). According to this view, living in harmony with nature is superior to beating nature through aggressive treatment (Nilchaikovit, Hill, & Holland, 1993). This attitude is sometimes associated with a generally fatalistic view of the world, which has been found to be more common among both Latinos and African Americans than non-Hispanic Whites, even when controlling for SES and education (C. E. Ross, Mirowsky, & Cockerham, 1983; Sugarek, Deyo, & Holmes, 1988).

Fatalistic attitudes may also be associated with cancer, specifically. In a comparison of older African Americans and Whites, Powe (1995) found that African Americans expressed more fatalistic views of cancer. Ethnicity, less education, and low income made significant, independent contributions to the prediction of cancer fatalism in multivariate analyses. Perez-Stable et al. (1992) surveyed Latino and White members of an urban HMO. Although the two groups agreed on many beliefs, Latinos reported a greater belief that cancer was a "death sentence," a view which the researchers attributed to *fatalismo*. With some sites of cancer, of course, this view may be accurate rather than a sign of fatalism. It appears that lower levels of acculturation, more than less education, may be associated with a sense of fatalism and lack of control with regard to cancer (Balcazar, Castro, & Krull, 1995).

These attitudes, although linked with cancer, have not been demonstrated to have a role in cancer-related adherence behaviors. There is some evidence that fatalistic beliefs may be linked to quality of life, however. Domino, Fragoso, and Moreno (1991) found that greater fatalism was associated with pessimism about cancer and with greater anxiety and depression. In qualitative interviews, Mathews et al. (1994) described how fatalistic views and distrust of physicians led to difficulties in adjustment for 26 rural southern African American patients with breast cancer. Further evidence of the relation between distress and fatalism was obtained by C. E. Ross et al. (1983). They found that the effects of SES and Mexican identity on psychological distress were mediated entirely through fatalism.

Familism.   Although all ethnic groups value the extended family, African Americans, Asians, and Latinos have been described as placing higher value on interdependence and strong family ties than do middle-class non-Hispanic White Americans (Guillory, 1987; Hartog & Hartog, 1983; Hogan-Garcia, Martinez, & Martinez, 1979; Kagawa-Singer, 1987; Keefe, 1984; Nilchaikovit et al., 1993; Trill & Holland, 1993). Sabogal, Marin, Otero-Sabogal, Oss-Marin, and Perez-Stable (1987) compared community samples of Latinos and Whites and found that Latinos reported stronger familism, regardless of level of acculturation.

Within some cultures, a cure is seen as requiring full family participation (Maduro, 1983). Although American health care providers may view such attitudes as inappropriately dependent (Inclan & Hernandez, 1992), familism may buffer patients from physical and emotional stressors (Sabogal et al., 1987). For example, Mindel (1980) found that both Mexican Americans and African Americans were significantly higher than Whites on several aspects of familism. Whites were more isolated from their kin and, therefore, less able to benefit from family support. There also is some evidence that family-based versus individually oriented interventions may be more effective for patients with high beliefs in familism (see Cousins et al., 1992).

It is not clear what the role of familism is specifically in the care of patients with cancer and how this differs among ethnic groups. There is evidence that some members of ethnic groups may prefer that the family rather than the individual make medical decisions. Blackhall, Murphy, Frank, Michel, and Azen (1995) found that Korean Americans and Mexican Americans were less likely than African Americans and White Americans to believe that patients should make decisions about life support in terminal cases and more likely to believe that the family should make those decisions. However, the fact that the cultural value of familism is higher in some ethnic groups does not necessarily mean that it will be mobilized when cancer is diagnosed or that it will be helpful in terms of informational, instrumental, or emotional support.

Other familial aspects of culture, such as gender and family roles, have been thought to influence treatment decisions. For example, in Latino culture, writers describe a traditional female gender role in which women are supposed to subordinate their own needs to those of the family. According to this view, the woman's emphasis should be on her spouse and children (Cox & Monk, 1993; Golding & Baezconde-Garbanati, 1990). When a woman holding such values is faced with a cancer treatment that may debilitate her and make her unable to carry out her domestic duties for some period of time, the assumption has been that she may delay or reject the treatment and perhaps limit her survival as a consequence. However, it is important to note that there is no evidence to support this speculation nor the claim that such cultural views lead family members to discourage women from obtaining necessary health care for cancer. In an interview study of older Latina women (Richardson et al., 1987), the researchers did not find that Latino men tried to prevent their wives from obtaining Pap smears. It is unclear whether these findings would generalize to younger women, who might have greater child care and household responsibilities and who might want, or be expected, to maintain reproductive capacity. Work in progress by Richardson and Hudson (1998) based on interviews with Latina patients with breast cancer indicates that in almost all cases, women believe that their partners and other family members would expect them to keep doctors appointments over family obligations.

Beliefs in folk medicine.   Considerable discussion and numerous case examples confirm the prevalence of three types of beliefs in "folk medicine" among persons of color. First, illnesses that are not recognized by "scientific," Western medicine have been described in several cultures: *susto* (fright), *mal de ojo* (evil eye), *empacho* (stomach congestion), and dirty blood (e.g., Mathews et al., 1994; Pachter, 1994). Respondents of Mexican heritage in Los Angeles (Castro, Furth, & Karlow, 1984) and in Texas (Trotter, 1991) reported significantly stronger beliefs in these diseases than Whites, regardless of level of acculturation.

A second area of folk beliefs involves the use of indigenous healers (Kleinman, Eisenberg, & Good, 1978). Although the specific names for and treatments provided by healers differ by culture, their importance outside the scientific medical community is widespread. *Curanderos* in Latino cultures (Maduro, 1983), voodoo practitioners among African Americans and Caribbean Islanders (Guillory, 1987), medicine men among Native Americans (Antle, 1987), and herbal healers and *shaman* within Asian cultures (Kagawa-Singer, 1987; Uba, 1992) continue to play integral roles in providing medical care for some individuals. For example, close to half of the Mexican American heads of household surveyed by Farge (1977) in Houston

(Texas) reported that folk healers were effective and 98% described physicians as effective. These beliefs were negatively correlated with SES and education but were unrelated to degree of acculturation.

The third area in which folk beliefs often differ from beliefs of standard Western medicine involves theories of illness and cure. For example, a prevalent conception in both traditional Latino and Asian cultures is the hot–cold theory of illness (Castro et al., 1984; Hartog & Hartog, 1983; Kleinman et al., 1978). According to this theory, illnesses, medications, and foods are either hot or cold. Individuals should take foods and medicines that counteract their condition, such that drinking a cold food (e.g., juice) for a cold condition (e.g., a cold) would be unacceptable (Harwood, 1971). Other common views include seeing illness as punishment from angry or evil spirits (Uba, 1992), as due to imbalances in the blood or energy systems (Mathews et al., 1994; Uba, 1992), or as a normal and acceptable part of life.

Less has been written about specific folk beliefs about cancer. Pachter (1994) suggested that "patients' beliefs and behaviors concerning illnesses such as asthma and cancer are often only slightly different than biomedical doctrine" (pp. 690–691). Cancer, for example, is typically not identified as a hot or cold illness, although symptoms of cancer or cancer treatments are individually categorized. Domino and his colleagues (Domino et al., 1991; Domino & Lin, 1991) developed the Cancer Metaphors Test to identify attitudes toward cancer among White Americans, Mexicans, and Chinese and found that the same general views of cancer were endorsed by all groups. However, as described earlier, fatalistic views of cancer may be more prevalent among African Americans and Latinos (Mathews et al., 1994; Perez-Stable et al., 1992).

It is important to note that high levels of folk belief do not tend to be associated with the underuse of standard medical care (Castro et al., 1984; Farge, 1977; Nall & Speilberg, 1967). As Maduro (1983) explained, "many believe that only a *curandero* can cure certain types or aspects of illnesses and only physicians can cure others" (p. 869). People who hold folk beliefs rarely hold them to the exclusion of acceptance of standard medical care but, rather, seem able to hold a dual belief system that allows for both types of interventions (Castro et al., 1984; Pachter, 1994). Therefore, these beliefs appear to be an instance of bicultural competence, and there is no reason to believe that they would negatively impact adherence. For example, Loehrer et al. (1991) found that poor African Americans were more likely than poor Whites to believe that alternative treatments, such as laetrile (an extract from apricot pits), could cure cancer. They found no racial differences in care-seeking behaviors, however, suggesting that these attitudes do not influence willingness to seek standard medical care. However, beliefs could affect quality of life if medical providers evidence misunderstanding or disdain toward patients' views.

Attitudes toward coping. The impact of these culture-specific beliefs may be mediated through coping. The prevalence of use of certain coping mechanisms may differ across cultures. For example, Draguns (1988) suggested that passive withdrawal may be more common and more adaptive among Latinos, whereas Americans from the majority culture may respond to stress with active coping efforts. The very few studies that are available suggest that coping may differ among patients with cancer, specifically. Kagawa-Singer (1993), for example, found that White and American-born Japanese patients had similar coping objectives but different coping styles. Whites were more likely to fight and use will power to stay upbeat, whereas

Japanese Americans were more likely to endure stoically and to avoid overt acceptance of the disease.

Use and accessibility of social support may differ as well. In interviews with a large sample of Latino and White patients with cancer drawn from a tumor registry, Goodwin, Hunt, and Samet (1991) found that Whites were less likely to have adequate social support networks. Insofar as appropriate social support appears to be related to willingness to accept treatment and to overall quality of life (see Meyerowitz, Leedham, & Hart, in press), strong social networks may benefit patients of color. It is likely that this social support will typically be drawn from family networks; White, middle-class patients are more likely to seek out support groups and other extrafamilial social resources (Taylor, Falke, Shoptaw, & Lichtman, 1986).

These differences in coping are consistent with the cultural attitudes discussed above. We now need research to determine if coping strategies that have been found to be helpful for majority culture patients would also be effective for patients of other ethnicities or if coping recommendations should be tailored to culture. For example, active involvement in medical decision making has been associated with better quality of life (see Meyerowitz et al., in press) but may conflict with views within some cultures regarding patient–physician relationships.

Access to adequate care and interactions with physicians. In our discussion of access to screening and follow-up, we documented that African Americans and Latinos tend to have less access to regular medical care than Whites. The difficulties that this lack of access creates for screening apply to cancer treatment as well. In addition, there is evidence that even when patients do have access to care, the care that they receive may differ by ethnicity. In general, for example, African Americans are admitted to hospitals with more severe cases of a disease, get sicker while hospitalized, and stay hospitalized for shorter periods than do Whites (Buckle, Horn, Oates, & Abbey, 1992). Cancer-specific care also seems to differ. African American patients are less likely to be treated aggressively and more likely to be untreated or treated nonsurgically, even when controlling for age and stage of disease (Mayer & McWhorter, 1989; McWhorter & Mayer, 1987). However, there is also some evidence that African Americans can be overtreated. Diehr et al. (1989) found that although African American women were less likely to have appropriate tumor assays or to be referred for postmastectomy rehabilitation, they were more likely to have inappropriate liver scans and radiation therapy. In addition to decreasing survival rates, inappropriate treatment may have an impact on quality of life. A recent study, for example, indicated that fewer African American than White women with operable breast cancer that had spread to the lymph nodes underwent breast conservation versus more disfiguring radical surgery (Muss et al., 1992).

In two recent studies, researchers examined the relation between race and prostate cancer when access to care and treatment were held constant. Participants were active duty military personnel (Optenberg et al., 1995) and men treated through the Veterans Affairs system (Powell, Schwartz, & Hussain, 1995) who have equal access to medical services. African Americans were more likely than Whites to present with metastatic disease in both studies. With regard to survival, Powell et al. concluded that equal access to care did not appear to influence survival because African American men under 70 years of age had worse survival rates than Whites, although older African American men had a survival advantage compared with Whites. Optenberg et al., however, compared survival by stage and found that African American men with metastatic disease had slightly longer survival than White men with similar diagnoses.

Regardless of the availability of optimal medical treatment, there may be ethnic differences in the nature of the interaction between physician and patient. Almost every writer who describes cross-cultural differences in reaction to the medical system stresses the importance of understanding different cultural attitudes toward medical authorities and toward the doctor–patient relationship (e.g., Hartog & Hartog, 1983). Although persons of color may hold attitudes different from middle-class non-Hispanic White Americans, there appears to be great variability across cultures in what is viewed as optimal. Writers have generalized, for example, that many Asians and Asian Americans may consider the physician an important authority who should be treated with deference (Kim et al., 1993; Uba, 1992) whereas many African Americans may be highly distrustful of the health care system due to its documented mistreatment of African Americans in the United States (Guillory, 1987). Similarly, patients may prefer different modes of interaction with the physician—differences in amount of touching, level of friendliness, extent of questioning, and willingness to express emotion have all been suggested (Antle, 1987; Maduro, 1983; Muecke, 1983; Nilchaikovit et al., 1993; Pachter, 1994). Moreover, monolingual staff have difficulty communicating with immigrant populations and understanding their special needs (Seijo, Gomez, & Freidenberg, 1991).

Physicians may also misjudge patient preferences for information. Blackhall et al. (1995) found that Korean Americans and Mexican Americans were less likely than European Americans or African Americans to believe that patients should be told of a diagnosis of metastatic or terminal cancer. Similar results were obtained by Perez-Stable et al. (1992), who found that Latinos were more likely than Whites to state that they would prefer not to be told if they had incurable cancer (33% of Latinos vs. 23% of Anglos). It is important to note, however, that a large majority of both groups of patients preferred to be told their prognosis. These findings highlight the importance of considering differences within ethnic groups.

The extent to which these attitudes and beliefs are factors in compliance or predict cancer outcomes is largely untested. Case studies, however, do highlight difficulties faced by patients when they prefer to reject treatment (viewed as "unacceptable fatalism" by the medical team in Lima & Cohen, 1991) or hold traditional beliefs about treatment (Eisenbruch & Handelman, 1990; Sawyers & Eaton, 1992).

Conclusion

In the consideration of survival and quality of life, as with screening and follow-up, the relations with ethnicity are complex. Research has established that ethnicity is correlated with survival, and the specific relation varies by ethnicity and site of disease. In general, African Americans have worse survival outcomes, and Japanese have better survival outcomes than most other ethnic groups. The impact of ethnicity on survival, though, appears to be mediated largely through other variables, such as SES, knowledge and attitudes, and, probably, differential access to optimal treatment. General information on the correlation between treatment adherence and survival suggests that adherence is likely to play a strong mediating role between ethnicity and survival as well. It is possible, as depicted in Figure 1, that low income predicts poor access, which, in turn, predicts poor adherence and, possibly, poor treatment. Similarly, study of the role of attitudinal variables in predicting adherence holds promise for future research. Unfortunately, few data are available on ethnic differences in adherence and possible mediators between ethnicity and adherence.

There is surprisingly little research on ethnicity and quality of life outcomes. The literature contains many articles that speculate about probable relations but almost no data. Research on quality of life will not be easy. A comprehensive program of research will require reliable and valid tools to measure general quality of life components and components specific to the cultural values of the individuals being studied. These tools will need to be carefully translated into multiple languages. Canales, Ganz, and Coscarelli (1995) described the difficulties inherent in translating and validating quality of life instruments. Even when psychometrically sound instruments are available, similar scores may have very different meanings due to cultural differences in how quality of life constructs are operationalized. Additionally, it is almost impossible to identify distinctive groups for study. Even subcultural breakdowns are inadequate, as Uba (1992) pointed out in a discussion of the many differences among newly immigrated Southeast Asians. However, without appropriate normative data for comparison, it will be very difficult to interpret quality of life data. Adopting a multidimensional approach to studying ethnicity as a psychological construct may help to lessen these methodological and conceptual problems.

Conclusions and Recommendations for Future Research

We have reviewed the research that addresses the links between ethnicity and cancer outcomes. The results of this research are neither direct nor obvious in all cases. For example, the common sense view that screening rates would be lower for African Americans given their lower survival rates is not supported by major national studies. However, the studies do indicate that Latina women have both the lowest rates of screening for precursors of cervical cancer and the highest incidence rates of the disease. Similarly, differences in cancer survival rates by ethnicity appear to be due to differences in stage of disease at time of diagnosis in some cases but not in others. With regard to quality of life outcomes, many writers have suggested that members of several minority groups have greater acceptance of death as an integral part of life, whereas others have reported findings suggesting that there may be less openness for some patients of color to information about a possible terminal prognosis.

There are several possible reasons for the lack of clear, consistent, and direct findings that these examples underscore. First, many important questions have not yet been addressed by research. An examination of Figure 1 indicates several areas that require greater attention. For example, we know little about quality of life following the detection of cancer for ethnic minority patients or about the possible links between attitudes and cancer outcomes. The literature is especially deficient in exploring multidimensional components of ethnicity in understanding cancer outcomes and mediators and in considering the interrelations among these components. Even those questions that have been studied extensively are often limited in their scope —as in the case of the narrow focus on breast and cervical cancer in African Americans, Whites, and Latinas in the screening literature.

Second, the research that has been conducted is often marred by methodological problems. Many of these problems are common in health psychology research, in general. For example, there is no consensus on the most appropriate, psychometrically sound approaches for assessing complex constructs such as adherence and attitudes. Studies are often designed in the absence of comprehensive, conceptual frameworks, and without attention to potentially confounding variables, allowing researchers to capitalize on chance findings. Also, many studies suffer from sample selection biases and cross-sectional designs that restrict generalizability. In the case of treatment adherence, for example, cross-sectional samples are likely to be those who like the clinic staff, have stayed in treatment, and are most likely to comply. Inception cohort studies are rare because they require repeat contacts to evaluate the consistency of behavior. Equally troublesome is the almost complete lack of experimental intervention studies designed to improve treatment adherence and measure biological and quality of life outcomes.

Other methodological problems are inherent in multicultural research. Researchers have not yet developed accurate and culturally sensitive translations for widely used measures, although there is evidence that language of assessment can have a strong effect on results (Angel & Guarnaccia, 1989; Canales et al., 1995). Moreover, there is a controversy over which variables should be included in studies: Will variables that have proven useful in research with non-Hispanic Whites also be of greatest value in multicultural research? It is also difficult to identify coherent and meaningful ethnic groupings. As this review indicated, there are considerable intergroup similarities and intragroup differences. Even definitions of non-Hispanic Whites are open to debate and differ across studies. The development of adequate tools for assessing ethnicity as a psychological construct as it relates to cancer will require considerable effort. In addition, poor or minority individuals may be reluctant to participate in research, leading to an exacerbation of other methodological problems such as sampling bias (Reid, 1993).

A third possible explanation for the complexity of findings reported here is that there may not be direct pathways from ethnicity to cancer outcomes. We suggest that factors that vary by ethnicity—socioeconomic variables, knowledge and attitudes, access to care, and adherence to treatment recommendations—hold greater explanatory value. By documenting these factors, researchers and clinicians may be in a better position to predict cancer outcomes than by knowing ethnicity per se. Research that simply compares ethnic groups is less likely to provide conceptually or clinically useful information than research based on models that seek to identify the active factors that underlie these differences. Such models also encourage a multidisciplinary approach to research. As the preceding literature review documented, social scientists have not yet integrated literatures that address similar questions from different disciplinary perspectives.

The framework that we presented is an effort to organize and integrate the existing empirical literature to help in understanding ethnic differences in cancer outcomes. Although the mediating variables that we proposed are relatively straightforward, they have not been adequately studied in comprehensive models with psychologically meaningful measurement of ethnicity. Until comprehensive models are tested, it is impossible to know whether the variables we proposed here will fully account for the ethnic differences in cancer outcomes. There are likely to be other routes as well. At several points, we have speculated about variables that have received so little empirical attention in the health psychology literature that we could not explore them fully. For example, issues such as the link between family–gender roles and health culture, the impact of racist attitudes on the part of medical staff, the role of affect in determining attitudes toward cancer and treatment access, and ethnic differences in the role of active coping all deserve further attention.

Ultimately, a comprehensive mediational model will require consideration of biological variables, in addition to the public health, behavioral, and psychosocial variables included in the proposed framework (see, e.g., the biobehavioral model of stress and cancer outcomes developed by Andersen, Kiecolt-Glaser, & Glaser, 1994). Ethnic differences in basic immunological and endocrinological functioning, as well as specific differences in response to cancer, should be considered. Further research will be necessary to determine the extent to which these differences are mediated through behaviors such as diet and exercise. For example, as Asians have acculturated to American dietary habits, their rates of cancer have shifted to approximate those of non-Hispanic Whites in the United States (Whittemore et al., 1990).

An additional advantage to a multidimensional, mediational model is that it can help to identify targets for intervention. A growing body of research documents that behavioral and psychosocial interventions can improve both survival and quality of life for non-Hispanic White patients with cancer (Andersen, 1992; Ironson, Antoni, & Lutgendorf, 1995). Determining whether these interventions are equally useful for ethnic minority patients requires investigation. It is possible, for example, that family-oriented programs, as compared with the more common individual and support group interventions, may be especially beneficial for some patients. Additionally, as Zeltzer and LeBaron (1985) noted, the medical staff's attitudes toward ethnic differences may be important in determining whether patients with cancer accept psychosocial interventions.

Clearly, this review suggested that much more research is needed to understand the links between ethnicity and cancer outcomes. Cancer is a leading cause of death and disability in this country. It is also among the most psychologically distressing illnesses for the hundreds of thousands of patients who have been diagnosed with cancer and for their families. An awareness of the importance of these issues has led social scientists to publish thousands of articles on the behavioral and psychosocial aspects of the disease. That this research has focused almost entirely on non-Hispanic Whites is a problem that must be addressed. The increasing ethnic diversity in this country coupled with the high cancer rates among some ethnic groups argue for the importance of understanding psychosocial and behavioral contributors to cancer outcomes among all major ethnic groups. This research will not be easy, nor is it likely to be as methodologically sound in its early stages as studies in more well-established research areas. Nonetheless, developing a multidisciplinary, conceptually based approach could yield important information for developing theory and clinical interventions relevant to all patients with cancer and, possibly, patients with other chronic illnesses.

References

Alagaratnam, T. T., & Kung, N. Y. (1986). Psychosocial effects of mastectomy: Is it due to mastectomy or the diagnosis of malignancy? *British Journal of Psychiatry, 149,* 296–299.

American Cancer Society. (1995). *Cancer facts and figures—1995*. Atlanta, GA: Author.

Andersen, B. L. (1992). Psychological interventions for cancer patients to enhance quality of life. *Journal of Consulting and Clinical Psychology, 60*, 552–568.

Andersen, B. L., Kiecolt-Glaser, J. K., & Glaser, R. (1994). A biobehavioral model of cancer stress and disease course. *American Psychologist, 49*, 389–404.

Angel, R., & Guarnaccia, P. J. (1989). Mind, body, and culture: Somatization among Hispanics. *Social Science and Medicine, 28*, 1229–1238.

Antle, A. (1987). Ethnic perspectives of cancer nursing: The American Indian. *Oncology Nursing Forum, 14*, 70–73.

Austin, J. P., Azia, H., Potter, L., Thelmo, W., Chen, P., Choi, K., Brandys, M., Macchia, R. J., & Rotman, M. (1990). Diminished survival of young Blacks with adenocarcinoma of the prostate. *American Journal of Clinical Oncology, 13*, 465–469.

Axtell, L., & Myers, M. (1978). Contrasts in survival of Black and White cancer patients 1960–73. *Journal of the National Cancer Institute, 60*, 1209–1215.

Balcazar, H., Castro, F. G., & Krull, J. L. (1995). Cancer risk reduction in Mexican American women: The role of acculturation, education, and health risk factors. *Health Education Quarterly, 22*, 61–84.

Bando, M. (1990). Experiences of breast reconstruction following mastectomy in cases of cancer and evaluation of psychological aspects of the patients. *Gan To Kagaku Ryoho, 17*, 804–810.

Baquet, C. R., Ringen, K., Pollack, E. S., Young, J. L., Horm, J. W., Ries, L. A. G., & Simpson, N. K. (1986). *Cancer among Blacks and other minorities: Statistical profiles* (National Institutes of Health Pub. No. 86-2785). Bethesda, MD: National Cancer Institute.

Bassett, M. T., & Krieger, N. (1986). Social class and Black–White differences in breast cancer survival. *American Journal of Public Health, 76*, 1400–1403.

Bastani, R., Marcus, A. C., & Hollatz-Brown, A. (1991). Screening mammography rates and barriers to use: A Los Angeles County survey. *Preventive Medicine, 20*, 350–363.

Berg, J., Ross, R., & Latourette, H. (1977). Economic status and survival of cancer patients. *Cancer, 39*, 467–477.

Berry, J. W., & Kim, U. (1988). Acculturation and mental health. In P. R. Dassen, J. W. Berry, & N. Sartorius (Eds.), *Health and crosscultural psychology: Toward application* (pp. 207–236). Newbury Park, CA: Sage.

Blackhall, L. J., Murphy, S. T., Frank, G., Michel, V., & Azen, S. (1995). Ethnicity and attitudes toward patient autonomy. *Journal of the American Medical Association, 274*, 820–825.

Blendon, R. J., Aiken, L. H., Freeman, H. E., & Corey, C. R. (1989). Access to medical care for Black and White Americans: A matter of continuing concern. *Journal of the American Medical Association, 261*, 278–281.

Bloom, J. R., Hayes, W. A., Saunders, F., & Flatt, S. (1987). Cancer awareness and secondary prevention practices in Black Americans: Implications for intervention. *Family and Community Health, 10*, 19–30.

Bonadonna, G., & Valagussa, P. (1981). Dose–response effect of adjuvant chemotherapy in breast cancer. *New England Journal of Medicine, 304*, 10–14.

Bowman, J. A., Redman, S., Dickinson, J. A., Gibberd, R., & Sanson-Fisher, R. W. (1991). The accuracy of Pap smear utilization self-report: A methodological consideration in cervical screening research. *Health Services Research, 26*, 97–107.

Breen, N., & Kessler, L. (1994). Changes in the use of screening mammography: Evidence from the 1987 and 1990 National Health Interview Surveys. *American Journal of Public Health, 84*, 62–67.

Brotzman, G. L., & Butler, D. J. (1991). Cross-cultural issues in the disclosure of a terminal diagnostic: A case report. *Journal of Family Practice, 32*, 426–427.

Buckle, J. M., Horn, S. D., Oates, V. M., & Abbey, H. (1992). Severity of illness and resource use differences among White and Black hospitalized elderly. *Archives of Internal Medicine, 152,* 1596–1603.

Burack, R. C., & Liang, J. (1989). The acceptance and completion of mammography by older Black women. *American Journal of Public Health, 79,* 721–726.

Burns, R. B., McCarthy, E. P., Freund, K. M., Marwill, S. L., Shwartz, M., Ash, A., & Moskowitz, M. A. (1996). Black women receive less mammography even with similar use of primary care. *Annals of Internal Medicine, 125,* 173–182.

Calle, E. E., Flanders, W. D., Thun, M. J., & Martin, L. M. (1993). Demographic predictors of mammography and Pap smear screening in US women. *American Journal of Public Health, 83,* 53–60.

Canales, S., Ganz, P. A., & Coscarelli, C. A. (1995). Translation and validation of a quality of life instrument for Hispanic American cancer patients: Methodological considerations. *Quality of Life Research, 4,* 3–11.

Caplan, L. S., Wells, B. L., & Haynes, S. (1992). Breast cancer screening among older racial/ethnic minorities and Whites: Barriers to early detection. *Journal of Gerontology, 47,* 101–110.

Castro, F., Furth, P., & Karlow, H. (1984). The health beliefs of Mexican, Mexican American and Anglo American women. *Hispanic Journal of Behavioral Sciences, 6,* 365–383.

Cella, D. F., Orav, E. J., Kornblith, A. B., Holland, J. C., Silberfarb, P. M., Lee, K. W., Comis, R. L., Perry, M., Cooper, R., Maurer, L. H., Hoth, D. F., Perloff, M., Bloomfield, C. D., McIntyre, O. R., Leone, L., Lesnick, G., Nissen, N., Glicksman, A., Henderson, E., Barcos, M., Crichlow, R., Faulkner, C. S., II, Eaton, W., North, W., Schein, P. W., Chu, F., King, G., & Chahinian, A. P. (1991). Socioeconomic status and cancer survival. *Journal of Clinical Oncology, 9,* 1500–1509.

Champion, V. L. (1992). Compliance with guidelines for mammography screening. *Cancer Detection and Prevention, 16,* 253–258.

Chavez, L. R., Cornelius, W. A., & Jones, O. W. (1985). Mexican immigrants and the utilization of U.S. health services: The case of San Diego. *Social Science and Medicine, 2,* 93–102.

Chavez, L. R., Hubbell, F. A., McMullin, J. M., Martinez, R. G., & Mishra, S. I. (1995). Structure and meaning in models of breast and cervical cancer risk factors: A comparison of perceptions among Latinas, Anglo women, and physicians. *Medical Anthropology Quarterly, 9,* 40–74.

Chesney, A. P., Chavira, J. A., Hall, R. P., & Gary, H. E. (1982). Barriers to medical care of Mexican Americans: The role of social class, acculturation and social isolation. *Medical Care, 20,* 883–891.

Coates, R. J., Bransfield, D. D., Wesley, M., Hankey, B., Eley, J. W., Greenberg, R. S., Flanders, D., Hunter, C. P., Edwards, B. K., Forman, M., Chen, V. W., Reynolds, P., Boyd, P., Austin, D., Muss, H., Blacklow, R. S., & Black/White Cancer Survival Study Group. (1992). Differences between Black and White women with breast cancer in time from symptom recognition to medical consultation. *Journal of the National Cancer Institute, 84,* 938–950.

Coates, R. J., Clark, W. S., Eley, J. W., Greenberg, R. S., Huguley, C. M., Jr., & Brown, R. L. (1990). Race, nutritional status, and survival from breast cancer. *Journal of the National Cancer Institute, 82,* 1684–1692.

Cockburn, J., White, V. M., Hirst, S., & Hill, D. (1992). Barriers to cervical screening in older women. *Australian Family Physician, 21,* 973–978.

Coreil, J. (1984). Ethnicity and cancer prevention in a tri-ethnic urban community. *Journal of the National Medical Association, 76,* 1013–1019.

Coronary Drug Project Research Group. (1980). Influence of adherence to treatment and response of cholesterol on mortality in the Coronary Drug Project. *New England Journal of Medicine, 303,* 1038–1041.

Cotugna, N., Subar, A. F., Heimendinger, J., & Kahle, L. (1992). Nutrition and cancer prevention knowledge, beliefs, attitudes and practices: The 1987 National Health Interview
Survey. *Journal of the American Dietetic Association, 92*, 963–968.

Cousins, J. H., Rubovits, D. S., Dunn, J. K., Reeves, R. S., Ramirez, A. G., & Foreyt, J. P.
(1992). Family versus individually oriented intervention for weight loss in Mexican
American women. *Public Health Reports, 107*, 549–555.

Cox, C., & Monk, A. (1993). Hispanic culture and family care of Alzheimer's patients. *Health
and Social Work, 18*, 92–99.

Daly, M. B., Clark, G. M., & McGuire, W. L. (1985). Breast cancer prognosis in a mixed
Caucasian–Hispanic population. *Journal of the National Cancer Institute, 74*, 753–757.

Dansey, R. D., Hessel, P. A., Browde, S., Lange, M., Derman, D., Nissenbaum, M., & Be-
zwoda, W. R. (1988). Lack of a significant independent effect of race on survival in
breast cancer. *Cancer, 61*, 1908–1912.

Dayal, H., Power, R., & Chiu, C. (1982). Race and socioeconomic status in survival from
breast cancer. *Journal of Chronic Disease, 35*, 675–683.

Degnan, D., Harris, R., Ranney, J., Quade, D., Earp, J., & Gonzalez, J. (1992). Measuring
the use of mammography: Two methods compared. *American Journal of Public Health,
82*, 1386–1388.

Demark-Whanefried, W., Strigo, T., Catoe, K., Conaway, M., Brunetti, M., Rimer, B. K., &
Robertson, C. N. (1995). Knowledge, beliefs, and prior screening behavior among Blacks
and Whites reporting for prostate cancer screening. *Urology, 46*, 346–351.

Diehr, P., Yergan, J., Chu, J., Feigl, P., Glaefke, G., Moe, R., Bergner, M., & Rodenbaugh, J.
(1989). Treatment modality and quality differences for Black and White breast cancer
patients treated in community hospitals. *Medical Care, 27*, 942–958.

Dietrich, A. J., Carney-Gersten, P., Holmes, D. W., McIntyre, O. P., Reed, S., Clauson, B., &
Zaso, K. (1989). Community screening for cervical cancer in New Hampshire. *Journal
of Family Practice, 29*, 319–323.

Domino, G., Fragoso, A., & Moreno, H. (1991). Cross-cultural investigations of the imagery
of cancer in Mexican nationals. *Hispanic Journal of Behavioral Sciences, 13*, 422–435.

Domino, G., & Lin, J. (1991). Images of cancer: China and the United States. *Journal of
Psychosocial Oncology, 9*, 67–78.

Douglas, M., Bartolucci, A., Waterbor, J., & Sirles, A. (1995). Breast cancer early detection:
Differences between African American and White women's health beliefs and detection
practices. *Oncology Nursing Forum, 22*, 835–837.

Draguns, J. G. (1988). Personality and culture: Are they relevant for the enhancement of
quality of mental life? In P. R. Dassen, J. W. Barry, & N. Sartorius (Eds.), *Health and
cross-cultural psychology: Toward applications* (pp. 141–161). Newbury Park, CA: Sage.

Duelberg, S. I. (1992). Preventive health behavior among Black and White women in urban
and rural areas. *Social Science and Medicine, 34*, 191–198.

Eisenbruch, M., & Handelman, L. (1990). Cultural consultation for cancer: Astrocytoma in a
Cambodian adolescent. *Social Science and Medicine, 31*, 1295–1299.

Estrada, A. L., Treviño, F. M., & Ray, L. A. (1990). Health care utilization barriers among
Mexican Americans: Evidence from HHANES 1982–84. *American Journal of Public
Health, 80*(Suppl.), 27–31.

Etzi, S., Lane, D. S., & Grimson, R. (1994). The use of mammography vans by low-income
women: The accuracy of self-reports. *American Journal of Public Health, 84*, 107–109.

Farge, E. J. (1977). A review of findings from "three generations" of Chicano health care
behavior. *Social Science Quarterly, 58*, 407–411.

Farley, T. A., & Flannery, J. T. (1989). Late stage diagnosis of breast cancer in women of
lower socioeconomic status: Public health implications. *American Journal of Public
Health, 79*, 1508–1512.

Feld, R., Rubinstein, L., & Thomas, P. A. (1993). Adjuvant chemotherapy with cyclophosphamide, doxorubicin, and cisplatin in patients with completely resected stage I non-
small-cell lung cancer. *Journal of the National Cancer Institute*, *85*, 299–306.

Fink, R., & Shapiro, S. (1990). Significance of increased efforts to gain participation in
screening for breast cancer. *American Journal of Preventive Medicine*, *6*, 34–41.

Fisher, E. R., Redmond, C., Fisher, B., & Bass, G. (1990). Pathologic findings from the
National Surgical Adjuvant Breast and Bowel Projects (NSABP): Prognostic discrimi-
nants for 8-year survival for node-negative invasive breast cancer patients. *Cancer*, *65*,
2121–2128.

Fletcher, S. W., Morgan, T. M., O'Malley, M. S., Earp, J. A., & Degnan, D. (1989). Is breast
self-examination predicted by knowledge, attitudes, beliefs, or sociodemographic characteristics? *American Journal of Preventive Medicine*, *5*, 207–215.

Formenti, S. C., Meyerowitz, B. E., Ell, K., Muderspach, L., Groshen, S., Leedham, B.,
Klement, V., & Morrow, P. C. (1995). Inadequate adherence to radiotherapy in Latina
immigrants with carcinoma of the cervix: Potential impact on disease free survival. *Cancer*, *75*, 1135–1140.

Fox, S. A., Klos, D. S., Worthen, N. J., Pennington, E., Bassett, L. W., & Gold, R. H. (1990).
Improving the adherence of urban women to mammography guidelines: Strategies for
radiologists. *Radiology*, *174*, 203–206.

Fox, S. A., Murata, P. J., & Stein, J. A. (1991). The impact of physician compliance on
screening mammography for older women. *Archives of Internal Medicine*, *151*, 50–56.

Fox, S. A., & Stein, J. A. (1991). The effect of physician–patient communication on mammography utilization by different ethnic groups. *Medical Care*, *29*, 1065–1082.

Frazier, T. G., & Cummings, P. D. (1990). Motivational factors for participation in breast
cancer screening. *Journal of Cancer Education*, *5*, 51–54.

Freeman, H. P., & Wasfie, T. J. (1989). Cancer of the breast in poor Black women. *Cancer*,
63, 2562–2569.

Fulton, J. P., Rakowski, W., & Jones, A. C. (1995). Determinants of breast cancer screening
among inner-city Hispanic women in comparison with other inner-city women. *Public
Health Reports*, *110*, 476–482.

Garcia, H. B., & Lee, P. C. (1988). Knowledge about cancer and use of health care services
among Hispanic- and Asian-American older adults. *Journal of Psychosocial Oncology*,
6, 157–177.

Gemson, D. H., Elinson, J., & Messeri, P. (1988). Differences in physician prevention practice
patterns for White and minority patients. *Journal of Community Health*, *13*, 53–64.

Golding, J. M., & Baezconde-Garbanati, L. A. (1990). Ethnicity, culture, and social resources.
American Journal of Community Psychology, *18*, 465–486.

Golding, J. M., & Burnam, M. A. (1990). Stress and social support as predictors of depressive
symptoms in Mexican Americans and non-Hispanic Whites. *Journal of Social and Clinical Psychology*, *9*, 268–286.

Goodwin, J. S., Hunt, W. C., & Samet, J. M. (1991). A population-based study of functional
status and social support networks of elderly patients newly diagnosed with cancer. *Archives of Internal Medicine*, *151*, 366–370.

Gordon, N. H., Crowe, J. P., Brumberg, D. J., & Berger, N. A. (1992). Socioeconomic factors
and race in breast cancer recurrence and survival. *American Journal of Epidemiology*,
135, 609–618.

Graham, M. V., Geitz, L. M., Byhardt, R., Asbell, S., Roach, M., III, Urtasun, R. C., Curran,
W. J., Jr., Lattin, P., Russell, A. H., & Cox, J. D. (1992). Comparison of prognostic
factors and survival among Black patients and White patients treated with irradiation for
non-small-cell lung cancer. *Journal of the National Cancer Institute*, *84*, 1731–1735.

Greenwald, H. P., & Henke, C. J. (1991). HMO membership, treatment, and mortality risk
among prostatic cancer patients. *American Journal of Public Health*, *82*, 1099–1104.

Guillory, J. (1987). Ethnic perspectives of cancer nursing: The Black American. *Oncology Nursing Forum, 14,* 66–69.

Hahn, R. A. (1992). The state of federal health statistics on racial and ethnic groups. *Journal of the American Medical Association, 267,* 268–271.

Hahn, R. A., & Stroup, D. F. (1994). Race and ethnicity in public health surveillance: Criteria for the scientific use of social categories. *Public Health Reports, 109,* 7–15.

Harlan, L. C., Bernstein, A. B., & Kessler, L. G. (1991). Cervical cancer screening: Who is not screened and why? *American Journal of Public Health, 81,* 885–890.

Harper, A. P. (1993). Mammography utilization in the poor and medically underserved. *Cancer, 72,* 1478–1482.

Hartog, J., & Hartog, E. A. (1983). Cultural aspects of health and illness behavior in hospitals. *Western Journal of Medicine, 139,* 910–916.

Harwood, A. (1971). The hot–cold theory of disease: Implications for treatment of Puerto Rican patients. *Journal of the American Medical Association, 216,* 1153–1158.

Hayward, R. A., Shapiro, M. F., Freeman, H. E., & Corey, C. R. (1988). Who gets screened for cervical and breast cancer? Results from a new national survey. *Archives of Internal Medicine, 148,* 1177–1181.

Hogan-Garcia, M. H., Martinez, J. L., Jr., & Martinez, S. (1979). The semantic differential: A tri-ethnic comparison of sex and familiar concepts. *Hispanic Journal of Behavioral Sciences, 1,* 135–149.

Holland, J. C., & Rowland, J. H. (Eds.). (1989). *The handbook of psychooncology.* New York: Oxford University Press.

Horm, J. W. (1987). *Cancer among minorities: A statistical profile.* Bethesda, MD: National Cancer Institute, Division of Cancer Prevention and Control.

Howe, H. L. (1992). Repeat mammography among women over 50 years of age. *American Journal of Preventive Medicine, 8,* 182–185.

Hubbell, F. A., Chavez, L. R., Mishra, S. I., Magana, J. R., & Valdez, R. B. (1995). From ethnography to intervention: Developing a breast cancer control program for Latinas. *Journal of the National Cancer Institute Monographs, 18,* 109–115.

Hubbell, F. A., Waitzkin, H., Mishra, S. I., Dombrink, J., & Chavez, L. R. (1991). Access to medical care for documented and undocumented Latinos in a southern California county. *Western Journal of Medicine, 154,* 414–417.

Inclan, J., & Hernandez, M. (1992). Cross-cultural perspectives and codependence: The case of poor Hispanics. *American Journal of Orthopsychiatry, 62,* 245–255.

Ironson, G., Antoni, M., & Lutgendorf, S. (1995). Can psychological interventions affect immunity and survival? Present findings and suggested targets with a focus on cancer and human immunodeficiency virus. *Mind/Body Medicine, 1,* 85–110.

Jacob, T. C., Penn, N. E., & Brown, M. (1989). Breast self-examination: Knowledge, attitudes, and performance among Black women. *Journal of the National Medical Association, 81,* 769–776.

Jenkins, C. N. H., McPhee, S. J., Bird, J. A., & Bonilla, N. H. (1990). Cancer risks and prevention practices among Vietnamese refugees. *Western Journal of Medicine, 153,* 34–39.

Jepson, C., & Chaiken, S. (1990). Chronic issue-specific fear inhibits systematic processing of persuasive communications. *Journal of Social Behavior and Personality, 5,* 61–84.

Kagawa-Singer, M. (1987). Ethnic perspectives of cancer nursing: Hispanics and Japanese-Americans. *Oncology Nursing Forum, 14,* 59–65.

Kagawa-Singer, M. (1993). Redefining health: Living with cancer. *Social Science and Medicine, 37,* 295–304.

Kang, S. H., & Bloom, J. R. (1993). Social support and cancer screening among older Black Americans. *Journal of the National Cancer Institute, 85,* 737–742.

Kaplan, K. M., Weinberg, B. B., Small, A., & Herndon, J. L. (1991). Breast cancer screening among relatives of women with breast cancer. *American Journal of Public Health, 81*, 1174–1179.

Karjalainen, S., & Pukkala, E. (1990). Social class as a prognostic factor in breast cancer survival. *Cancer, 66*, 819–826.

Keefe, S. E. (1984). Real and ideal extended familism among Mexican Americans and Anglo Americans: On the meaning of "close" family ties. *Human Organization, 43*, 65–70.

Kim, H. S., Holter, I. M., Lorensen, M., Inayoshi, M., Shimaguchi, S., Shimazaki-Ryder, R., Kawaguchi, Y., Hori, R., Takezaki, K., Leino-Kilpi, H., & Munkki-Utunen, M. (1993). Patient–nurse collaboration: A comparison of patients' and nurses' attitudes in Finland, Japan, Norway, and the U.S.A. *International Journal of Nursing Studies, 30*, 387–401.

Kimmick, G., Muss, H. B., Case, L. D., & Stanley, V. (1991). A comparison of treatment outcomes for Black patients and White patients with metastatic breast cancer: The Piedmont Oncology Association experience. *Cancer, 67*, 2850–2854.

King, E. S., Rimer, B. K., Trock, B., Balshem, A., & Engstrom, P. (1990). How valid are mammography self-reports? *American Journal of Public Health, 80*, 1386–1388.

Kleinman, A., Eisenberg, L., & Good, B. (1978). Culture, illness and care. *Annals of Internal Medicine, 88*, 251–258.

Lackland, D. T., Dunbar, J. B., Keil, J. E., Knapp, R. G., & O'Brien, P. H. (1991). Breast cancer screening in a biracial community: The Charleston tricounty experience. *Southern Medical Journal, 84*, 862–866.

Laedtke, T. W., & Dignan, M. (1992). Compliance with therapy for cervical dysplasia among women of low socioeconomic status. *Southern Medical Journal, 85*, 5–8.

LaFromboise, T., Coleman, H. L. K., & Gerton, J. (1993). Psychological impact of biculturalism: Evidence and theory. *Psychological Bulletin, 114*, 395–412.

Lauver, D. (1994). Care-seeking behavior with breast cancer symptoms in Caucasian and African-American women. *Research in Nursing and Health, 17*, 421–431.

Lauver, D., Barsevick, A., & Rubin, M. (1990). Spontaneous causal searching and adjustment to abnormal Papanicolaou test results. *Nursing Research, 39*, 305–308.

LaVeist, T. A. (1994). Beyond dummy variables and sample selection: What health services researchers ought to know about race as a variable. *Health Services Research, 29*, 1–16.

Lebovitz, A. H., Strain, J. J., Schleifer, S. J., Tanaka, J. S., Bhardwaj, S., & Messe, M. R. (1990). Patient noncompliance with self-administered chemotherapy. *Cancer, 65*, 17–22.

LeMarchand, L. (1991). Ethnic variation in breast cancer survival: A review. *Breast Cancer Research and Treatment, 18*, S119–S126.

LeMarchand, L., Kolonel, L. N., & Nomura, A. M. Y. (1984). Relationship of ethnicity and other prognostic factors to breast cancer survival patterns in Hawaii. *Journal of the National Cancer Institute, 73*, 1259–1265.

Lerman, C., Hanjani, P., Caputo, C., Miller, S., Delmoor, E., Nolte, S., & Engstrom, P. (1992). Telephone counseling improves adherence to colposcopy among lower-income minority women. *Journal of Clinical Oncology, 10*, 330–333.

Levine, A. M., Richardson, J. L., Marks, G., Chan, K., Graham, J., Selser, J. N., Kisbaugh, C., Shelton, D. R., & Johnson, C. A. (1987). Compliance with oral drug therapy in patients with hematologic malignancy. *Journal of Clinical Oncology, 5*, 1469–1476.

Lewin-Epstein, N. (1991). Determinants of regular source of health care in Black, Mexican, Puerto Rican, and non-Hispanic White populations. *Medical Care, 29*, 543–557.

Lima, J., & Cohen, M. A. (1991). Treatment decisions in end-stage bladder cancer. *General Hospital Psychiatry, 13*, 209–212.

Lipid Research Clinics Program. (1984). The Lipid Research Clinics Coronary Primary Prevention Trial results: II. The relationship of reduction in incidence of coronary heart disease to cholesterol lowering. *Journal of the American Medical Association, 251*, 365–374.

Lipworth, L., & Parker, P. (1972). Prognosis of nonprivate cancer patients. *Journal of the National Cancer Institute, 48,* 11–16.

Loehrer, P. J., Sr., Greger, H. A., Weinberger, M., Musick, B., Miller, M., Nichols, C., Bryan, J., Higgs, D., & Brock, D. (1991). Knowledge and beliefs about cancer in a socioeconomically disadvantaged population. *Cancer, 68,* 1665–1671.

Longman, A. J., Saint-Germain, M. A., & Modiano, M. (1992). Use of breast cancer screening by older Hispanic women. *Public Health Nursing, 9,* 118–124.

Maduro, R. (1983). *Curanderismo* and Latino views of disease and curing. *Western Journal of Medicine, 139,* 868–874.

Mah, Z., & Bryant, H. (1992). Age as a factor in breast cancer knowledge, attitudes and screening behaviour. *Canadian Medical Association Journal, 146,* 2167–2174.

Mamon, J. A., Shediac, M. C., Crosby, C. B., Sanders, B., Matanoski, G. M., & Celentano, D. D. (1990). Inner-city women at risk for cervical cancer: Behavioral and utilization factors related to inadequate screening. *Preventive Medicine, 19,* 363–376.

Mandelblatt, J., Andrews, H., Kerner, J., Zauber, A., & Burnett, W. (1991). Determinants of late stage diagnosis of breast and cervical cancer: The impact of age, race, social class and hospital type. *American Journal of Public Health, 81,* 646–649.

Mandelblatt, J., Traxler, M., Lakin, P., Kanetsky, P., & Kao, R. (1992). Mammography and Papanicolaou smear use by elderly poor Black women. *Journal of the American Geriatrics Society, 40,* 1001–1007.

Mandelblatt, J., Traxler, M., Lakin, P., Kanetsky, P., Thomas, L., Chauhan, P., Matseoane, S., Ramsey, E., & the Harlem Study Team. (1993). Breast and cervical cancer screening of poor, elderly, Black women: Clinical results and implications. *American Journal of Preventive Medicine, 9,* 133–138.

Manfredi, C., Warnecke, R. B., Graham, S., & Rosenthal, S. (1977). Social psychological correlates of health behavior: Knowledge of breast self-examination techniques among Black women. *Social Science and Medicine, 11,* 433–440.

Marcus, A. C., Crane, L. A., Kaplan, C. P., Reading, A. E., Savage, E., Gunning, J., Bernstein, G., & Berek, J. S. (1992). Improving adherence to screening follow-up among women with abnormal Pap smears. *Medical Care, 30,* 216–230.

Mathews, H. F., Lannin, D. R., & Mitchell, J. P. (1994). Coming to terms with advanced breast cancer: Black women's narratives from eastern North Carolina. *Social Science and Medicine, 38,* 789–800.

Mayer, W. J., & McWhorter, W. P. (1989). Black/White differences in non-treatment of bladder cancer patients and implications for survival. *American Journal of Public Health, 79,* 772–775.

McCurtis, J. W. (1979). Social contact factors in the diffusion of cervical cytology among Mexican-Americans in Los Angeles County, CA. *Social Science and Medicine, 13A,* 807–811.

McKenney, N. R., & Bennett, C. E. (1994). Issues regarding data on race and ethnicity: The census bureau experience. *Public Health Reports, 109,* 16–25.

McWhorter, W. P., & Mayer, W. J. (1987). Black/White differences in type of initial breast cancer treatment and implications for survival. *American Journal of Public Health, 77,* 1515–1517.

McWhorter, W. P., Schatzkin, A. G., Horm, J. W., & Brown, C. C. (1989). Contribution of SES to Black/White differences in cancer incidence. *Cancer, 63,* 982–987.

Meyerowitz, B. E., Formenti, S. C., Ell, K. O., & Leedham, B. (1997). *Predictors of adjustment among indigent, Latina cervical cancer patients receiving radiotherapy.* Unpublished manuscript, University of Southern California.

Meyerowitz, B. E., Leedham, B., & Hart, S. (in press). Psychosocial considerations for breast cancer patients and their families. In J. Kavanagh, S. E. Singletary, N. Einhorn,

A. D. DePetrillo, & S. Pecorelli (Eds.), *Cancer in women*. Cambridge, MA: Blackwell Science.

Michielutte, R., & Diseker, R. A. (1982). Racial differences in knowledge of cancer: A pilot study. *Social Science and Medicine, 16*, 245–252.

Michielutte, R., Diseker, R., Young, L., & May, W. J. (1985). Noncompliance in screening follow-up among family planning clinic patients with cervical dysplasia. *Preventive Medicine, 14*, 248–258.

Mickey, R. M., Durski, J., Worden, J. K., & Danigelis, N. L. (1995). Breast cancer screening and associated factors for low-income African-American women. *Preventive Medicine, 24*, 467–476.

Miller, B. A., Gloeckler Ries, L. A., Hankey, B. F., Kosary, C. L., Harras, A., Devesa, S. S., & Edwards, B. K. (Eds.). (1993). *SEER cancer statistics review 1973–1990* (National Institutes of Health Publication No. 93-2789). Bethesda, MD: U.S. Department of Health and Human Services, Public Health Service, and National Institutes of Health, National Cancer Institute.

Miller, B. A., Kolonel, L. N., Bernstein, L., Young, J. L., Swanson, G. M., West, D., Key, C. R., Liff, J. M., Glover, C. S., & Alexander, G. A. (Eds.). (1996). *Racial/ethnic patterns of cancer in the United States 1988–1992* (National Institutes of Health Publications No. 96-4104). Bethesda, MD: U.S. Department of Health and Human Services, Public Health Service, and National Institutes of Health, National Cancer Institute.

Mindel, C. H. (1980). Extended familism among urban Mexican Americans, Anglos and Blacks. *Hispanic Journal of Behavioral Sciences, 2*, 21–34.

Mo, B. (1992). Modesty, sexuality, and breast health in Chinese-American women. *Western Journal of Medicine, 157*, 260–264.

Morrow, G. R., Leirer, V., & Sheikh, J. (1988). Adherence and medication instructions: Review and recommendations. *Journal of the American Geriatrics Society, 36*, 1147–1160.

Muecke, M. A. (1983). Caring for Southeast Asian refugee patients in the USA. *American Journal of Public Health, 73*, 431–438.

Muss, H. B., Hunter, C. P., Wesley, M., Correa, P., Chen, V. W., Greenberg, R. S., Eley, J. W., Austin, D. F., Korman, R., & Edwards, B. K. (1992). Treatment plans for Black and White women with stage II node-positive breast cancer: The National Cancer Institute Black/White Cancer Survey Study experience. *Cancer, 70*, 2460–2467.

Nall, F. C., II, & Speilberg, J. (1967). Social and cultural factors in the responses of Mexican-Americans to medical treatment. *Journal of Health and Social Behavior, 8*, 299–308.

Natarajan, N., Nemoto, T., Mettlin, C., & Murphy, G. P. (1985). Race-related differences in breast cancer patients. *Cancer, 56*, 1704–1709.

National Center for Health Statistics. (1993). *Healthy people 2000 review: Health, United States, 1992*. Hyattsville, MD: Public Health Service.

Nemcek, M. A. (1989). Factors influencing Black women's breast self-examination practice. *Cancer Nursing, 12*, 339–343.

Neves-Arruda, E. N., Larson, P. J., & Meleis, A. I. (1992). Comfort: Immigrant Hispanic cancer patients' views. *Cancer Nursing, 15*, 387–394.

Ngan, H. T. S., & Tang, G. (1988). Further study of sexual functioning following treatment of carcinoma of the cervix in Chinese patients. *Journal of Psychosomatic Obstetrics and Gynaecology, 9*, 117–129.

Nickens, H. W. (1995, April). The role of race/ethnicity and social class in minority health status (Pt. II). *Health Services Research, 30*, 151–162.

Nilchaikovit, T., Hill, J. M., & Holland, J. C. (1993). The effects of culture on illness behavior and medical care: Asian and American diferences. *General Hospital Psychiatry, 15*, 41–50.

O'Hare, P. A., Malone, D., Lusk, E., & McCorkle, R. (1993). Unmet needs of Black patients with cancer posthospitalization: A descriptive study. *Oncology Nursing Forum, 20*, 659–664.

O'Hoy, K. M., & Tang, G. W. (1985). Sexual function following treatment for carcinoma of cervix. *Journal of Psychosomatic Obstetrics and Gynaecology, 4*, 51–58.

Optenberg, S. A., Thompson, I. M., Friedrichs, P., Wojcik, B., Stein, C. R., & Kramer, B. (1995). Race, treatment, and long-term survival from prostate cancer in an equal-access medical care delivery system. *Journal of the American Medical Association, 274*, 1599–1605.

Osborne, N. G., & Feit, M. D. (1992). The use of race in medical research. *Journal of the American Medical Association, 267*, 275–279.

Pachter, L. M. (1994). Culture and clinical care: Folk illness beliefs and behaviors and their implications for health care delivery. *Journal of the American Medical Association, 271*, 690–694.

Paskett, E. D., Carter, W. B., Chu, J., & White, E. (1990). Compliance behavior in women with abnormal Pap smears: Developing and testing a decision model. *Medical Care, 28*, 643–656.

Payne, B. D., Smith, J. E., & Payne, D. A. (1983). Sex and ethnic differences in relationships of test anxiety to performance in science examinations by fourth and eighth grade students: Implications for valid interpretations of achievement test scores. *Educational and Psychological Measurement, 43*, 267–270.

Perez-Stable, E. J., Sabogal, F., & Otero-Sabogal, R. (1995). Use of cancer-screening tests in the San Francisco Bay area: Comparison of Latinos and Anglos. *Journal of the National Cancer Institute Monographs, 18*, 147–153.

Perez-Stable, E. J., Sabogal, F., Otero-Sabogal, R., Hiatt, R. A., & McPhee, S. J. (1992). Misconceptions about cancer among Latinos and Anglos. *Journal of the American Medical Association, 268*, 3219–3223.

Peters, R. K., Bear, M. B., & Thomas, D. (1989). Barriers to screening for cancer of the cervix. *Preventive Medicine, 18*, 133–146.

Pham, C. T., & McPhee, S. J. (1992). Knowledge, attitudes, and practices of breast and cervical cancer screening among Vietnamese women. *Journal of Cancer Education, 7*, 305–310.

Phinney, J. S. (1996). When we talk about American ethnic groups, what do we mean? *American Psychologist, 51*, 918–927.

Pizzo, P. A., Robichaud, K. J., Edwards, B. K., Schumaker, C., Kramer, B. S., & Johnson, A. (1983). Oral antibiotic prophylaxis in patients with cancer: A double-blind randomized placebo controlled trial. *Journal of Pediatrics, 102*, 125–133.

Powe, B. D. (1995). Cancer fatalism among elderly Caucasians and African Americans. *Oncology Nursing Forum, 22*, 1355–1359.

Powell, I. J., Schwartz, K., & Hussain, M. (1995). Removal of the financial barrier to health care: Does it impact on prostate cancer at presentation and survival? A comparative study between Black and White men in a Veterans Affairs system. *Urology, 46*, 825–830.

Price, J. H., Colvin, T. L., & Smith, D. (1993). Prostate cancer: Perceptions of African-American males. *Journal of the National Medical Association, 85*, 941–947.

Price, J. H., Desmond, S. M., Slenker, S., Smith, D., & Stewart, P. W. (1992). Urban Black women's perceptions of breast cancer and mammography. *Journal of Community Health, 17*, 191–204.

Price, J. H., Desmond, S. M., Wallace, M., Smith, D., & Stewart, P. W. (1988a). Black Americans' perceptions of cancer: A study utilizing the health belief model. *Journal of the National Medical Association, 80*, 1297–1304.

Price, J. H., Desmond, S. M., Wallace, M., Smith, D., & Stewart, P. W. (1988b). Differences in Black and White adolescents' perceptions about cancer. *Journal of School Health, 58*, 66–70.

Ragland, K. E., Selvin, S., & Merrill, D. W. (1991). Black–White differences in stage-specific cancer survival: Analysis of seven selected sites. *American Journal of Epidemiology, 133*, 672–682.

Rakowski, W., Rimer, B. K., & Bryant, S. A. (1993). Integrating behavior and intention regarding mammography by respondents in the 1990 National Health Interview Survey of Health Promotion and Disease Prevention. *Public Health Reports, 108*, 605–624.

Reid, P. T. (1993). Poor women in psychological research: Shut up and shut out. *Psychology of Women Quarterly, 17*, 133–150.

Richardson, J. L., & Hudson, S. (1998). Adherence to chemotherapy regimens after the diagnosing of breast cancer in Hispanic women [unpublished data]. University of Southern California.

Richardson, J. L., Langholz, B., Bernstein, L., Burciaga, C., Danley, K., & Ross, R. K. (1992). Stage and delay in breast cancer diagnosis by race, socioeconomic status, age and year. *British Journal of Cancer, 65*, 922–926.

Richardson, J. L., Marks, G., Solis, J. M., Collins, L. M., Birba, L., & Hisserich, J. C. (1987). Frequency and adequacy of breast cancer screening among elderly Hispanic women. *Preventive Medicine, 16*, 761–774.

Richardson, J. L., Shelton, D. R., Krailo, M., & Levine, A. (1990). The effect of compliance with treatment on survival among patients with hematologic malignancies. *Journal of Clinical Oncology, 8*, 356–364.

Rimer, B. K., Keintz, M. K., Kessler, H. B., Engstrom, P. F., & Rosan, J. R. (1989). Why women resist screening mammography: Patient-related barriers. *Radiology, 172*, 243–246.

Rimer, B. K., Ross, E., Cristinzio, C. S., & King, E. (1992). Older women's participation in breast screening. *Journal of Gerontology, 47*, 85–91.

Robinson, R. G., Kessler, L. G., & Naughton, M. D. (1991). Cancer awareness among African Americans: A survey assessing race, social status, and occupation. *Journal of the National Medical Association, 83*, 491–497.

Rogler, L. H., Cortes, D. E., & Malgady, R. G. (1991). Acculturation and mental health status among Hispanics: Convergence and new directions for research. *American Psychologist, 46*, 585–597.

Ross, C. E., Mirowski, J., & Cockerham, W. C. (1983). Social class, Mexican culture and fatalism: Their effects on psychological distress. *American Journal of Community Psychology, 11*, 383–399.

Ross, R. K., Burnstein, L., Lobo, R. A., Shimizu, H., Stanczyk, F. Z., Pike, M. C., & Henderson, B. E. (1992). 5-alpha-reductose activity and risk of prostate cancer among Japanese and U.S. White and Black males. *Lancet, 339*, 887–889.

Rubel, A. J., & Garro, L. C. (1992). Social and cultural factors in the successful control of tuberculosis. *Public Health Reports, 107*, 626–636.

Ruiz, M. S., Marks, G., & Richardson, J. L. (1992). Language acculturation and screening practices of elderly Hispanic women: The role of exposure to health-related information from the media. *Journal of Aging and Health, 4*, 268–281.

Sabogal, F., Marin, G., Otero-Sabogal, R., Van Oss-Marin, B., & Perez-Stable, E. J. (1987). Hispanic familism and acculturation: What changes and what doesn't. *Hispanic Journal of Behavioral Sciences, 9*, 397–412.

Sackett, D. L., Haynes, R. B., Gibson, E. S., & Johnson, A. (1976). The problem of compliance with antihypertensive therapy. *Practical Cardiology, 2*, 35–39.

Sackett, D. L., & Snow, J. C. (1979). Compliance and noncompliance. In R. B. Haynes, D. W. Taylor, & D. L. Sackett (Eds.), *Compliance in health care* (pp. 11–23). Baltimore: Johns Hopkins University Press.

Sawyer, J. A., Earp, J. A., Fletcher, R. H., Daye, F. F., & Wynn, T. M. (1989). Accuracy of women's self-report of their last Pap smear. *American Journal of Public Health, 79*, 1036–1037.

Sawyer, J. A., Earp, J., Fletcher, R. H., Daye, F. F., & Wynn, T. M. (1990). Pap tests of rural Black women. *Journal of General Internal Medicine, 5*, 115–119.

Sawyers, J. E., & Eaton, Ł. (1992). Gastric cancer in the Korean-American: Cultural implications. *Oncology Nursing Forum, 19,* 619–623.

Schulman, K. A., Rubenstein, L. E., Chesley, F. D., & Eisenberg, J. M. (1995). The roles of race and socioeconomic factors in health services research. *Health Services Research, 30,* 179–195.

Scott, S., & Suagee, M. (1992). *Enhancing health statistics for American Indian and Alaskan Native communities: An agenda for action—A report to the National Center for Health Statistics.* St. Paul, MN: American Indian Health Care Association.

Seijo, R., Gomez, H., & Freidenberg, J. (1991). Language as a communication barrier in medical care for Hispanic patients. *Hispanic Journal of Behavioral Sciences, 13,* 363–376.

Shope, J. T. (1981). Medication compliance. *Pediatric Clinics of North America, 28,* 5–21.

Skinner, C. S., Strecher, V. J., & Hospers, H. (1994). Physicians' recommendations for mammography: Do tailored messages make a difference? *American Journal of Public Health, 84,* 43–49.

Smith, S. D., Rosen, D., Trueworthy, R. C., & Lowman, J. T. (1979). A reliable method for evaluating drug compliance in children with cancer. *Cancer, 43,* 169–173.

Solis, J. M., Marks, G., Garcia, M., & Shelton, D. (1990). Acculturation, access to care, and use of preventive services by Hispanics: Findings from HHANES 1982–84. *American Journal of Public Health, 80*(Suppl.), 11–19.

Spurlock, C., Nadel, M., & McMannon, E. (1992). Age and Pap smear history as a basis for intervention strategy. *Journal of Community Health, 17,* 97–107.

Stanaway, L., Lambie, D. G., & Johnson, R. H. (1985). Noncompliance with anti-convulsant therapy as a cause of seizures. *New Zealand Medical Journal, 98,* 150–152.

Stanford, J. L., & Greenberg, R. S. (1989). Breast cancer incidence in young women by estrogen receptor status and race. *American Journal of Public Health, 79,* 71–73.

Stein, J. A., & Fox, S. A. (1990). Language preference as an indicator of mammography use among Hispanic women. *Journal of the National Cancer Institute, 82,* 1715–1716.

Stein, J. A., Fox, S. A., & Murata, P. J. (1991). The influence of ethnicity, socioeconomic status, and psychological barriers on use of mammography. *Journal of Health and Social Behavior, 32,* 101–113.

Stein, J. A., Fox, S. A., Murata, P. J., & Morisky, D. E. (1992). Mammography usage and the health belief model. *Health Education Quarterly, 19,* 447–462.

Stewart, D. E., Buchegger, P. M., Lickrish, G. M., & Sierra, S. (1994). The effect of educational brochures on follow-up compliance in women with abnormal Pap smears. *Obstetrics and Gynecology, 83,* 583–585.

Stone, A. J., & Siegel, J. M. (1986). Correlates of accurate knowledge of cancer. *Health Education Quarterly, 13,* 39–50.

Struewing, J. P., Abeliovich, D., Peretz, T., Avishai, N., Kaback, M. M., Collins, F. S., & Brody, L. C. (1995). The carrier frequency of the BRCA1 185delAG mutation is approximately 1 percent in Ashkenazi Jewish individuals. *Nature Genetics, 11,* 198–200.

Suarez, L. (1994). Pap smear and mammogram screening in Mexican-American women: The effects of acculturation. *American Journal of Public Health, 84,* 742–746.

Suarez, L., & Pulley, L. (1995). Comparing acculturation scales and their relationship to cancer screening among older Mexican-American women. *Journal of the National Cancer Institute Monographs, 18,* 41–47.

Sugarek, N. J., Deyo, R. A., & Holmes, B. C. (1988). Locus of control and beliefs about cancer in a multi-ethnic clinic population. *Oncology Nursing Forum, 15,* 481–486.

Sutherland, C. M., & Mather, F. J. (1986). Long-term survival and prognostic factors in breast cancer patients with localized (no skin, muscle, or chest wall attachment) disease with and without positive lymph nodes. *Cancer, 57,* 622–629.

Szapocznik, J., & Kurtines, W. M. (1993). Family psychology and cultural diversity: Opportunities for theory, research, and application. *American Psychologist, 48,* 400–407.

Taylor, S. E., Falke, R. L., Shoptaw, S. J., & Lichtman, R. R. (1986). Social support, support groups, and the cancer patient. *Journal of Consulting and Clinical Psychology, 54,* 608–615.

Trill, M. D., & Holland, J. (1993). Cross-cultural differences in the care of patients with cancer: A review. *General Hospital Psychiatry, 15,* 21–30.

Trotter, R. T. (1991). A survey of four illnesses and their relationship to intracultural variation in a Mexican-American community. *American Anthropologist, 93,* 115–125.

Uba, L. (1992). Cultural barriers to health care for Southeast Asian refugees. *Public Health Reports, 107,* 544–548.

U.S. Bureau of the Census. (1990a). 1990 census of population, social and economic characteristics (1990CP-2-1). Washington, DC: U.S. Government Printing Office.

U.S. Bureau of the Census. (1990b). Persons of Hispanic origin in the United States, 1990 census of population (1990CP-3-3). Washington, DC: U.S. Government Printing Office.

Vaz, R. M., Best, D. L., & Davis, S. W. (1988). Testicular cancer: Adolescent knowledge and attitudes. *Journal of Adolescent Health Care, 9,* 474–479.

Vega, W. A. (1992). Theoretical and pragmatic implications of cultural diversity for community research. *American Journal of Community Psychology, 20,* 375–391.

Vernon, S. W., Tilley, B. C., Neale, A. V., & Steinfeldt, L. (1985). Ethnicity, survival and delay in seeking treatment for symptoms of breast cancer. *Cancer, 55,* 1563–1571.

Vernon, S. W., Vogel, V. G., Halabi, S., Jackson, G. L., Lundy, R. O., & Peters, G. N. (1992). Breast cancer screening behaviors and attitudes in three racial/ethnic groups. *Cancer, 69,* 165–174.

Villar, H. V., & Menck, H. R. (1994). The national cancer data base report on cancer in Hispanics: Relationships between ethnicity, poverty and the diagnosis of some cancers. *Cancer, 74,* 2386–2395.

Vogel, V. G., Graves, D. S., Coody, D. K., Winn, R. J., & Peters, G. N. (1990). Breast screening compliance following a statewide low-cost mammography project. *Cancer Detection and Prevention, 14,* 573–576.

Wagner, E. H., Truesdale, R. A., & Warner, J. R. (1981). Compliance treatment practices and blood pressure control: Community and survey findings. *Journal of Chronic Disease, 34,* 519–525.

Walter, S. D., Clarke, E. A., Hatcher, J., & Stitt, L. W. (1988). A comparison of physician and patient reports of Pap smear histories. *Journal of Clinical Epidemiology, 41,* 401–410.

Weinberger, M., Saunders, A. F., Samsa, G. P., Bearon, L. B., Gold, D. T., Brown, J. T., Booher, P., & Loehrer, P. J. (1991). Breast cancer screening in older women: Practices and barriers reported by primary care physicians. *Journal of the American Geriatric Society, 39,* 22–29.

Weissman, J. S., Stern, R., Fielding, S. L., & Epstein, A. M. (1991). Delayed access to health care: Risk factors, reasons and consequences. *Annals of Internal Medicine, 114,* 325–331.

Wells, K. B., Golding, J. M., Hough, R. L., Burnam, M. A., & Karno, M. (1988). Factors affecting the probability of use of general and medical health and social/community services for Mexican Americans and non-Hispanic Whites. *Medical Care, 26,* 441–452.

Wells, K. B., Hough, R. L., Golding, J. M., Burnam, M. A., & Karno, M. (1987). Which Mexican-Americans underutilize health services? *American Journal of Psychiatry, 144,* 918–922.

Whittemore, A., Wu-Williams, A., Lee, M., Zheng, S., Gallagher, R., Jiao, D. A., Zhou, L., Wang, X., Chen, K., Jung, D., Teh, C. Z., Ling, C., Xu, J. Y., Paffenbarger, R., & Henderson, B. E. (1990). Diet, physical activity and colorectal cancer among Chinese in North America and the People's Republic of China. *Journal of the National Cancer Institute, 82,* 915–926.

Wilkinson, D. Y., & King, G. (1987). Conceptual and methodological issues in the use of race as a variable: Policy implications. *The Milbank Quarterly, 65,* 56–71.

Williams, D. R., Lavizzo-Mourey, R., & Warren, R. C. (1994). The concept of race and health status in America. *Public Health Reports, 109,* 26–41.

Wilson, W. J. (1987). *The truly disadvantaged: The inner city, the underclass and public policy.* Chicago: University of Chicago Press.

Young, J. L., Jr., Ries, L. G., & Pollack, E. S. (1984). Cancer patient survival among ethnic groups in the United States. *Journal of the National Cancer Institute, 73,* 341–352.

Yu, E. (1993). Measurement and use of ethnicity in public health surveillance. *Morbidity and Mortality Weekly Report, 42,* 73.

Zapka, J. G., Stoddard, A., Barth, R., Costanza, M. E., & Mas, E. (1989). Breast cancer screening utilization by Latina community health center clients. *Health Education Research, 4,* 461–468.

Zeltzer, L. K., & LeBaron, S. (1985). Does ethnicity constitute a risk factor in the psychological distress of adolescents with cancer? *Journal of Adolescent Health Care, 6,* 8–11.

(Appendixes follow)

Appendix A

Average Annual Age-Adjusted Cancer Incidence Rates per 100,000 (1988–1992)

Type of cancer	Non-Hispanic White	Black	White Hispanic	Japanese	Chinese	Hawaiian	Native American
Women							
Breast	115.7	95.4	73.5	82.3	55.0	105.6	31.6
Colon–rectum	39.2	45.5	25.9	39.5	33.6	30.5	15.3
Lung–bronchus	43.7	44.2	20.4	15.2	25.3	43.1	a
Cervix uteri	7.5	13.2	17.1	5.8	7.3	9.3	9.9
Corpus uteri	23.0	14.4	14.5	14.5	11.6	23.9	10.7
Stomach	3.9	7.6	8.4	15.3	8.3	13.0	a
Ovary	16.2	10.2	12.1	10.1	9.3	11.8	17.5
Men							
Prostate	137.9	180.6	92.8	88.0	46.0	57.2	52.5
Colon–rectum	57.6	60.7	40.2	64.1	44.8	42.4	18.6
Lung–bronchus	79.0	117.0	44.0	43.0	52.1	89.0	14.4
Stomach	9.6	17.9	16.2	30.5	15.7	20.5	a
Urinary–bladder	33.1	15.2	16.7	13.7	13.0	a	a
Non-Hodgkin's lymphoma	19.1	13.2	15.0	11.6	12.4	12.5	a

Note. Data from *Racial/Ethnic Patterns of Cancer in the United States 1988–1992* (National Institutes of Health Publication No. 96-4104), by B. A. Miller, L. N. Kolonel, L. Bernstein, J. L. Young, G. M. Swanson, D. West, C. R. Key, J. M. Liff, C. S. Glover, and G. A. Alexander (Eds.), 1996, Bethesda, MD: U.S. Department of Health and Human Services, Public Health Service, and National Institutes of Health, National Cancer Institute.

[a]Rate is based on fewer than 25 cases and may be subject to greater variability than other rates, which are based on larger numbers.

Appendix B
Average Annual Age-Adjusted Cancer Mortality Rates per 100,000 (1988–1992)

Type of cancer	Non-Hispanic White	Black	White Hispanic	Japanese	Chinese	Hawaiian	Native American
Women							
Breast	27.7	31.4	15.7	12.5	11.2	25.0	8.7[a]
Colon–rectum	15.6	20.4	8.6	12.3	10.5	11.4	[b]
Lung–bronchus	32.9	31.5	11.2	12.9	18.5	44.1	[b]
Cervix uteri	2.5	6.7	3.6	1.5	2.6	[b]	8.0[a]
Corpus uteri	3.3	6.0	2.4	1.9	2.2	8.4	[b]
Stomach	2.7	5.6	4.4	9.3	4.8	12.8	7.3[a]
Ovary	8.2	6.6	5.1	5.0	4.0	7.3	[b]
Pancreas	7.0	10.4	5.4	6.7	5.1	9.1	7.4[a]
Men							
Prostate	24.4	53.7	15.9	11.7	6.6	19.9	16.2
Colon–rectum	23.4	28.2	13.4	20.5	15.7	23.7	8.5[a]
Lung–bronchus	74.2	105.6	33.6	32.4	40.1	88.9	10.4[a]
Stomach	2.7	5.6	8.8	17.4	10.5	14.4	11.2[a]
Urinary bladder	6.0	4.8	2.9	2.0	2.0	[b]	[b]
Non-Hodgkin's lymphoma	8.2	5.8	5.6	4.8	5.2	8.8	[b]
Pancreas	9.8	14.4	7.4	8.5	6.7	12.8	[b]

Note. Data from *Racial/Ethnic Patterns of Cancer in the United States 1988–1992* (National Institutes of Health Publication No. 96-4104), by B. A. Miller, L. N. Kolonel, L. Bernstein, J. L. Young, G. M. Swanson, D. West, C. R. Key, J. M. Liff, C. S. Glover, and G. A. Alexander (Eds.), 1996, Bethesda, MD: U.S. Department of Health and Human Services, Public Health Service, and National Institutes of Health, National Cancer Institute.

[a] Rate is based on fewer than 25 deaths and may be subject to greater variability than other rates, which are based on larger numbers.

[b] Rate is not provided due to a small number of deaths.

Chapter 9
ETIOLOGY AND TREATMENT OF THE PSYCHOLOGICAL SIDE EFFECTS ASSOCIATED WITH CANCER CHEMOTHERAPY:
A Critical Review and Discussion

Michael P. Carey and Thomas G. Burish

Chemotherapy is the treatment of choice for hundreds of thousands of cancer patients diagnosed each year in the United States (Silverberg & Lubera, 1986). Its frequent use with cancer patients is the result of recent advances in antineoplastic medication; new and more effective medications have increased the life expectancy for many patients and, in some cases, have resulted in remission and cure. Unfortunately, such long-term gain can come at considerable short-term cost to the cancer patient in the form of aversive and debilitating side effects. Among the more common drug-induced side effects are alopecia, stomatitis, immunosuppression, anorexia, nausea, and vomiting. In addition to these pharmacological side effects, chemotherapy patients also experience psychological side effects.

Psychological side effects, which should not necessarily be regarded as abnormal or indicative of psychopathology, are those that cannot be attributed directly to the antineoplastic medications; instead, such symptoms are believed to result from psychological processes (e.g., learning) that occur in the chemotherapy context. These symptoms can occur before chemotherapy (in which case they are referred to as anticipatory side effects) as well as during and after the actual chemotherapy infusion. When they occur after chemotherapy has been administered (and while the drugs remain pharmacologically active within the system), it is practically impossible to distinguish such psychological side effects from their pharmacological counterparts. Unfortunately, there has been much inconsistency in the literature concerning the definition of these symptoms and the terminology used to describe them. For the most part, however, research with humans has focused on three symptoms, namely, nausea, vomiting, and dysphoria. However, it should be noted that considerable animal research and recent human research have also focused on other side effects of cancer treatments, especially learned side effects such as conditioned taste and food aversions (e.g., Bernstein & Borson, 1986; Smith, Blumsack, & Bilek, 1985) and conditioned immunosuppression (e.g., Ader, 1981; Ader & Cohen, 1985). These phenomena may develop through mechanisms that are similar to those that are the focus of this article.

Symptoms such as nausea, vomiting, and dysphoria are not only frequent among cancer chemotherapy patients but can also be extremely stressful. In addition to the

Reprinted from *Psychological Bulletin, 104*(3), 307–325. (1988). Copyright © 1988 by the American Psychological Association. Used with permission of the author.

The authors wish to thank Kate B. Carey and the anonymous reviewers for their many helpful suggestions on an earlier draft of this review. The writing of this manuscript was supported in part by Grant No. 25516 from the National Cancer Institute, Grant No. PBR-29 from the American Cancer Society, and Grant No. 24 from Syracuse University.

physical and affective distress they cause, many patients are embarrassed by their display of symptoms (e.g., anticipatory vomiting), and others even fear for their sanity. In fact, some patients eventually discontinue chemotherapy, abandoning the hope for remission and cure rather than suffer from such symptoms (Wilcox, Fetting, Nettesheim, & Abeloff, 1982). It has been suggested that still other patients will turn to ineffective and expensive "quack" treatments rather than tolerate the paradoxical worsening quality of life that chemotherapy can bring. Consequently, oncologists (e.g., Laszlo & Lucas, 1981), oncology nurses (e.g., Oberst, 1978), and cancer patients themselves (e.g., Cohn, 1982) have all implored researchers to identify an effective treatment for the side effects associated with cancer chemotherapy.

Pharmacological agents (e.g., prochlorperazine, delta-9-tetrahydrocannabinol) have been used to control the psychological responses to chemotherapy, but standard antiemetics have been found largely ineffective for this type of symptom (Laszlo, 1983; Morrow, Arseneau, Asbury, Bennett, & Boros, 1982). In addition, there is evidence that these medications can actually worsen the symptomatology under some conditions (Zeltzer, LeBaron, & Zeltzer, 1984a). Moreover, even when antiemetics provide some relief, they often have side effects of their own (e.g., sedation, dystonic reactions) or administration demands (e.g., the need for inpatient hospitalization) that limit their acceptance or usefulness among some patients. The ineffectiveness, the paradoxical worsening of symptoms, and the practical limitations of pharmacological agents have all prompted researchers to consider psychological treatments as an alternative method of controlling such symptoms.

In recent years, research on the etiology and treatment of anticipatory and exacerbatory side effects of cancer chemotherapy has burgeoned and has attracted researchers from several health-care disciplines. This increasingly widespread interest is based on at least two primary factors. First, from a theoretical point of view, the psychological side effects of cancer chemotherapy present an unusual opportunity to study the natural development of reactions to repeated aversive treatment within a clinical population. As we shall see, these reactions share some commonalities with other aversive responses but also appear to have some notable differences. Second, from a clinical point of view, these side effects are quite prevalent and can be aversive and debilitating. As a result, they represent an important clinical problem.

The primary purpose of this article is to review the research evidence on the etiology and treatment of the most common psychological side effects associated with cancer chemotherapy, namely, nausea, vomiting, and dysphoria. We begin with an overview and evaluation of the etiological formulations that have been preferred to explain the development of such symptoms. After this discussion of etiology, we review and critique the treatment literature, focusing on investigations that provide quantitative outcome data. We discuss the implications of this research, paying particular attention to patient factors associated with outcome, hypothesized mechanisms by which the treatments may exert their impact, and clinical issues in the application of such interventions.

Etiology of Psychological Side Effects Associated With Cancer Chemotherapy

Psychological side effects are believed to be relatively common. For example, prevalence data obtained from prospective, longitudinal studies indicate that approximately 45% of adult cancer patients experience nausea, vomiting, or both in the 24 hr preceding their chemotherapy (Burish & Carey, 1986). Although precise estimates of the prevalence of postchemotherapy psychological side effects in adults are not available, they are believed to be even more common (Burish & Carey, 1986).

Several causal explanations have been offered to explain the development of psychological side effects. One hypothesis is that these symptoms "may be surfacing manifestations of underlying psychological readjustment problems, associated with life-threatening illness" (Chang, 1981, p. 707). This view suggests that nonpharmacological symptoms represent the negative affect that patients harbor toward their chemotherapy treatments. To date, no data are available to support this assertion. A second hypothesis is that patients may display such symptoms in order to gain attention and sympathy. Inconsistent with this hypothesis, however, is the observation that the punishing side effects of chemotherapy far outweigh any secondary gains that may be realized by cancer patients; moreover, there are no data to support the notion that removal of attention can reduce nonpharmacological symptoms. A third hypothesis is that the observed symptoms may "be produced by brain metastasis or local cancer involvement of the gastrointestinal tract" (Chang, 1981, p. 707). Although this explanation may be accurate for a few patients, it has been ruled out as an explanation for most patients (e.g., Morrow, 1982).

In contrast with the first three hypotheses, which are speculative and lack empirical support, the fourth hypothesis has been supported by the research literature. This hypothesis holds that nonpharmacological or psychological side effects develop through an associative learning process. According to the most widely accepted conditioning viewpoint, after one or more pairings, an association is established between the pharmacological side effects (the unconditioned responses; UCRs) caused by the chemotherapy (the unconditioned stimulus; UCS) and various stimuli (e.g., sights, smells, thoughts; the conditioned stimuli; CSs) associated with the chemotherapy setting. As a result of repeated associations, the CSs begin to elicit nausea, vomiting, and dysphoria (the conditioned responses; CRs), even in the absence of the UCS. Two variations of the conditioning model have also been suggested. The first, proposed by Leventhal, Easterling, Nerenz, and Love (1988), is that postchemotherapy nausea and vomiting might occasionally serve as the UCS, with responses to this nausea and vomiting (e.g., anxiety and secondary nausea occurring later in time) being the UCRs. These UCRs then become conditioned to various stimuli in the chemotherapy environment and thereby take the form of CRs. Thus, in this first variation of the conditioning model, the morphology of the CS and CR is similar to that of the original model, but the UCS and UCR are not. The second variation was suggested by Garcia y Robertson and Garcia (1985), who believe that conditioned responses to cancer chemotherapy may develop through a process that closely resembles taste aversion learning. Although the published literature on conditioned responses to cancer chemotherapy has been based almost exclusively on the first model of conditioning, it should be noted that these two variations do provide viable conceptualizations of alternative, though not necessarily mutually exclusive, processes.

There are several sources of data that converge to support the hypothesis that associative learning is the primary phenomenon underlying the etiology of psychological symptoms. In no case were the data generated by experimental research that was designed deliberately to induce conditioned nausea and vomiting in cancer chemotherapy patients through controlled experimental manipulations, a procedure that would be ethically unacceptable. Rather, the data are based on analogous phenomena or experimental outcomes that consistently, logically, or exclusively point to associative learning as the most reasonable explanation. At least four sources of supporting data can be identified.

First, the symptoms that are displayed by chemotherapy patients have several topographical similarities to those of laboratory animals that ingest a gastrotoxic substance or that are irradiated while eating a certain food. The animals subsequently avoid that substance or food during future feedings, a phenomenon referred to as learned taste aversion (for an extended discussion of the similarities of conditioned nausea and vomiting in cancer patients and learned taste aversions, see Garcia y Robertson & Garcia, 1985). The symptoms have been shown to result from a learning process that is associative in nature, although it deviates, as does the conditioned response of chemotherapy patients, from the traditional classical conditioning paradigm in some interesting respects (e.g., the symptoms often develop after only one or a few associations and despite the fact that there may be several hours between the UCS and USR). Another example of documented animal conditioning that bears even closer resemblance to the chemotherapy situation was demonstrated by Collins and Tatum (1925) and Pavlov (1927). These investigators showed that dogs repeatedly injected with an emetic drug developed conditioned vomiting in response to stimuli associated with the injection.

Second, several human studies provide data that support an associative learning explanation. For example, I. L. Bernstein and her colleagues (e.g., I. L. Bernstein, 1978; I. L. Bernstein & Webster, 1980) demonstrated experimentally that taste aversions can develop in chemotherapy patients as a result of the emetic properties of the infused drugs. For example, in one study the investigators assigned pediatric cancer patients receiving emetogenic chemotherapy agents to one of two groups: to an experimental group that received a novel-flavored ice cream shortly before their scheduled drug treatment or to a control group that did not receive the ice cream. A second control group of patients receiving nonemetic chemotherapy drugs was also included. After 2 or more weeks, patients in all groups were offered either some of the novel-flavored ice cream or an opportunity to play with a game. Patients in the two control groups overwhelmingly chose the ice cream; patients in the experimental group showed an aversion to the ice cream, generally preferring the game. Similar results were subsequently demonstrated in adult cancer patients (see I. L. Bernstein & Webster, 1985, for a review).

Third, there have been reports of cancer chemotherapy patients becoming conditioned to antiemetic treatments. In these situations, the antiemetic was apparently given each time the patient became nauseated or was vomiting; as a result, it became associated with nausea and vomiting and later was able to elicit, on its own, nausea and vomiting. For example, Kutz, Borysenko, Come, and Benson (1980) reported the case of a patient with neurofibrosarcoma who smoked marijuana to alleviate severe nausea and vomiting. After chemotherapy was discontinued, the smell of marijuana in social situations elicited nausea and vomiting. In another case reported by the same authors, the marijuana was administered in brownies and cookies. For a year after the chemotherapy was discontinued, the taste or sight of these foods produced nausea. Similar conditioning to antiemetics has been reported by other investigators (e.g., Morrow et al., 1982).

Fourth, research has shown that factors related to the development of conditioned symptoms in cancer chemotherapy patients conform to the principles of associative learning. For example, Andrykowski et al. (in press) and Andrykowski, Redd, and Hatfield (1985) conducted two longitudinal studies of the development of anticipatory nausea in cancer chemotherapy patients. In these investigations, which together involved the study of over 150 patients, the authors found that anticipatory nausea never occurred without the prior occurrence of postchemotherapy nausea, that is, consistent with the principles of associative learning, the presence of a UCR was necessary for the acquisition of a CR. Moreover, after a careful analysis of other factors that contributed to the development of anticipatory symptoms, the authors concluded that, consistent with an associative learning model, "all of the factors that reliably predicted the development of AN [anticipatory nausea] were either directly or indirectly linked to the magnitude" of the unconditioned symptoms (Andrykowski et al., in press, p. 11). As has been noted elsewhere (Burish & Carey, 1986), other descriptive data on the development and nature of conditioned responses in cancer chemotherapy patients also consistently conform, in prospective as well as retrospective studies, to the principles of associative learning.

In addition to supporting the conditioning model, the available data suggest that several factors can serve to mediate or potentiate the learning process and thereby produce considerable variation in symptom development. These individual difference factors may arise independently of, but nontheless contribute to, the development of conditioned responses.

One major individual difference may be proneness to nausea and vomiting. Research has suggested that patients who have a history of motion sickness or of experiencing nausea and vomiting to various foods or situations (e.g., pregnancy) are more likely to report posttreatment and anticipatory nausea and vomiting in response to cancer chemotherapy (Jacobsen et al., 1988; Morrow, 1985). Morrow (1985) has suggested that there is a neurological basis for this relationship. The experience of nausea and vomiting is thought to result from activation of the "vomiting center," located in the lateral reticular formation of the medulla oblongata (Borison & McCarthy, 1983). The vomiting center has four major inputs, including one from the vestibular system, which is thought to play a role in motion sickness. It has been suggested that in addition to affecting the other major inputs, chemotherapy may affect the vestibular system, which in patients with a susceptibility to motion sickness may lead to additional stimulation of the vomiting center and therefore an increased likelihood of nausea and vomiting (Morrow, 1985). Redd and his colleagues (Jacobsen et al., 1988; Andrykowski et al., in press) have suggested that there may be constitutional differences in cancer patients' susceptibility to gastrointestinal distress, including that due to chemotherapy. Patients with a greater constitutional vulnerability to gastrointestinal distress may be more likely to respond to chemotherapy with high levels of posttreatment nausea and vomiting, which in turn increases the likelihood that they will develop conditioned nausea and vomiting, in comparison with patients without this diathesis. In summary, the data suggest that patients with a past history of nausea and vomiting resulting from motion sickness, certain foods, or other experiences are more likely to develop conditioned nausea and vomiting in response to cancer chemotherapy.

A second major factor that appears to affect the development of conditioned responses to chemotherapy is a patient's anxiety level.[1] Specifically, state anxiety levels have been positively related to the presence of conditioned responses in a number of retrospective studies (e.g., Ingle, Burish, & Wallston, 1984; van Komen & Redd, 1985) and prospective investigations (e.g., Andrykowski et al., 1985, in press; Nerenz, Leventhal, Easterling, & Love, 1986). For example, Nerenz et al. (1986) interviewed cancer patients before each of their first six treatment cycles. The authors found that the incidence of anticipatory nausea was related to the level of pretreatment anxiety: for mildly anxious patients the incidence averaged 9.8%; for highly anxious patients the incidence was approximately twice as much, averaging 18.1%. Andrykowski et al. (1985) found that a patient's self-reported anxiety level before treatments accounted for more variance (13.6%) than any other single variable except posttreatment nausea in determining whether a patient developed anticipatory nausea.

Although data from numerous studies appear to suggest that heightened anxiety levels facilitate the development of conditioned symptoms, two questions remain. First, what are the temporal parameters that determine the relationship between state anxiety and the development of conditioned responses? That is, exactly when during the course of chemotherapy do elevated anxiety levels produce this relationship? Second, why is heightened anxiety associated with conditioned symptoms? A number of possible answers have been discussed, although none have been tested in the chemotherapy context. In most cases, investigators have speculated that anxiety directly or indirectly affects the associative learning process in ways that lead to enhanced conditioning. For example, some of the explanations suggest that anxiety levels directly affect conditioning by influencing the speed with which associative learning takes place. According to this explanation, highly anxious patients condition more quickly than do less anxious patients (e.g., Spence, 1958). Data recently reported by Andrykowski and Redd (1987) conflict with this explanation, however. These authors interviewed patients before each of their chemotherapy treatments to determine pretreatment anxiety levels and pre- and posttreatment nausea levels. They found that patients who developed anticipatory symptoms late in the course of chemotherapy (i.e., after their seventh treatment) generally had higher anxiety levels during all treatments than did patients who developed anticipatory symptoms early in the treatment course. Andrykowski and Redd (1987) also noted that late-onset patients generally had lower posttreatment nausea levels until the session just before they developed anticipatory nausea, at which time their posttreatment levels increased substantially. The authors speculated that the heightened pretreatment anxiety levels eventually led to the increased posttreatment nausea and that once posttreatment nausea increased, patients were more likely to develop anticipatory symptoms (i.e.,

---

[1]For the sake of completeness, it should be noted that in addition to anxiety level, a number of other individual difference factors have been found to be correlated with the presence of anticipatory symptoms, for example, experiencing taste sensations during chemotherapy, having an inhibitive rather than facilitative coping style, being treated in a large group room rather than in a small private room, being younger rather than older, experiencing itching sensations during chemotherapy, and receiving chemotherapy treatments through long infusions rather than through short push injections (see Burish & Carey, 1986, for a review). However, most of these factors have been reported in retrospective investigations exclusively, have been found in only one or two studies and not in others, and have not been linked causally to the development of conditioned symptoms.

the greater the intensity of the unconditioned response, the more likely the development of a conditioned response).

Others have focused on different parameters in trying to explain the relationship between anxiety and conditioning. Dolgin, Katz, McGinty, and Siegel (1985), for example, have suggested that highly anxious patients tend to show high levels of vigilance to their environments and, as a result, tend to notice more closely various stimuli in the clinic setting. Such attention increases the likelihood that these stimuli will develop into CSs. They found that consistent with this hypothesis, pediatric cancer patients with anticipatory symptoms attended to and processed more stimuli in their environments, and habituated to these stimuli more slowly, than did matched patients without anticipatory symptoms.

Although most of the speculation about the relationship between anxiety and conditioned symptoms focuses on the role of anxiety within the learning paradigm, J. H. Fetting (personal communication, March 1, 1988) has suggested a neurologically based explanation that involves the relationship between anxiety and neurotransmitter changes. In the first stage of a hypothesized two-stage process, a cancer patient's propensity for experiencing nausea and vomiting is increased as a result of either a decreased nausea/vomiting threshold or enhanced neuronal firings, either or both of which might be caused by repeated bouts of nausea and vomiting during periods of high anxiety. As a result of this enhanced propensity, a variety of stimuli will more readily cause gastrointestinal upset in the future.

In the second stage, increased noradrenergic activity, caused by the heightened anxiety or stress levels, contributes to the development of anticipatory nausea and vomiting in patients with the increased propensity. The process by which the increased noradrenergic activity leads to these effects is as yet undetermined, but J. H. Fetting (personal communication, March 1, 1988) speculated that with repeated exposure to emetogenic chemotherapy, the noradrenergic terminals in areas adjacent to the vomiting center in the cortex may show increased activity, leading to greater stimulation of the vomiting center. In an initial test of this hypothesis, Fetting et al. (1987) administered clonidine, a drug that reduces noradrenergic activity, to 8 chemotherapy patients who displayed anticipatory symptoms to their chemotherapy. After one trial of clonidine, the anticipatory symptoms were completely eliminated in 4 (50%) of the patients. Postchemotherapy nausea and vomiting appeared to be unaffected.

Overall, then, it appears that the psychological symptoms that occur during cancer chemotherapy, particularly the nausea and vomiting that occur prior to drug infusion, are acquired through an associative learning process; moreover, the data suggest that the development of such symptoms is moderated by one's prior experience with gastrointestinal upset from factors such as motion sickness or certain foods and by one's treatment-related anxiety level. Thus many writers have concluded that the psychological symptoms that occur in the chemotherapy setting are conditioned responses. In this regard, it is important to note that conditioned responses to cancer chemotherapy are similar, developmentally and phenomenologically, to conditioned aversive responses that develop routinely in other clinical contexts. For example, Garcia y Robertson and Garcia (1985) have related the animal and human literature on learned taste aversions to the research on conditioned nausea and vomiting in cancer chemotherapy patients. Conditioned responses to cancer chemotherapy can also be viewed as a subset of other conditioned drug responses (e.g., to morphine or alcohol; Siegel, 1979). Although the review of the extensive literature on conditioned aversive responses is beyond the scope of this article, it is important to keep these similarities in mind when reviewing the treatment literature because many of the procedures that have been used to ameliorate or prevent conditioned responses in cancer chemotherapy patients are similar to or are based on the same principles as those that have been used with other types of conditioned aversive responses. Many of the treatment advances that have been made in the cancer area are, therefore, potentially applicable to other areas as well.

Although associative learning appears to play an important role in the etiology of psychological side effects, we propose that side effects in the chemotherapy context might also result from, or be exacerbated by, a fifth mechanism, namely, psychological stress (i.e., the process that occurs when a person appraises a situation or stimulus as taxing his or her resources and endangering his or her well-being; Lazarus & Folkman, 1984). Thus, we hypothesize that a person who appraises the chemotherapy process as threatening or who is unprepared to cope with its demands might experience negative outcomes (e.g., dysphoria, nausea). It is important to emphasize that by *psychological stress* we are referring broadly to the appraisal and coping process, not solely to an affective state that results from that process (e.g., increased anxiety). In addition to initiating symptoms, psychological stress can worsen already existing (i.e., pharmacological and conditioned) symptoms. Thus, stress can play a role at almost any stage in the development and expression of psychological symptoms to cancer chemotherapy. Support for the role of stress in psychological symptoms comes both from the general stress literature (e.g., Lazarus, 1966; Lazarus & Folkman, 1984; Selye, 1976) and from empirical work conducted specifically in the chemotherapy context (e.g., Nerenz, Leventhal, & Love, 1982; Nerenz, Leventhal, Love, & Ringler, 1984). Unfortunately, most investigators have focused either on the role of associative learning or on the role of stress in accounting for the development of psychological symptoms, although there have been exceptions (e.g., Nerenz et al., 1982). In the end, however, we suspect that both processes are implicated, perhaps in a synergistic way.

In summary, five explanations have been put forward to explain the development of psychological symptoms in the chemotherapy context. Our review and interpretation of the literature leads us to conclude that many of these symptoms, especially those that occur prior to chemotherapy, are the result of associative learning. Furthermore, we have proposed that psychological stress may cause a variety of difficulties, or it may exacerbate existing symptoms. Thus we conclude that at least two factors contribute to the development and expression of psychological symptoms in the chemotherapy context: associative learning and psychological stress. Both can occur prior to, during, or after chemotherapy administration. It is likely that these two mechanisms co-occur with each other and perhaps with pharmacological factors to produce symptoms or symptom clusters. Next, we turn to an evaluation of interventions used to treat these side effects.

Review of Research on the Treatment of Psychological Side Effects

Five different psychological interventions have been investigated as techniques to ameliorate the conditioned and stress-related side effects associated with cancer chemotherapy: hypnosis, progressive muscle relaxation training with guided imagery, systematic desensitization, biofeedback, and distraction.[2] For each intervention, we provide a brief description of the technique and then review the research evaluating that technique. Although other techniques have been used clinically (e.g., stress inoculation training; see Moore & Altmaier, 1981), we do not include such interventions in our review because they have not yet been subjected to controlled research.

Hypnosis

Hypnosis was probably the first psychological technique used to control the side effects associated with chemotherapy and is still the most widely used procedure with children and adolescents. Our review of this literature suggests that the term *hypnosis* does not describe a specific technique as much as it refers to a number of induction procedures that require that the patient be completely attentive and absorbed in an activity prescribed or directed by the therapist. This activity may be purely cognitive, or it may include both cognitive and behavioral components. Hypnotic induction procedures may involve psychological quiescence (i.e., relaxation) and augmented suggestibility (cf. Wadden & Anderton, 1982), although these characteristics have not been reported universally in the cancer chemotherapy literature. For example, when used with children, hypnosis is usually characterized by a heavy reliance upon the use of playful fantasy rather than on the more passive images of natural beauty that are frequently used with adults; moreover, hypnotic imagery with children is often accompanied by physical movement and the use of toys and dolls, both of which may actually increase physiological arousal (Zeltzer & LeBaron, 1986). In contrast, when used with adult patients, hypnosis typically involves an induction procedure that is designed to produce deep physiological relaxation (e.g., Redd, Andersen, & Minagawa, 1982) and often employs imagery and suggestions related to natural beauty and serenity. Operationally, Redd (1985/1986) has noted that "the procedures for inducing passive relaxation are identical to those frequently used by many professionals who identify their procedures as hypnosis" (p. 21).

The early research on hypnosis with children (e.g., LaBaw, Holton, Tewell, & Eccles, 1975), adolescents (e.g., Ellenberg, Kellerman, Dash, Higgins, & Zeltzer, 1980), and adults (e.g., Dempster, Balson, & Whalen, 1976) suggested that hypnosis could reduce nausea, vomiting, pain, and the negative emotions associated with chemotherapy. Though encouraging, this early research was more heuristically than empirically valuable because it did not report objective data, use statistical analyses, or employ adequate methodological controls.

The controlled work with hypnosis is summarized in Table 1; the most programmatic set of studies has been conducted by Zeltzer and her colleagues with pediatric patients. These studies have either used hypnosis patients as their own controls (LeBaron & Zeltzer, 1984; Zeltzer, Kellerman, Ellenberg, & Dash, 1983) or compared them to patients receiving supportive counseling (Zeltzer, LeBaron, & Zeltzer,

---

[2]It is possible that the treatments reviewed decrease pharmacological side effects as well as conditioned and stress-related symptoms; however, it is practically impossible to separate out these differential effects when measuring postchemotherapy outcome measures. Many researchers who use psychological interventions have assumed, conservatively, that postchemotherapy symptom reductions resulting from these interventions reflect only the diminuation of psychologically produced symptoms.

Table 1—Summary of Controlled Research on the Use of Hypnosis With Conditioned Side Effects

Study	Patients	Study design	Treatment protocol	Assessment instruments	Results
Redd, Andresen, & Minagawa (1982)	N = 6 adults; Dx = varied: 4 breast, 1 lung, 1 hematologic; CP = varied	Single-subject multiple baseline	7–14 baseline, and 5–7 treatment sessions	RN observation of BP; Pt ratings of N	Decreased N and V during all treatment sessions for all patients
Zeltzer, Kellerman, Ellenberg, & Dash (1983)	N = 12 adolescents; Dx = varied; CP = varied	Single-subject, pre- and post-intervention	1 baseline, and 1 treatment session	Pt record of frequency duration and severity of V; Pt report of anxiety, health locus of control, illness impact, and self-esteem	8 of 12 Pts reduced frequency and severity of V; 6 of 12 Pts reduced duration of V. 1 Pt did not benefit; 3 Pts rejected hypnosis
LeBaron & Zeltzer (1984)	N = 8 adolescents; Dx = 6 hematologic, 2 bone; CP = varied	Single-subject, multiple baseline	2–3 baseline, and 2–3 treatment sessions	Pt ratings of N, V, bother, and disruption; parent ratings of N, V, bother, and disruption	Reduced, N, V, bother, and disruption of activities
Zeltzer, LeBaron, & Zeltzer (1984b)	N = 19 adolescents; Dx = 14 hematologic, 5 bone; CP = varied	Group comparison: hypnosis vs. supportive counseling	2 baseline, 2 treatment, and 1 follow-up session	Pt ratings of N, V, and bother; parent ratings of N, V, and bother	Reduced N, V, and bother for both groups during training and follow-up. No differences were found between the two interventions
Cotanch, Hockenberry, & Herman (1985)	N = 12 children and adolescents; Dx = 8 pediatric sarcomas, 2 hematologic, 2 other	Group comparison: self-hypnosis vs. standard treatment control	No baseline session, 1 training session, and 2 follow-up sessions	Pt ratings of N, V, and bother; RN ratings of N and bother; RN observation of V and oral intake	In comparison with controls, hypnosis Pts experienced decreased frequency, amount, severity, and duration of V; decreased intensity and duration of N; decreased bother during chemotherapy; and greater oral intake following chemotherapy

Note. N = nausea; V = vomiting; RN = registered nurse; Pt = patient; Dx = diagnosis; CP = chemotherapy protocol; BP = blood pressure.

1984b). Overall, this series of studies suggests that after one to three training sessions, patients receiving hypnosis reported reduced levels of postchemotherapy nausea and vomiting and that any postchemotherapy side effects that did remain were less bothersome than they were prior to training. Moreover, these benefits continued after training when the therapist was no longer present. No data on anticipatory symptoms were reported.

In the only hypnosis study to include a no-treatment control group, Cotanch, Hockenberry, and Herman (1985) compared 6 children given hypnosis plus standard antiemetic treatment with 6 children who received the standard antiemetic treatment alone. Results indicated that patients receiving hypnosis experienced reductions in the intensity and severity of both nausea and vomiting and an increase in food intake after chemotherapy, in comparison with patients receiving standard procedures.

Finally, in the only controlled study to use hypnosis with adults, Redd et al. (1982) studied 6 patients who had experienced anticipatory nausea and vomiting prior to at least their last three chemotherapy treatments. After completing two training sessions, the patients underwent chemotherapy while hypnotized. All 6 patients reported decreased nausea and were observed by nurses to have ceased all vomiting prior to and during the chemotherapy sessions in which hypnosis was used. When the patients did not use hypnosis during subsequent chemotherapy sessions, the anticipatory symptoms returned. No data on postchemotherapy symptoms were reported.

Overall, it appears that hypnotic procedures are an effective intervention for reducing both anticipatory and postchemotherapy nausea and vomiting and the negative affects associated with chemotherapy. Continued research is needed to replicate these findings, especially in adults. In this regard, it is important that investigators state explicitly which induction techniques and procedures they have used. Moreover, two points should be made regarding the use of hypnosis with cancer patients. First, not all patients will accept hypnosis (Hendler & Redd, 1986; Redd & Andrykowski, 1982; Zeltzer et al., 1983). Reasons for rejection typically have involved misperceptions about the process of hypnosis and potential posthypnotic effects. In an attempt to sidestep such concerns, Redd and his colleagues now refer to their hypnosis procedure as passive relaxation training with guided imagery, and they report greater acceptance by patients as a result of this change (W. H. Redd, personal communication, January 22, 1988). Second, in the only study that has compared hypnosis to an alternate treatment, it was found that adolescent patients who received hypnosis did not improve more than patients who received supportive counseling (Zeltzer et al., 1984b). Thus, although hypnosis may be effective, some people may not accept it, and others may be treated as effectively with alternate procedures.

Progressive Muscle Relaxation Training With Guided Imagery

Although hypnosis was probably the first psychological technique to be used in the chemotherapy context, progressive muscle relaxation training (PMRT) is the most widely researched technique.[3] PMRT is based on a series of muscle tensing and

---

[3]*Relaxation* is a broad term that has been used to refer to a disparate array of activities, including watching television, taking a cruise, and lying on a beach. These pleasurable activities may or may not result in physiological quiescence, the hallmark of progressive muscle relaxation training.

relaxing exercises developed by Jacobson (1938) and later modified by D. A. Bernstein and Borkovec (1973), among others. This procedure is sometimes referred to as *active* relaxation training because it includes a muscle tensing component. Relaxation training procedures that do not include a tensing component have also been used in the chemotherapy context and are generally referred to as *passive* relaxation procedures. In the cancer chemotherapy context, PMRT has usually been supplemented with guided imagery during the infusion period; guided imagery involves the use of a sequence of thoughts and mental pictures to facilitate relaxation (see Turk, Meichenbaum, & Genest, 1983, pp. 285–291, for examples of relaxation imagery). In most of the research reported in this area, the imagery is individualized to each patient on the basis of a preintervention interview.

As with hypnosis, uncontrolled case reports of the use of PMRT and guided imagery with cancer chemotherapy patients are available (e.g., Hamberger, 1982; Scott, Donahue, Mastrovito, & Hakes, 1983). These reports provide little more than suggestive evidence for the efficacy of relaxation training and guided imagery. Fortunately, controlled research on PMRT and guided imagery has been ample and provides stronger data.

The controlled research on PMRT and guided imagery is summarized in Table 2; this research has been conducted almost exclusively with adults and has focused on the psychological side effects and distress that occur during and after chemotherapy injections. Burish and his colleagues have completed five studies on the effectiveness of PMRT and guided imagery. The initial report was a single-subject investigation (Burish & Lyles, 1979), which was followed by a series of four group comparison designs (Burish, Carey, Krozely, & Greco, 1987; Burish & Lyles, 1981; Carey & Burish, 1987; Lyles, Burish, Krozely, & Oldham, 1982). In all of these studies, patients were trained in PMRT and guided imagery during the 30 min just prior to the chemotherapy injections and underwent chemotherapy while relaxed. Patients were asked to practice PMRT and guided imagery at home between treatments. Measurement of patient benefit included a number of physiological, self-report, and nurse-observation measures, which were collected during three to five training and follow-up sessions.

Overall, the research has demonstrated that training in PMRT and guided imagery can reduce physiological arousal, patient reports of nausea and dysphoria, and nurse reports of nausea and anxiety. In some studies, PMRT-related reductions in vomiting frequency were also observed, although this has not been a consistent finding, largely because of the low baseline frequency of this symptom (e.g., see Lyles et al., 1982). The gains achieved with PMRT and guided imagery have been observed in comparison with untreated control patients (e.g., Burish & Lyles, 1981) and with placebo control patients (Lyles et al., 1982). Typically, these effects were most salient during and after the chemotherapy infusions as opposed to before the infusions. Moreover, the benefits obtained during therapist-guided training were usually stronger than those achieved during follow-up (i.e., maintenance) sessions when the patient was asked to relax him or herself. Finally, PMRT and guided imagery were shown to be effective not only in ameliorating distress in veteran chemotherapy patients (e.g., Lyles et al., 1982) but also in preventing or at least delaying the apparent development of psychological side effects in new patients (Burish et al., 1987).

Cotanch and her associates have also conducted research that supports the efficacy of PMRT and guided imagery. The first study (Cotanch, 1983) used an own-control design in which 12 adult patients underwent one baseline chemotherapy session followed by five chemotherapy sessions during which they were trained in PMRT with guided imagery. Results indicated that PMRT and guided imagery produced reductions in physiological arousal, nausea, vomiting, and anxiety in 9 of 12 patients. In a follow-up study (Cotanch & Strum, 1985), PMRT and guided imagery delivered by audiotaped instructions were compared to a placebo treatment (therapist present while patient listened to music). The relaxation procedure was found to be more effective than the placebo tape in lowering physiological arousal and trait anxiety and in increasing postchemotherapy caloric intake. Unfortunately, no standard treatment control group was included in this study, making evaluation of the audiotaped instructions difficult.

Finally, Dahlquist, Gil, Armstrong, Ginsberg, and Jones (1985) reported on the use of cue-controlled muscle relaxation, controlled breathing, pleasant imagery, and positive self-statements with 3 children in a multiple baseline design. After this treatment, behavioral distress as observed by trained assistants was reduced 46–68% from baseline levels. Medical staff ratings of the patient's distress and patient self-reports of distress were also reduced as a result of treatment.

In summary, PMRT and guided imagery have been shown in several well-controlled investigations to be effective for the reduction of nausea, physiological arousal, and negative affect and for increasing food intake during the days after chemotherapy. Reductions in vomiting have not been consistently reported, although this may reflect less severe baseline symptoms in the patients studied. Finally, the effects of PMRT and guided imagery appear to be strongest during training, although modest benefits have also been observed during follow-up.

Systematic Desensitization

Systematic desensitization (SD) is a procedure that has been used widely in the treatment of phobias, sexual dysfunctions, and other anxiety-related disorders (Wolpe, 1958). The procedure basically consists of teaching a patient a relaxation skill, commonly some form of relaxation training, and then exposing the patient to progressively more anxiety-provoking stimuli. The goal is to have these stimuli elicit or be accompanied by a relaxation response rather than the anxiety response heretofore elicited by them. The underlying process responsible for the effectiveness of SD has been a topic of considerable recent debate; hypothesized mechanisms of action include counterconditioning, extinction, habituation, attentional control, and several others (see Masters, Burish, Hollon, & Rimm, 1987, for a review).

Support for the use of SD with cancer chemotherapy patients comes from both uncontrolled case studies (e.g., Hailey & White, 1983; Hoffman, 1982–1983; West & Piccionne, 1982) and from controlled research (summarized in Table 3). Morrow and Morrell (1982) studied 60 patients within a group comparison format to determine the relative efficacy of a self-control version of systematic desensitization, supportive counseling, and no treatment. Patients in the SD condition were taught PMRT and instructed to imagine themselves staying calm and relaxed in a number of situations, beginning with the day before chemotherapy and progressing through the actual chemotherapy infusion. Patients were seen twice in the therapist's office

Table 2—*Summary of Controlled Research on the Use of Progressive Muscle Relaxation Training With Conditioned Side Effects*

Study	Patients	Study design	Treatment protocol	Assessment instruments	Results
Burish & Lyles (1979)	N = 1 adult female; Dx = hematologic; CP = not reported	Single-subject, multiple-phase	1 baseline, 2 training, 2 follow-up, 2 more training, and 4 more follow-up sessions	BP; PR; Pt ratings of anxiety, depression, and N; RN ratings of anxiety, N, and V	During training, booster, and second follow-up, Pt reduced N, anxiety, depression, PR, BP, and frequency of V
Burish & Lyles (1981)	N = 16 adults; Dx = varied; CP = varied	Group comparison: PMRT plus GI vs. no treatment	1 baseline, 2 training, and 2 follow-up sessions	BP; PR; Pt ratings of anxiety, hostility, depression, and N; RN ratings of anxiety, N, and V	PMRT Pts reduced hostility, anxiety, depression, N, and PR during follow-up in comparison with controls; no differences between groups on V
Lyles, Burish, Krozely, & Oldham (1982)	N = 50 adults; Dx = varied; CP = varied	Group comparison: PMRT plus GI vs. placebo control vs. no-treatment control	1 baseline, 3 training, and 1 follow-up session	During chemotherapy: BP; PR; Pt ratings of anxiety, hostility, depression, and N; RN ratings of anxiety, N, and V Following chemotherapy: Pt ratings of anxiety, N and V for 3 days	In comparison with placebo and no-treatment controls, PMRT Pts reported less anxiety, depression, and N and had lower PRs and SBPs during chemotherapy; PMRT Pts also reported less N at home following chemotherapy
Cotanch (1983)	N = 12 adults; Dx = varied; CP = varied	Single subject, pre- and post-intervention design	1 baseline and 5 training sessions	During chemotherapy: BP; PR; RR; Pt ratings of anxiety, N, and V; RN/family ratings of N and V	In comparison with baseline, 9 of 12 Pts showed some decrease in N and V; caloric intake increase in all Pts; PR, RR, and trait anxiety were also reduced
Cotanch & Strum (1985)	N = 60 adults; Dx = varied; CP = varied	Group comparison: PMRT plus GI vs. placebo control vs. no-treatment control	1 baseline and 3–4 follow-up sessions. PMRT and placebo control (music) were both provided by audiotapes	During chemotherapy: BP; PR; RR; Pt ratings of both state and trait anxiety, N and V Following chemotherapy: Caloric count, skin fold measurement, body weight	In comparison with placebo controls, PMRT Pts evinced lower SBP, DBP, PR, RR, V, and trait anxiety; PMRT Pts also increased caloric intake. Data for no-treatment controls were not reported

Study	Sample	Design	Treatment	Measures	Results
Dahlquist, Gil, Armstrong, Ginsberg, & Jones (1985)	$N = 3$ children, aged 11–14; Dx = 1 Burkitts lymphoma, 2 osteosarcoma of the femur	Multiple baseline across subjects	Baseline: 2–15 preintervention venipunctures; treatment: 5–12 sessions of relaxation training combined with pleasant imagery and positive self-talk	Observational Scale of Behavioral Distress; parent, medical staff, and Pt ratings of distress	46–68% reductions from baseline levels of observed behavioral distress during venipunctures were found during intervention; medical staff and Pt ratings of distress during venipunctures also decreased during intervention
Burish, Carey, Krozely, & Greco (1987)	$N = 24$ adults; Dx = 9 breast, 4 lung, 10 gynecologic, 1 hematologic; CP = varied	Group comparison: PMRT plus GI vs. no-treatment control	3 training and 2 follow-up sessions. N.B.: Intervention initially delivered before Pt's first chemotherapy treatment	During chemotherapy: BP; PR; Pt ratings of anxiety, hostility, depression, and N; RN ratings of anxiety, N, and V Following chemotherapy: Pt ratings of anxiety, N, and V for 3 days	PMRT Pts, in comparison with controls, reported less severe and prolonged N; less anxiety, depression, and hostility and lower PRs and BPs. These differences were most salient during Sessions 4 and 5
Carey & Burish (1987)	$N = 45$ adults; Dx = varied; CP = varied	Group comparison: PMRT plus GI; delivered by (a) professionals, (b) volunteers, or (c) audiotape vs. no-treatment control	1 baseline, 3 training, and 1 follow-up session	During chemotherapy: BP; PR; RR; Pt ratings of dysphoria and N; RN ratings of anxiety, N, and V Following chemotherapy: Pt ratings of anxiety, N, V, and food intake	Overall, Pts trained in PMRT by professional therapists experienced less distress than did Pts trained by volunteers, Pts who used videotaped PMRT, and control Pts

Note. N = nausea; V = vomiting; RN = registered nurse; Pt = patient; Dx = diagnosis; CP = chemotherapy protocol; PMRT = progressive muscle relaxation training; GI = guided imagery; BP = blood pressure; PR = pulse rate; RR = respiration rate; SBP = systolic blood pressure; DBP = diastolic blood pressure.

Table 3—*Summary of Controlled Research on the Use of Systematic Desensitization With Conditioned Side Effects*

Study	Patients	Study design	Treatment protocol	Assessment instruments	Results
Morrow & Morrell (1982)	$N = 60$ adults; Dx = varied; CP = varied	Group comparison: SD vs. counseling vs. no-treatment counseling	2 baseline and 2 follow-up sessions. SD and counseling occurred between Pts' fourth and fifth chemotherapy sessions	Pt report of N, V, anxiety, and helplessness	SD Pts reported less frequent and severe AN and AV than did Pts in other groups. No differences were observed in anxiety or helplessness across conditions
Morrow (1986)	$N = 92$ adults; Dx = varied; CP = varied	Group comparison: SD vs. PMRT vs. counseling vs. no-treatment control	2 baseline and 2 follow-up sessions. SD, PMRT, and counseling occurred between Pts' fourth and fifth chemotherapy sessions	Pt report of N state anxiety, trait anxiety	SD Pts reported less AN, state anxiety, and trait anxiety than did Pts in other groups; SD and PMRT Pts reported less post-treatment N than did Pts in other groups

Note. N = nausea; V = vomiting; AN = anticipatory nausea; AV = anticipatory vomiting; RN = registered nurse; Pt = patient; Dx = diagnosis; CP = chemotherapy protocol; PMRT = progressive muscle relaxation training; SD = systematic desensitization.

and were then followed for two subsequent chemotherapy sessions. During follow-up, the patients receiving SD reported reduced frequency and severity, and a shortened duration, of both anticipatory nausea and vomiting, in comparison with counseling and control patients.

In a subsequent report, Morrow (1986) compared patients who received SD, counseling, or no treatment (most of the patients in these groups were the same as those participating in the Morrow & Morrell, 1982, study) with a new group of patients that received PMRT only. The procedures used for the first three groups were identical to those used in the Morrow and Morrell study; the PMRT group followed procedures identical to those of the SD group except that no cognitive hierarchy was used. The results suggested that SD reduced anticipatory nausea, state anxiety, and trait anxiety[4] more than the other three treatments did; these other treatments did not differ from each other on these variables. SD and PMRT produced changes in posttreatment nausea and vomiting that were comparable and significantly greater than those produced by the counseling or no treatment groups, which did not differ from each other. Because Morrow (1986) used different procedures to administer PMRT from those of other researchers (e.g., guided imagery was not given, and relaxation was not provided during chemotherapy treatments, nor were patients specifically told to use the relaxation during their treatments), he appropriately cautioned against viewing this study as a direct comparison of SD and PMRT. However, the data do suggest that SD is less effective without the cognitive hierachy.

In summary, Morrow's research on SD suggests that this procedure can provide an effective procedure for reducing conditioned responses to cancer chemotherapy.

Biofeedback Combined With PMRT and Guided Imagery

Biofeedback, a commonly used treatment method in behavioral medicine, involves training an individual to control physiological responses, such as systolic blood pressure or heart rate, by using external monitoring devices. Such devices indicate when a desired change occurs, and the patient seeks to learn and then to bring under conscious control the behaviors associated with the desired change. The combined use of biofeedback, PMRT, and guided imagery with cancer chemotherapy patients has been evaluated in two studies (summarized in Table 4).

Burish, Shartner, and Lyles (1981) implemented a multiple baseline design to study the combined effectiveness of an electromyograph (EMG) biofeedback and PMRT intervention with an adult patient who had developed psychological symptoms in response to her chemotherapy. During the four chemotherapy sessions in which the patient received the intervention and during three subsequent follow-up sessions, she showed reductions from baseline in physiological arousal and reported less anxiety and nausea. In a follow-up study, Shartner, Burish, and Carey (1985) randomly assigned 12 adults to (a) EMG biofeedback and PMRT, (b) thermal biofeedback and PMRT, or (c) a control condition. Patients were studied over five sessions. The results indicated that both forms of biofeedback, when combined with PMRT, reduced the negative affect and nausea associated with chemotherapy. Taken together, these two

---

[4]It is not clear why trait anxiety would change as a result of a short-term behavioral intervention, though it has been reported in several studies.

Table 4—*Summary of Controlled Research on the Use of Biofeedback With Conditioned Side Effects*

Study	Patients	Study design	Treatment protocol	Assessment instruments	Results
Burish, Shartner, & Lyles (1981)	N = 1 adult; Dx = adenocarcinoma; CP = not reported	Single-subject multiple baseline	3 baseline, 4 training, and 3 follow-up sessions. Intervention involved PMRT and multiple-site EMG biofeedback training	BP; PR; EMG activity; Pt ratings of anxiety, N, and V	In comparison with baseline, the Pt reduced PR, BP, EMG levels, and reported less anxiety and N. These improvements were obtained during both training and follow-up
Shartner, Burish, & Carey (1985)	N = 12; Dx = varied; CP = varied	Group comparison: thermal biofeedback with PMRT vs. EMG biofeedback with PMRT vs. control	4 training and 1 follow-up session	During chemotherapy: BP; PR; Pt ratings of anxiety, hostility, depression, and N; RN ratings of anxiety, N, and V / Following chemotherapy: Pt ratings of anxiety, N, and V for 3 days	In comparison with the control group, treated Pts reported less anxiety, hostility, depression, and N during and after chemotherapy. No differences in V among groups.

Note. N = nausea; V = vomiting; RN = registered nurse; Pt = patient; Dx = diagnosis; CP = chemotherapy protocol; PMRT = progressive muscle relaxation training; BP = blood pressure; PR = pulse rate; EMG = electromyograph.

reports suggest that the combined use of biofeedback with PMRT and guided imagery appears to be a promising intervention. Future research might study larger samples of patients and employ a dismantling strategy (Lang, 1969) so that biofeedback can be assessed independently of PMRT and guided imagery.

Distraction Techniques

A recent innovation in the treatment of psychological side effects has involved the use of attentional diversion/cognitive distraction techniques. This treatment approach was considered because of related research in the treatment of acute pain (see McCaul & Malott, 1984), as well as interest in the mechanism or mechanisms by which the other behavioral interventions exerted their impact (this point is addressed more fully in the Discussion section). Distraction techniques attempt to focus patients' attention on pleasant stimuli or activities, thereby directing attention away from unpleasant sensations and from potential CSs. Distraction might be achieved by any of a large number of tasks (e.g., pleasant imagery, music, focal point attention), but in the chemotherapy context, it has been most commonly accomplished by the use of external devices, particularly video games. The research using distraction to reduce the side effects of chemotherapy is described in Table 5.

In the first published study of distraction, Kolko and Rickard-Figueroa (1985) used a multiple baseline design to study the efficacy of video games in 3 adolescent cancer patients. When the patients used the video games, they experienced a reduction in the number of general anticipatory symptoms (e.g., nausea, insomnia, cold hands) displayed during the 24 hr prior to chemotherapy and a decrease in the aversiveness of the postchemotherapy side effects. When the games (distraction) were not available, the number of anticipatory symptoms returned to baseline levels.

Redd et al. (1987) conducted two studies to evaluate a video game-based distractor in 26 pediatric patients undergoing chemotherapy. In the first study, which used a group comparison design, these authors found a significant decrease in the intensity of nausea for those patients who employed distraction in comparison with control patients who did not. In a subsequent study, using a repeated measures reversal design (i.e., no distraction baseline, introduction to distraction, return to no distraction, return to distraction), Redd et al. found additional evidence for the efficacy of distraction, both for nausea and for anxiety. Interestingly, Redd et al. reported that the introduction and withdrawal of the opportunity to play video games did not consistently influence physiological indices of arousal.

In the only study of distraction reported thus far with adults, Greene, Seime, and Smith (1985) compared the efficacy of video games with relaxation training for the reduction of anticipatory nausea and vomiting. These authors implemented a complex, multiple-baseline design that included five phases: (a) no intervention, (b) video distraction, (c) removal of the distraction device (i.e., no intervention), (d) video distraction, and (e) relaxation training. This single-subject study took place over 18 chemotherapy sessions during a 9-month period. The results were consistent with earlier reports in that video distraction initially inhibited anticipatory nausea and vomiting and that these gains were not maintained when the distractor was unavailable. In contrast with previous work, however, the authors reported that the efficacy of distraction was attenuated with continued use (i.e., during Phase 4); more-

Table 5—*Summary of Controlled Research on the Use of Distraction With Conditioned Side Effects*

Study	Patients	Study design	Treatment protocol	Assessment instruments	Results
Kolko & Rickard-Figueroa (1985)	N = 3 adolescent males; Dx = acute lymphocitic leukemia; CP = not reported	Single subject, multiple baseline (ABAB)	3–5 baseline, 3 intervention, 3 withdrawal and intervention sessions. Intervention involved a cognitive distractor, i.e., access to video games	Pt report of general distress, anxiety, and chemotherapy-related symptoms; observer rating of distress	In comparison with baseline, distraction led to reduced number of anticipatory symptoms and to reduced severity of postchemotherapy side effects
Redd, Jacobsen, Die-Trill, Dermatis, McEvoy, & Holland (1987)	Study 1 N = 26 children and adolescents; Dx = varied; CP = varied Study 2 N = 15 children and adolescents; Dx = varied; CP = varied	Group comparison: video distraction vs. placebo control Single subject, multiple baseline (ABAB) design	1 baseline and 1 intervention session 1 session with 10 min baseline, 10 min distraction, 10 min no distraction 10 min distraction	Pt rating of N Pt rating of N; Pt rating of anxiety; PR; SBP; DBP	In comparison with control Pts, Pts using distraction experienced decreased N Use of distraction associated with decreased N and anxiety; PR and BP were not consistently affected
Greene, Seime, & Smith (1985)	N = 1 adult; Dx = adenocarcinoma of the stomach; CP = Fluorouracil, Adriomycin, and Mitomycin	Single subject, multiple baseline (ABABC)	3 baseline, 3 video distraction, 2 withdrawal, 3 video distraction, 6 relaxation training	Pt report of N and V; PR; SBP; DBP	Initially, video distraction reduced ANV; treatment effects not maintained with distraction. Relaxation reduced ANV and effect maintained.

Note. N = nausea; V = vomiting; ANV = anticipatory nausea and vomiting; Pt = patient; Dx = diagnosis; CP = chemotherapy protocol; BP = blood pressure; PR = pulse rate; RR = respiration rate; SBP = systolic blood pressure; DBP = diastolic blood pressure.

over, the subsequent use of relaxation was associated with a reduction in anticipatory symptoms. Although a single-subject study of this sort does not warrant firm conclusions, these results do suggest that (a) the effectiveness of distraction may lessen with extended use and (b) the benefits of relaxation may be more permanent. It may be that the poor maintenance of this distractor was related to its lessening novelty, whereas the comparatively better transfer of treatment gains with PMRT (and related techniques) may result from the fact that they provide patients with a self-control technique that is more permanent (see Thoresen & Mahoney, 1974).

Overall, preliminary research suggests that interventions that use external distractors (e.g., video games) do appear to reduce chemotherapy-related responses, at least initially, as long as the distracting stimuli are available. However, these results need to be accepted with caution until they have been replicated in controlled studies using larger patient samples. Moreover, at least four important questions are unresolved and warrant further investigation. First, does repeated use of an external distractor (e.g., video games) reduce that distractor's novelty and, therefore, efficacy over time? Second, can treatment gains achieved with external distraction be maintained after the distractor is withdrawn and the patient is left to his or her own resources? Third, is an internally generated distractor, which can change over time and retain its novelty, be more effective than an externally provided distractor, which may be more stable? And finally, how does the use of an internally generated distractor differ, if at all, from hypnosis or guided imagery?

Summary

Within the past 10 years, a number of case reports and controlled studies have assessed the efficacy of psychological interventions for reducing the side effects resulting from cancer chemotherapy. Controlled investigations have been completed for five interventions: hypnosis, progressive muscle relaxation training with guided imagery, systematic desensitization, EMG and thermal biofeedback, and cognitive distraction. This research suggests that hypnosis, PMRT and guided imagery, and SD can successfully reduce the psychological side effects that accompany cancer chemotherapy, including nausea, vomiting, and negative affect, and perhaps can also increase caloric intake in the days after chemotherapy. The studies on biofeedback and cognitive distraction are also positive in outcome, but because of the small number of subjects observed, these studies are only suggestive in nature. Overall, the data suggest that psychological interventions can effectively reduce much of the distress associated with cancer chemotherapy.

Discussion

Most of the investigations on the psychological treatment of chemotherapy-related side effects have focused on the relatively simple question, Are psychological interventions efficacious? As the foregoing review suggests, an affirmative answer to this question appears warranted. Increasingly, therefore, research will be devoted to subtler questions such as, With whom do such interventions work? How do the interventions exert their impact? How can we maximize the clinical utility and availability of these interventions? We now focus our attention on these questions.

Factors Associated With Treatment Acceptance and Outcome

Although psychological interventions for reducing chemotherapy-related side effects are effective with many patients, they are not effective with all patients. At least two types of factors might contribute to this fact. First, not all cancer chemotherapy patients are willing to try or to continue trying psychological interventions. For example, Zeltzer et al. (1983) reported that 25% (3 of 12) of the adolescents they studied rejected hypnosis for cultural reasons. Hendler and Redd (1986) found that many chemotherapy patients believed that the hypnotic state is an unconscious, powerful state involving loss of control and that given a choice, they prefer an intervention not labeled "hypnosis." Although the other psychological interventions are less likely than hypnosis to be rejected because of misconceptions about the technique or its goals, in our research we have found that a minority of patients do not pursue these other techniques because they are perceived to involve too much effort or time. This is especially likely for patients who are very ill or weak. In some cases we believe it is possible and clinically beneficial to gently encourage such patients, using the same clinical sensitivity and skill necessary in other treatment contexts, to use the intervention.

Second, not all patients who do try psychological interventions will profit from them. For example, Lyles et al. (1982) reported that even though the majority of their patients profited from PMRT and guided imagery, some showed no change, and a few evinced increased distress on some measures. Research designed to determine whether individual patient characteristics might predict treatment outcome has helped to explain such results. In a reanalysis of data collected in an earlier series of studies, Carey and Burish (1985) found that patients who had high and moderate baseline levels of anxiety were less likely than were low-anxious patients to benefit from PMRT and biofeedback. For such persons, the task of practicing a behavioral intervention such as PMRT may be appraised as an additional stressor that increases, rather than decreases, their discomfort during chemotherapy. In a related study, Burish et al. (1984) reported that cancer chemotherapy patients with an external health locus of control, in comparison with patients without such an orientation, were also more likely to profit from relaxation training. In contrast, no relationship has been found between hypnotic susceptibility and the degree of symptom reduction achieved with hypnosis (Zeltzer et al., 1984b) nor between pretreatment expectancies and outcome on systematic desensitization (Morrow & Morrell, 1982) or on PMRT (Carey & Burish, 1987). Although these results should be accepted cautiously because of the small number of patients studied, it appears that cancer chemotherapy patients who have low levels of pretreatment anxiety or who exhibit an external locus of control benefit more than do their high-anxious and nonexternally oriented counterparts. Unfortunately, no research has assessed the contribution of individual difference factors using a multivariate model in which the combined and interactive effects of several variables can be determined. It is possible that such an approach will allow us to account for a greater share of the variance in treatment outcome.

Mechanisms of Action

Given that psychological techniques can indeed be effective in reducing the conditioned and stress-induced symptoms associated with cancer chemotherapy, it is worthwhile to determine the means by which these techniques exert their impact. The identification of unique and common causal factors across interventions would be theoretically interesting and would also allow for more precise and cost-effective treatment planning. Unfortunately, few studies have provided the comparative and componential analyses required to address directly these issues in a convincing empirical fashion. Despite this lacuna in the research literature, it is possible to describe five hypotheses that may explain, at least in part, the mechanism or mechanisms by which psychological interventions reduce chemotherapy-related distress. We preface our descriptions by acknowledging that these represent hypotheses to be evaluated rather than conclusions to be drawn.

Nonspecific Factors

The first hypothesis, which must be considered in any discussion of possible mechanisms, is that the effectiveness of the treatment results from the various nonspecific factors associated with the treatment's delivery (Kazdin & Wilcoxon, 1976). Such nonspecific factors are likely to include positive expectancies of the patient (i.e., the placebo effect; Frank, 1973) as well as the empathy and social support provided by a therapist. Another nonspecific factor, especially relevant with regard to the use of video games with children, is the unconventional nature of the intervention; such an unusual intervention (from a traditional medical perspective) may communicate to patients that despite the rather serious, sterile medical environment, the professionals working with them are indeed interested in their psychological welfare as well as in treating their disease. This message may allay medically related anxieties and prevent common hospital fears from being exacerbated.

In order to test this hypothesis, several studies have included plausible attention-placebo procedures to control for nonspecific factors (e.g., Cotanch & Strum, 1985; Lyles et al., 1982; Morrow & Morrell, 1982). In each of these investigations the specific intervention was clearly superior to the placebo condition, which in turn did not differ from the nontreatment control. Moreover, investigators who have studied antiemetic medications (see Siegel & Longo, 1981) or alternative behavior interventions (e.g., Carey & Burish, 1987) have demonstrated that positive expectancies and increased attention alone cannot account for treatment efficacy. Thus, although nonspecific factors probably do contribute to the overall impact of the treatments, it is unlikely that these factors account for much of the observed effect.

Physiological Relaxation

An alternative explanation for the beneficial effects observed in the chemotherapy context is that such improvements may be attributable to deep somatic restfulness, sometimes called the *relaxation response* (Benson, 1975). This effect would appear to be produced by four of the five interventions just reviewed (viz., hypnosis, PMRT, SD, and EMG biofeedback).[5] In this regard, previous clinical research suggests that despite some differences in their effects, these stress-management procedures are quite similar in that they produce "a large *global* relaxation response" (Lehrer & Woolfolk, 1984, p. 463; emphasis added).

Within the chemotherapy context, relaxation may exert its effect through one or more of several related pathways, with the degree of relaxation achieved related to level of effectiveness. First, relaxation may reduce symptoms indirectly by reducing generalized physiological arousal; that is, it can be hypothesized that the side effects of chemotherapy often lead to arousal, which in turn may (a) become a conditioned stimulus for those same side effects, (b) be associated with neurotransmitter changes that contributre to conditioned responses, or (c) exacerbate pharmacological, conditioned, or other stress-related symptoms by adding to the overall stressfulness of the situation. Thus, by minimizing general physiological arousal, the interventions may be effective in reducing chemotherapy-related side effects. Second, relaxation may directly inhibit the muscular contractions in the gastrointestinal tract that accompany nausea and vomiting or may indirectly influence such activity by affecting neurochemical changes in the brain that in turn control gastrointestinal activity. Finally, relaxation may produce its effects by increasing the threshold (i.e., decreasing the sensitivity) of the chemoreceptor trigger zone, which is believed to coordinate the vomiting response (Borison & McCarthy, 1983).

Although these hypotheses are speculative, indirect support for their validity is provided by the following general findings. First, many antiemetic medications (e.g., prochlorperazine) are effective in reducing emesis in part because they produce a physiological sedation effect (Borison & McCarthy, 1983) that may be similar to, although stronger than, that produced by behavioral relaxation techniques (cf. Lader, 1984). Second, there is ample evidence from other clinical contexts that relaxation produces a general decrease in sympathetic arousal and EMG activity (Borkovec & Sides, 1979). Finally, Hoffman et al. (1982) have reported that relaxation can result in augmented plasma norepinephrine levels, particularly under conditions of stress. These authors speculated that individuals skilled at deep relaxation are physiologically less responsive to stress, with reduced adrenergic end-organ responsivity. Overall, therefore, the data suggest that deep physiological relaxation may be an active ingredient contributing to the reduction of conditioned and stress-related responses to chemotherapy.

Despite this support for the relaxation mechanism, some research suggests that physiological relaxation cannot explain completely the effectiveness of all the interventions that have been used. Specifically, Kolko and Rickard-Figueroa (1985) and Redd et al. (1987) reported that even patients who exhibited none of the signs of deep relaxation were able to reduce chemotherapy-related symptoms by becoming actively involved in video games. In addition, research by Morrow (1986) suggests that relaxation training alone is not as effective as training that included imagery components.

---

[5]This phenomenon has also been labeled *cognitive distraction, attentional control*, or *absorption*.

Counterconditioning

A third explanation for the efficacy of the various treatments, given that many of the symptoms experienced in the chemotherapy setting probably develop through an associative learning process, is counterconditioning. According to this explanation, the pairing of conditioned stimuli (e.g., the sight of the nurse) that formerly elicited nausea and vomiting with feelings of relaxation and comfort counterconditions these stimuli so that in the future they will elicit relaxation, or at least a less stressful state, rather than nausea and vomiting. Direct support for this hypothesis comes from research on SD (Morrow & Morrell, 1982); indirect support can be gleaned from research on the other interventions (viz., hypnosis, PMRT, and biofeedback), but only if one makes the assumption that patients were aware of the conditioned stimuli present in the chemotherapy environment while they were undergoing the various psychological treatments. If this assumption is valid, it is possible to construe these alternative interventions as a form of in vivo desensitization, whereas Morrow and Morrell's (1982) use of SD can be viewed as the traditional Wolpean version of desensitization.

Although it is an attractive explanation, several problems can be raised with the counterconditioning hypothesis. First, the assumption that patients are attending to the conditioned stimuli present in the chemotherapy context while undergoing hypnosis or PMRT seems dubious; if they are not attending to such conditioned stimuli, then it is less likely that they are being counterconditioned. Second, from a theoretical perspective, it would seem difficult to establish a new association between the CS and the new response (e.g., relaxation) when a host of negative pharmacological side effects (i.e., the UCR) continue to occur after each chemotherapy treatment. Finally, even if these problems were not present, the effects of SD, even in the well-controlled laboratory setting, cannot be attributed completely to counterconditioning, because there are numerous other mechanisms, including those presented here, that appear to be operative (cf. Masters et al., 1987; McGlynn, Mealiea, & Landau, 1981).

Attentional Diversion or Redirection

All five of the behavioral interventions reviewed earlier require that patients participate cognitively in the intervention, usually by attending to relaxing or at least nonanxiety-producing situations. It may be that such attentional diversion or redirection may be mediating the therapeutic effect of the various interventions; that is, with patients attending to interesting external (e.g., video games) or internal (e.g., pleasant imagery) stimuli, there is less attention available to focus on unpleasant internal sensations (e.g., nausea) or potential CSs (e.g., drug taste). Such attentional diversion might also be understood from a "stress and coping" perspective (e.g., Lazarus & Folkman, 1984); that is, if the distracting task is enjoyable (as with pleasant imagery or the use of video games), then appraisal of the overall aversiveness (i.e., threat) of chemotherapy may be lessened, resulting in less dysphoria. This is true even if the distractor produces increased physiological arousal, which results from video games (Redd et al., 1987). Such arousal is believed to result from positive emotions, such as excitement, or from physical effort that is part of the game rather than from a distressing situation (although, conceivably, an improperly chosen distractor could become distressing, such as a video game that was too difficult or produced feelings of failure). Thus, even though some distractors may increase physiological arousal, they can focus attention on a pleasant task and thereby decrease distress.

Direct empirical support for the distraction hypothesis comes from the three reports described earlier (i.e., Greene et al., 1985; Kolko & Rickard-Figueroa, 1985; Redd et al., 1987). Indirect support for the distraction hypothesis comes from research with other procedures (i.e., hypnosis, PMRT with guided imagery, biofeedback, and systematic desensitization), which all require that the patient attend to specific instructions or actively participate in certain procedures while undergoing chemotherapy.[6] These instructions and procedures are typically quite absorbing of cognitive capacity, especially to the extent that patients are motivated and interested. Morrow's (1986) study can be seen as supporting this position in that he found that PMRT was not effective when guided imagery was not used during the infusion time; that is, Morrow's version of PMRT may have required less of the patients' attention during their chemotherapy and was, as a result, less efficacious than was this procedure in other studies in which patients did use imagery during the infusion (e.g., Lyles et al., 1982). There is one study that did not support the use of distraction: Cotanch and Strum (1985) reported that listening to audiotapes of music was not successful in reducing the aversiveness of chemotherapy. Perhaps the distractor used in this study was not sufficiently engaging; that is, listening to music may not have occupied completely the patients' cognitive capacity, which is a necessary characteristic of effective cognitive distractors (see McCaul & Malott, 1984). In summary, attentional diversion or cognitive distraction may play an important role in reducing psychological side effects.

Enhanced Perception of Self-Efficacy and Mastery

In one way or another, all of the treatments discussed afford patients an active coping strategy (cf. Goldfried, 1971; Goldfried & Trier, 1974) and may produce in patients an increased sense of self-efficacy or of perceived mastery (see Bandura, 1977). Morrow and Morrell's (1982) modified SD procedure, for example, has patients imagining themselves staying relaxed and calm in situations that formerly caused considerable anxiety. PMRT and hypnosis procedures show patients how to relax in the midst of a busy chemotherapy treatment room, seated in the treatment chair, with the tray of syringes at their side. Attentional diversion techniques illustrate how the patients can control their attention so as to virtually ignore and thereby render impotent the conditioned stimuli in the environment. The confidence developed when a person believes that the use of an intervention will allow control over a stressful situation may, in the chemotherapy context as in many other contexts, be an important ingredient of the treatment package.

---

[6]Systematic desensitization may be thought to involve cognitive participation only during training; because SD training has typically occurred outside of the chemotherapy context, it would appear that SD does not involve a distracting component during the actual chemotherapy infusion. Alternatively, however, SD may involve a distraction component during chemotherapy if patients are actively using the relaxation procedures that they learned during training as a way of managing discomfort, distress, or both resulting from venipuncture, the infusion, or other chemotherapy procedures. In this case, SD would appear to involve an active distraction component.

It may be said that the data on health locus of control, a concept related to perceived mastery, do not support the enhanced self-efficacy explanation. For example, Morrow and Morrell (1982) found that reductions in anticipatory nausea and vomiting were not accompanied by corresponding changes in health locus of control. Also, we (Burish et al., 1984) have found that chemotherapy patients with a high external health locus of control orientation are more likely to benefit from a treatment intervention than are patients low on this dimension. Although our data appear to weaken the perceived mastery explanation (Burish et al., 1984), upon reflection, this may not be so: health locus of control measures a person's view of where the locus of control lies, not whether there is control or whether one desires or has control. Indeed, even if the control lies in a source external to one's self (e.g., in a videotape or a psychologist's suggestions), by availing oneself of that source of control, one could clearly come to believe that mastery can be achieved. Although the role of perceived mastery and self-efficacy is hypothetical at this point, it warrants continued empirical investigation.

Conclusion

Five different mechanisms have been proposed in order to explain the efficacy of psychological interventions for the reduction of conditioned and stress-related responses in cancer chemotherapy. At this stage, the comparative research needed to answer the question, "How do these treatments exert their impact?", is incomplete. Nonetheless, on the basis of the limited research that has addressed this question, either directly or indirectly, we conclude that it is unlikely that any single mechanism adequately accounts for the beneficial effects that have been observed in this context. Rather, we suggest that these different mechanisms should be viewed as cooperating and interacting to produce an effect rather than as competing hypotheses. A related interpretation is that the different mechanisms proposed herein reflect different levels of analysis in a biopsychosocial framework (cf. Engel, 1977; Schwartz, 1982).

Clinical Issues

In previous reviews of the literature (e.g., Burish & Carey, 1984; Redd & Andrykowski, 1982), several important clinical issues were discussed, including (a) choosing among the various interventions, (b) promoting maintenance of treatment gains, and (c) identifying individuals at risk for not profiting from psychological interventions and developing approaches to meet their special needs. These issues continue to be important, but in this article we discuss four additional issues that have emerged in recent years.

First, to date, most work concerned with nausea and vomiting in cancer patients has been either biomedical or psychosocial in nature. Many psychosocial researchers regard pharmacological (i.e., antiemetic) treatments as nuisance variables requiring methodological control. Similarly, biomedical researchers have neglected important psychosocial issues (Carey, Burish, & Brenner, 1983). The time has come for biomedical and psychosocial research on nausea and vomiting to be integrative and complementary, with the goal being to develop the best possible treatment package. A psychological intervention that commences prior to the initiation of chemotherapy, combined with an effective drug protocol that balances antiemetic protection with toxic side effects, may be able to prevent or substantially reduce most nausea and vomiting associated with chemotherapy. Interdisciplinary (i.e., biopsychosocial; Engel, 1977; Schwartz, 1982) research of this nature is clearly desirable.

Second, in order for psychological interventions to be used widely in cancer clinics and hospitals throughout the country, a more favorable cost-effectiveness ratio is needed. Most cancer clinics do not use psychological interventions, even though they may be aware of their efficacy, because of the monetary costs and time involved (usually several hours per patient) or the lack of available and trained therapists. We recently completed a study to determine whether our PMRT and guided imagery intervention could be delivered as effectively by audiotapes or by trained paraprofessionals as by experienced psychologists (Carey & Burish, 1987). Unfortunately, our data suggest that the experienced therapists were significantly more effective than the other service delivery techniques, which dampens our enthusiasm for these alternate approaches as cost-effective solutions. The modified SD procedure used by Morrow and Morrell (1982) requires perhaps the least amount of intervention time (about 2 hr), but outcome data are not available beyond two postintervention sessions. Distraction has the potential of being a cost-effective approach, although it may be necessary to insure that external distractors are always available to patients, at home and in the clinic. Clearly, low-cost delivery techniques are needed in order to make the current technology available to the majority of chemotherapy patients who could benefit from it.

Third, in some settings and for some types of chemotherapy treatment protocols, nausea and vomiting have become less problematic in recent years. For example, Stefanek, Sheidler, and Fetting (1988) compared the prevalence and severity rates of anticipatory symptoms reported by adult patients in their clinic in 1987 with those of approximately 5 years earlier. In general, they found that while the prevalence rates were similar, the severity ratings were lower; that is, there was a significant decrease in severity from the first to the second sampling, with the more recent ratings indicating that anticipatory nausea and vomiting were no longer "a significant clinical problem" for patients receiving parenteral chemotherapy. We have also noticed a decline in the severity of these side effects, as well as a decreased prevalence, in adult patients seen in our clinic (Carey & Burish, 1987). Moreover, we anticipate that this trend may continue, at least in adults, largely because of the development of antiemetic drugs that are less toxic and more effective and because of the increased availability of these medications beyond major medical centers. If we assume that this trend is occurring and does continue, will this mean that in the future there will be less need for psychological interventions with chemotherapy patients? We believe the answer is no. But these data and observations, and reports of the side effects of newer forms of cancer treatments (e.g., interleukin-2), do suggest that the focus of the psychological interventions may need to change. As this review has shown, most of the psychological research with chemotherapy patients has focused on nausea and vomiting as the only or the primary outcome measures. However, psychological interventions can have a positive effect on a number of other symptoms that chemotherapy patients experience, including negative emotional states (Lyles et al., 1982), reduced food intake (Campbell, Dixon, Sanderford, & Denicola, 1984), and pain (Spiegel, 1985). Future researchers might do well to broaden both the symptoms that are targeted and the outcome measures that are assessed. We suspect that such an approach will ultimately provide even stronger support for the use of psychological interventions with cancer patients.

Finally, research on the treatment of psychological responses to cancer chemotherapy has progressed to a point at which oneshot, noncontrolled studies will usually contribute little, empirically or heuristically, to the area. Advances will depend increasingly upon controlled studies that build upon prior findings. Comparative studies, and studies using a dismantling design in order to clarify treatment mechanisms, hold much promise. And, as indicated earlier, continued research on the etiology of conditioned and stress-related responses to cancer chemotherapy is warranted.

Conclusion

On the basis of the data reviewed, it can be concluded that the psychological symptoms that result from cancer chemotherapy appear to be the product of both associative learning and the stress associated with chemotherapy. Moreover, these side effects can, in many instances, be prevented or ameliorated with psychological techniques. This conclusion is based on research conducted in a vareity of clinics, on children and adults, by independent research teams, using poorly controlled as well as well-controlled methodological designs. Overall, therefore, these findings can be considered robust.

Although considerable knowledge has been generated in a short period of time, and although the rate of publications continues to increase, we believe that research on the psychological treatment of the side effects of cancer chemotherapy is at a critical point in its development. The use of progressively less toxic and more effective antiemetic drugs, the increased emphasis on cost-effectiveness, and the methodological and scientific evolution of the field will demand changes in the strategies and approaches used by psychosocial investigators. For example, a focus on why some people do not benefit from psychological treatments might prove useful theoretically and clinically, as might more integrative, comprehensive treatment packages that include pharmacological components and that attempt to do more than reduce anticipatory nausea and vomiting. Such studies will help to insure that research on the treatment of psychological side effects of cancer chemotherapy continues to make significant theoretical and clinical advances.

References

Ader, R. (1981). *Psychoneuroimmunology*. Orlando, FL: Academic Press.

Ader, R., & Cohen, N. (1985). CNS–immune system interactions: Conditioning phenomena. *Behavioral and Brain Sciences, 8,* 379–394.

Andrykowski, M. A., Jacobsen, P. B., Marks, E., Gorfinkle, K., Hakes, T., Kaufman, R. J., Currie, V. E., Holland, J. C., & Redd, W. H. (in press). Prevalence, predictors, and course of anticipatory nausea in women receiving adjuvant chemotherapy for breast cancer. *Cancer*.

Andrykowski, M. A., & Redd, W. H. (1987). Longitudinal analysis of the development of anticipatory nausea. *Journal of Consulting and Clinical Psychology, 55,* 36–41.

Andrykowski, M. A., Redd, W. H., & Hatfield, A. K. (1985). Development of anticipatory nausea: A prospective analysis. *Journal of Consulting and Clinical Psychology, 53,* 447–454.

Bandura, A. (1977). Self-efficacy: Toward a unifying theory of behavioral change. *Psychological Review, 85,* 191–215.

Benson, H. (1975). *The relaxation response.* New York: Avon.

Bernstein, D. A., & Borkovec, T. D. (1973). *Progessive relaxation training: A manual for the helping professions.* Champaign, IL: Research Press.

Bernstein, I. L. (1978). Learned taste aversions in children receiving chemotherapy. *Science, 200,* 1302–1303.

Bernstein, I. L., & Borson, S. (1986). Learned food aversion: A component of anorexia syndromes. *Psychological Review, 93,* 462–472.

Bernstein, I. L., & Webster, M. M. (1980). Learned taste aversions in humans. *Physiology and Behavior, 25,* 363–366.

Bernstein, I. L., & Webster, M. M. (1985). Learned food aversions: A consequence of cancer chemotherapy. In T. G. Burish, S. M. Levy, & B. E. Meyerowitz (Eds.), *Cancer, nutrition, and eating behavior: A biobehavioral perspective* (pp. 103–116). Hillsdale, NJ: Erlbaum.

Borison, H. L., & McCarthy, L. E. (1983). Neuropharmacologic mechanisms of emesis. In J. Laszlo (Ed.), *Antiemetics and cancer chemotherapy* (pp. 6–20). Baltimore, MD: Williams & Wilkins.

Borkovec, T. D., & Sides, J. K. (1979). Critical procedural variables related to the physiological effects of progressive relaxation: A review. *Behaviour Research and Therapy, 17,* 119–126.

Burish, T. G., & Carey, M. P. (1984). Conditioned responses to cancer chemotherapy: Etiology and treatment. In B. H. Fox & B. H. Newberry (Eds.), *Impact of psychoendocrine systems in cancer immunity* (pp. 147–178). Toronto: Hogrefe.

Burish, T. G., & Carey, M. P. (1986). Conditioned aversive responses in cancer chemotherapy patients: Theoretical and developmental analysis. *Journal of Consulting and Clinical Psychology, 54,* 593–600.

Burish, T. G., Carey, M. P., Krozely, M. G., & Greco, F. A. (1987). Conditioned nausea and vomiting induced by cancer chemotherapy: Prevention through behavioral treatment. *Journal of Consulting and Clinical Psychology, 55,* 42–48.

Burish, T. G., Carey, M. P., Wallston, K. A., Stein, M. J., Jamison, R. N., & Lyles, J. N. (1984). Health locus of control and chronic disease: An external orientation may be advantageous. *Journal of Social and Clinical Psychology, 2,* 326–332.

Burish, T. G., & Lyles, J. N. (1979). Effectiveness of relaxation training in reducing the aversiveness of chemotherapy in the treatment of cancer. *Journal of Behavior Therapy and Experimental Psychiatry, 10,* 357–361.

Burish, T. G., & Lyles, J. N. (1981). Effectiveness of relaxation training in reducing adverse reactions to cancer chemotherapy. *Journal of Behavioral Medicine, 4,* 65–78.

Burish, T. G., Shartner, C. D., & Lyles, J. N. (1981). Effectiveness of multiple-site EMG biofeedback and relaxation in reducing the aversiveness of cancer chemotherapy. *Biofeedback and Self-Regulation, 6,* 523–535.

Campbell, D. F., Dixon, J. F., Sanderford, L. D., & Denicola, M. D. (1984). Relaxation: Its effect on the nutritional status and performances status of clients with cancer. *Journal of the American Dietetic Association, 84,* 201–204.

Carey, M. P., & Burish, T. G. (1985). Anxiety as a predictor of behavioral therapy outcome for cancer chemotherapy patients. *Journal of Consulting and Clinical Psychology, 53,* 860–865.

Carey, M. P., & Burish, T. G. (1987). Providing relaxation training to cancer chemotherapy patients: A comparison of three methods. *Journal of Consulting and Clinical Psychology, 55,* 732–737.

Carey, M. P., Burish, T. G., & Brenner, D. E. (1983). Delta-9-tetrahydrocannabinol in cancer chemotherapy: Research problems and issues. *Annals of Internal Medicine, 99,* 106–114.

Chang, J. C. (1981). Nausea and vomiting in cancer patients: An expression of psychological mechanisms? *Psychosomatics, 22,* 707–709.

Cohn, K. H. (1982). Chemotherapy from an insider's perspective. *Lancet, 1,* 1006–1009.

Collins, K. H., & Tatum, A. L. (1925). A conditioned salivary reflex established by chronic morphine poisoning. *American Journal of Physiology, 74,* 14–15.

Cotanch, P. (1983). Relaxation training for control of nausea and vomiting in patients receiving chemotherapy. *Cancer Nursing, 6,* 277–283.

Cotanch, P., Hockenberry, M., & Herman, S. (1985). Self-hypnosis antiemetic therapy in children receiving chemotherapy. *Oncology Nursing Forum, 12,* 41–46.

Cotanch, P., & Strum, S. (1985). *Progressive muscle relaxation as antiemetic therapy for cancer patients: A controlled study.* Unpublished manuscript, Duke University, Durham, NC.

Dahlquist, L. M., Gil, K. M., Armstrong, F. D., Ginsberg, A., & Jones, B. (1985). Behavioral management of children's distress during chemotherapy. *Journal of Behavior Therapy and Experimental Psychiatry, 16,* 325–329.

Dempster, C. R., Balson, P., & Whalen, B. T. (1976). Supportive hypnotherapy during the radical treatment of malignancies. *International Journal of Clinical and Experimental Hypnosis, 24,* 1–9.

Dolgin, M. J., Katz, E. R., McGinty, K., & Siegel, S. E. (1985). Anticipatory nausea and vomiting in pediatric cancer patients. *Pediatrics, 75,* 547–552.

Ellenberg, L., Kellerman, J., Dash, J., Higgins, G., & Zeltzer, L. (1980). Use of hypnosis for multiple symptoms in an adolescent girl with leukemia. *Journal of Adolescent Health Care, 1,* 132–136.

Engel, G. L. (1977). The need for a new medical model: A challenge for biomedicine. *Science, 196,* 129–136.

Fetting, J. H., Sheidler, V. R., Stefanek, M. E., & Enterline, J. P. (1987). Clonidine for anticipatory nausea and vomiting: A pilot study examining dose–toxicity relationships and potential for further study. *Cancer Treatment Reports, 71,* 409–410.

Frank, J. D. (1973). *Persuasion and healing* (2nd ed.). Baltimore, MD: Johns Hopkins University.

Garcia y Robertson, R., & Garcia, J. (1985). X-rays and learned taste aversions: Historical and psychological ramifications. In T. G. Burish, S. M. Levy, & B. E. Meyerowitz (Eds.), *Cancer, nutrition, and eating behavior: A biobehavioral perspective* (pp. 11–41). Hillsdale, NJ: Erlbaum.

Goldfried, M. R. (1971). Systematic desensitization as training in self-control. *Journal of Consulting and Clinical Psychology, 37,* 228–234.

Goldfried, M. R., & Trier, C. S. (1974). Effectiveness of relaxation as an active coping skill. *Journal of Abnormal Psychology, 83,* 348–355.

Greene, P. G., Seime, R. J., & Smith, M. E. (1985). *Distraction and relaxation training in the treatment of anticipatory nausea and vomiting: A single subject intervention.* Manuscript submitted for publication.

Hailey, B. J., & White, J. G. (1983). Systematic desensitization for anticipatory nausea associated with chemotherapy. *Psychosomatic, 24,* 289–291.

Hamberger, L. K. (1982). Reduction of generalized aversive responding in a posttreatment cancer patient: Relaxation as an active coping skill. *Journal of Behavior Therapy and Experimental Psychiatry, 13,* 229–233.

Hendler, C. S., & Redd, W. H. (1986). Fear of hypnosis: The role of labeling in patients' acceptance of behavioral interventions. *Behavior Therapy, 17,* 2–13.

Hoffman, J. W., Benson, H., Arns, P. A., Stainbrook, G. L., Landsberg, L., Young, J. B., & Gill, A. (1982). Reduced sympathetic nervous system responsivity associated with the relaxation response. *Science, 215,* 190–192.

Hoffman, M. L. (1982–1983). Hypnotic desensitization for the management of anticipatory emesis in chemotherapy. *American Journal of Clinical Hypnosis, 25,* 173–176.

Ingle, R. J., Burish, T. G., & Wallston, K. A. (1984). Conditionability of cancer chemotherapy patients. *Oncology Nursing Forum, 11,* 97–102.

Jacobsen, P. B., Andrykowski, M. A., Redd, W. H., Die-Trill, M., Hakes, T. B., Kaufman, R. J., Currie, V. E., & Holland, J. C. (1988). Nonpharmacologic factors in the development of posttreatment nausea with adjuvant chemotherapy for breast cancer. *Cancer, 61,* 379–385.

Jacobson, E. (1938). *Progressive relaxation.* Chicago, IL: University of Chicago.

Kazdin, A. E., & Wilcoxon, L. A. (1976). Systematic desensitization and nonspecific treatment effects: A methodological evaluation. *Psychological Bulletin, 83,* 729–758.

Kolko, D. J., & Rickard-Figueroa, J. L. (1985). Effects of video games on the adverse corollaries of chemotherapy in pediatric oncology patients: A single-case analysis. *Journal of Consulting and Clinical Psychology, 53,* 223–228.

Kutz, I., Borysenko, J. Z., Come, S. E., & Benson, H. (1980). Paradoxical emetic response to antiemetic treatment in cancer patients. *New England Journal of Medicine, 303,* 1480.

LaBaw, W., Holton, C., Tewell, K., & Eccles, D. (1975). The use of self-hypnosis by children with cancer. *American Journal of Clinical Hypnosis, 17,* 233–238.

Lader, M. (1984). Pharmacological methods. In R. L. Woolfolk & P. M. Lehrer (Eds.), *Principles and practice of stress management* (pp. 306–333). New York: Guilford.

Lang, P. J. (1969). The mechanics of desensitization and the laboratory study of fear. In C. M. Franks (Ed.), *Behavior therapy: Appraisal and status.* New York: McGraw-Hill.

Laszlo, J. (1983). *Antiemetics and cancer chemotherapy.* Baltimore, MD: Williams & Wilkins.

Laszlo, J., & Lucas, V. S. (1981). Emesis as a critical problem in chemotherapy. *New England Journal of Medicine, 305,* 948–949.

Lazarus, R. S. (1966). *Psychological stress and the coping process.* New York: McGraw-Hill.

Lazarus, R. S., & Folkman, S. (1984). *Stress, appraisal, and coping.* New York: Springer.

LeBaron, S., & Zeltzer, L. K. (1984). Behavioral intervention for reducing chemotherapy-related nausea and vomiting in adolescents with cancer. *Journal of Adolescent Health Care, 5,* 178–182.

Lehrer, P. M., & Woolfolk, R. L. (1984). Are stress reduction techniques interchangeable, or do they have specific effects? A review of the comparative empirical literature. In R. L. Woolfolk & P. M. Lehrer (Eds.), *Principles and practice of stress management* (pp. 404–477). New York: Guilford.

Leventhal, H., Easterling, D. V., Nerenz, D. R., & Love, R. R. (1988). The role of motion sickness in predicting anticipatory nausea. *Journal of Behavioral Medicine, 11,* 117–130.

Lyles, J. N., Burish, T. G., Krozely, M. G., & Oldham, R. K. (1982). Efficacy of relaxation training and guided imagery in reducing the aversiveness of cancer chemotherapy. *Journal of Consulting and Clinical Psychology, 50,* 509–524.

Masters, J. C., Burish, T. G., Hollon, S. D., & Rimm, D. C. (1987). *Behavior therapy* (3rd ed.). New York: Harcourt Brace Jovanovich.

McCaul, K. D., & Malott, J. M. (1984). Distraction and coping with pain. *Psychological Bulletin, 95,* 516–533.

McGlynn, F. D., Mealiea, W. L., Jr., & Landau, D. L. (1981). The current status of systematic desensitization. *Clinical Psychology Review, 1,* 149–179.

Moore, K., & Altmaier, E. M. (1981). Stress inoculation training with cancer patients. *Cancer Nursing, 4,* 389–393.

Morrow, G. R. (1982). Prevalence and correlates of anticipatory nausea and vomiting in chemotherapy patients. *Journal of the National Cancer Institute, 68,* 484–488.

Morrow, G. R. (1985). The effect of a susceptibility to motion sickness on the side effects of cancer chemotherapy. *Cancer, 55,* 2766–2770.

Morrow, G. R. (1986). Effect of the cognitive hierarchy in the systematic desensitization treatment of anticipatory nausea in cancer patients: A component comparison with relaxation only, counseling and no treatment. *Cognitive Therapy and Research, 10,* 421–446.

Morrow, G. R., Arseneau, J. C., Asbury, R. F., Bennett, J. M., & Boros, L. (1982). Anticipatory nausea and vomiting with chemotherapy. *New England Journal of Medicine, 306,* 431–432.

Morrow, G. R., & Morrell, C. (1982). Behavioral treatment for the anticipatory nausea and vomiting induced by cancer chemotherapy. *New England Journal of Medicine, 307,* 1476–1480.

Nerenz, D. R., Leventhal, H., Easterling, D. V., & Love, R. R. (1986). Anxiety and drug taste as predictors of anticipatory nausea in cancer chemotherapy. *Journal of Clinical Oncology, 4,* 224–233.

Nerenz, D. R., Leventhal, H., & Love, R. R. (1982). Factors contributing to emotional distress during cancer chemotherapy. *Cancer, 50,* 1020–1027.

Nerenz, D. R., Leventhal, H., Love, R. R., & Ringler, K. E. (1984). Psychological aspects of cancer chemotherapy. *International Journal of Applied Psychology, 33,* 521–529.

Oberst, M. T. (1978). Priorities in cancer nursing research. *Cancer Nursing, 1,* 281.

Pavlov, I. P. (1927). *Conditioned reflexes: An investigation of physiological activity of the cerebral cortex (Lecture III).* Oxford, England: Oxford University Press.

Redd, W. H. (1985/1986). Use of behavioral methods to control the aversive effects of chemotherapy. *Journal of Psychosocial Oncology, 3,* 17–22.

Redd, W. H., Andresen, G. V., & Minagawa, R. Y. (1982). Hypnotic control of anticipatory emesis in patients receiving cancer chemotherapy. *Journal of Consulting and Clinical Psychology, 50,* 14–19.

Redd, W. H., & Andrykowski, M. A. (1982). Behavioral intervention in cancer treatment: Controlling aversion reactions to chemotherapy. *Journal of Consulting and Clinical Psychology, 50,* 1018–1029.

Redd, W. H., Jacobsen, P. B., Die-Trill, M., Dermatis, H., McEvoy, M., & Holland, J. C. (1987). Cognitive/attentional distraction in the control of conditioned nausea in pediatric cancer patients receiving chemotherapy. *Journal of Consulting and Clinical Psychology, 55,* 391–395.

Schwartz, G. E. (1982). Testing the biopsychosocial model: The ultimate challenge facing behavioral medicine. *Journal of Consulting and Clinical Psychology, 50,* 1040–1053.

Scott, D. W., Donahue, D. C., Mastrovito, R. C., & Hakes, T. B. (1983). The antiemetic effect of clinical relaxation: Report of an exploratory pilot study. *Journal of Psychosocial Oncology, 1,* 71–84.

Selye, H. (1976). *The stress of life* (rev. ed.). New York: McGraw-Hill.

Shartner, C. D., Burish, T. G., & Carey, M. P. (1985). Effectiveness of biofeedback with progressive muscle relaxation training in reducing the aversiveness of cancer chemotherapy: A preliminary report. *Japanese Journal of Biofeedback Research, 12,* 33–40.

Siegel, L. J., & Longo, D. L. (1981). The control of chemotherapy-induced emesis. *Annals of Internal Medicine, 95,* 352–359.

Siegel, S. (1979). The role of conditioning in drug tolerance and addiction. In J. D. Keehn (Ed.), *Psychopathology in animals: Research and clinical applications* (pp. 143–168). Orlando, FL: Academic Press.

Silverberg, E., & Lubera, J. (1986). Cancer statistics, 1986. *CA–A Journal for Clinicians, 36,* 9–25.

Smith, J. C., Blumsack, J. T., & Bilek, F. S. (1985). Radiation-induced taste aversions in rats and humans. In T. G. Burish, S. M. Levy, & B. E. Meyerowitz (Eds.), *Cancer, nutrition, and eating behavior: A biobehavioral perspective* (pp. 77–101). Hillsdale, NJ: Erlbaum.

Spence, K. W. (1958). A theory of emotionally based drive (D) and its relation to performance in simple learning situations. *American Psychologist, 13,* 131–141.

Spiegel, D. (1985). The use of hypnosis in controlling cancer pain. *CA—A Cancer Journal for Clinicians, 35,* 221–231.

Stefanek, M. E., Sheidler, V. R., & Fetting, J. H. (1988). *Anticipatory nausea and vomiting: Does it remain a significant clinical problem?* Unpublished manuscript, Johns Hopkins University, Baltimore, MD.

Thoresen, C. E., & Mahoney, M. J. (1974). *Behavioral self-control.* New York: Holt, Rinehart & Winston.

Turk, D. C., Meichenbaum, D., & Genest, M. (1983). *Pain and behavioral medicine: A cognitive–behavioral perspective.* New York: Guilford.

van Komen, R. W., & Redd, W. H. (1985). Personality factors associated with anticipatory nausea/vomiting in patients receiving cancer chemotherapy. *Health Psychology, 4,* 189–202.

Wadden, T. A., & Anderton, C. H. (1982). The clinical use of hypnosis. *Psychological Bulletin, 91,* 215–243.

West, B. L., & Piccionne, C. (1982). Cognitive–behavioral techniques in treating anorexia and depression in a cancer patient. *The Behavior Therapist, 5,* 115–117.

Wilcox, P. M., Fetting, J. H., Nettesheim, K. M., & Abeloff, M. D. (1982). Anticipatory vomiting in women receiving cyclophosphamide, methotrexate, and 5-FU (CMF) adjuvant chemotherapy for breast carcinoma. *Cancer Treatment Reports, 66,* 1601–1604.

Wolpe, J. (1958). *Psychotherapy by reciprocal inhibition.* Stanford, CA: Stanford University.

Zeltzer, L. K., Kellerman, J., Ellenberg, L., & Dash, J. (1983). Hypnosis for reduction of vomiting associated with chemotherapy and disease in adolescents with cancer. *Journal of Adolescent Health Care, 4,* 77–84.

Zeltzer, L. K., & LeBaron, S. (1986). Assessment of acute pain and anxiety and chemotherapy related nausea and vomiting in children and adolescents. *Hospice Journal, 2*(3), 75–98.

Zeltzer, L. K., LeBaron, S., & Zeltzer, P. (1984a). Paradoxical effects of prophylactic phenothiazine antiemetics in children receiving chemotherapy. *Journal of Clinical Oncology, 2,* 930–936.

Zeltzer, L. K., LeBaron, S., & Zeltzer, P. (1984b). The effectiveness of behavioral intervention for reducing nausea and vomiting in children receiving chemotherapy. *Journal of Clinical Oncology, 2,* 683–690.

Chapter 10
PSYCHOSOCIAL OUTCOMES OF BREAST-CONSERVING SURGERY VERSUS MASTECTOMY:
A Meta-Analytic Review

Anne Moyer

Recently, increasing awareness of psychosocial difficulties associated with breast cancer has put a new emphasis on quality of life (Derogatis, 1986). Efforts to improve quality of life have increased the use of less mutilating types of breast surgery (Fallowfield, Baum, & Maguire, 1986). Developments in medical knowledge, such as the demonstration of similar effectiveness of tumor excision plus radiation versus mastectomy for early disease (Early Breast Cancer Trialists' Collaborative Group, 1995; Fisher et al., 1989, 1995; Jacobson et al., 1995) and a new understanding of cancer's spread, have also encouraged this trend (Cady & Stone, 1990; Fisher, 1992; Henderson, 1995; Rowland & Holland, 1989). Either breast-conserving surgery with radiation or mastectomy is now considered appropriate for patients with stage I and II disease (tumors up to 5 cm, with or without axillary node metastases, and no distant metastases) of all ages, barring circumstances that would indicate mastectomy for cosmetic or medical reasons—for example, a large tumor relative to the size of the breast, multiple primary tumors, or a high risk of subsequent new or recurrent tumors (Coon, 1988; Kennedy, 1989). Thus, today many women with breast cancer may be successfully treated with either surgical treatment and may be offered a choice, by law in some states.

As breast-conserving surgical techniques became more widely available, a literature comparing their psychosocial effects to those of mastectomy developed, summarized in Table 1. (A table with more detail regarding study design, specific measures used, and results is available from the author.) Unexpectedly, many of the findings have been equivocal and typically show a lack of substantial benefits for breast-conserving surgery as compared with mastectomy. For example, Pozo et al. (1992) studied 63 women longitudinally, with assessments at 10 days and at 3, 6, and 12 months postoperatively. Although conservatively treated patients reported better sexual adjustment at 6 and 12 months, no other group differences were found in mood disturbance, perceptions of social support, marital satisfaction, life satisfaction, quality of life, or self-rated adjustment. Previous reviewers have concluded that although there may be some advantage for body image and to some extent for sexual functioning (Kiebert, de Haes, & van de Velde, 1991), there is little solid evidence for considerable superior psychological adjustment after breast-conserving treatment

Reprinted from *Health Psychology, 16*(3), 284–298. (1997). Copyright © 1997 by the American Psychological Association. Used with permission of the author.

Preparation of this article was supported by National Institute of Mental Health Training Grant MH19391.

The author is grateful to Nancy Adler, AnnJanette Alejano-Steele, Halle Brown, Turhan Canli, Marilee Coriell, Philip Moore, Lauri Pasch, Cynthia Rosengard, and Peter Salovey for helpful comments on earlier versions of this article.

Table 1—Summary of Studies Comparing Psychosocial Outcomes of Breast-Conserving Surgeries Versus Those of Mastectomy

Study	Participants and design[a]	Dependent variables	Results
Sanger and Reznikoff (1981)	20 BCT + RT, 20 MRM Not randomized 2 months to 4.5 years postsurgery	BI, MS, PA	BCT group had more intactness of body boundaries, less change in overall body satisfaction; no group differences in body anxiety, marital satisfaction, or psychological adjustment.
Beckman, Johansen, Richardt, and Blichert-Toft (1983)	11 BCT + RT, 11 M Not randomized 7–12 months postsurgery	BI, FC, MS	BCT group had better preserved body image, fewer problems showing themselves naked, earlier resumption of sexual activity, and preserved feelings of sexual attractiveness; no group difference in fear of recurrence.
Schain et al. (1983)	18 BCT + RT ± CT, 20 M ± CT Randomized 56–610 days postsurgery	BI, FC, MS, PA, SA	Only difference was that M group had a more negative reaction to their bodies nude.
Ashcroft, Leinster, and Slade (1985) and Ashcroft, Leinster, and Slade (1986)	40 total: BCT + RT, M ± RC Some patients randomized, some given choice Before surgery, 3 months and 1 year postsurgery	BI, MS, PA, SA	Very little difference between groups.
Bartelink, van Dam, and van Dongen (1985)	114 BCT + RT ± CT, 58 RM ± CT BCT randomized, RM not randomized 1–2 years postsurgery	BI, FC	BCT group had more positive body image and less fear of recurrence.
de Haes and Welvaart (1985) and de Haes, van Oostrom, and Welvaart (1986)	21 BCT + RT, 18 MRM Randomized 11 and 18 months postsurgery	BI, FC, GA, MS, PA	At both time points, BCT group had less change in body image; no group differences in fear of recurrence and death, global quality of life, changes in life patterns, sexual functioning, or psychological discomfort.

Study	Sample and design	Measures	Results
Steinberg, Juliano, and Wise (1985)	21 BCT + RT ± CT, 46 MRM ± CT; Half of BCT group had choice of treatment, remainder not randomized; 14 months postsurgery	BI, MS, PA, SA	MRM group felt less attractive and less feminine, was more concerned with dress and appearance and had more severe sexual dysfunction; no group differences in mood or depression; BCT group felt more supported.
S. E. Taylor et al. (1985)	26 BCT ± RT ± CT, 31 SM and MRM ± RT ± CT, 9 RM ± RT ± CT; Not randomized; 2–60 months postsurgery	BI, MS, PA, SA	Extensiveness of surgery and overall psychosocial adjustment were correlated; no relation between extent of surgery and support or change in social life; RM group had larger decline in the quality of affectional and sexual relationships.
Baider, Rizel, and Kaplan De-Nour (1986)	32 BCT + RT ± CT, 32 M ± CT; Not randomized; About 1.5 years postsurgery	GA, PA	Practically no group differences.
Fallowfield, Baum, and Maguire (1986)	48 BCT + RT ± CT, 53 M ± RT ± CT; Randomized; 4–32 months postsurgery	MS, PA	Anxiety state or depressive illness or both evident in 33% of M group and 38% of BCT group.
Ganz, Schag, Polinsky, Heinrich, and Flack (1987)	19 BCT + RT, 31 MRM; Not randomized; 3–5 weeks postsurgery	BI, FC, GA, MS, PA, SA	BCT group had less difficulty with clothing and showing scar to others; MRM group more likely to experience a decline in quality of life; BCT group tended to have difficulty asking partners for care; no difference in sexual difficulties or psychological problems.
Lasry et al. (1987)	44 BCT ± CT, 36 BCT + RT ± CT, 43 TM ± CT; Randomized; <1–9 years postsurgery	BI, FC, PA	M group had worse body image than BCT and BCT + RT groups; no group differences in fear of cancer recurrence or global depression score.

Table 1—(Continued)

Study	Participants and design[a]	Dependent variables	Results
Aaronson, Bartelink, van Dongen, and van Dam (1988)	44 BCT ± RT ± CT, 31 RM ± RT ± CT Randomized 2–4 years postsurgery	BI, FC, MS, PA	BCT group had better body image, greater acceptance of bodily change, and fewer sexual problems; fear of recurrence more frequent in the RM group; no differences in quality of marital relationship or psychological distress.
Kemeny, Wellisch, and Schain (1988)	25 BCT ± RT ± CT, 27 M ± CT Randomized 6 months to 4 years postsurgery	BI, FC, MS, PA, SA	BCT group had fewer negative changes in body image, less apprehension about cancer recurrence, fewer sexual problems, and a less troubled emotional response.
Holmberg, Omne-Pontén, Burns, Adami, and Bergström (1989)	37 BCT ± RT, 62 MRM ± RT ± CT Not randomized 4 and 13 months postsurgery	GA, MS, PA	No group differences in global rating of overall adjustment or sexual adjustment; at 13 months, proportion of those rated globally as disturbed was higher in MRM group.
Levy, Herberman, Lee, Lippman, and d'Angelo (1989)	71 and 40 BCT + RT ± CT, 27 and 53 M ± CT Two samples: one not randomized, one randomized 5 days and 3 months postsurgery	PA, SA	In the first sample, BCT group was more distressed and depressed and experienced a decrease in emotional support over time; in the second sample, there were few group differences.
Maunsell, Brisson, and Deschênes (1989)	80 BCT ± RT ± CT, 147 TM ± RT ± CT Not randomized 3 and 18 months postsurgery	PA	Three months after initial treatment, BCT group had higher psychiatric symptoms even after controlling for potential confounding variables; 18 months postsurgery, the two groups were identical.

Study	Sample / Design	Measures	Results
Meyer and Aspegren (1989)	28 BCT + RT, 30 MRM; Not randomized; 5 years postsurgery	BI, FC, MS, PA, SA	BCT group had better female identity and body acceptance; no group differences in fear of cancer recurrence, marital adjustment, mental symptoms, or psychiatric state.
van Heeringen, van Moffaert, and de Cuypere (1989)	18 BCT + RT, 84 M + RT; Not randomized; During postsurgery period	PA	No group differences in depression scores.
Wellisch et al. (1989)	22 BCT + RT ± CT, 15 M + RC ± CT, 14 M ± CT; Not randomized; 1–3 years postsurgery (reported on feelings before surgery, 6 months postsurgery, and present)	BI, FC, MS, PA, SA	BCT group had best body image; no group differences in concerns about cancer recurrence or psychiatric symptoms; few differences in sexual functioning.
Wolberg, Romsaas, Tanner, and Malec (1989)	41 BCT ± RT ± CT, 78 M ± RT ± CT, 72 benign breast biopsy; Not randomized; Before diagnosis, 4–8 and 16 months posttreatment	BI, GA, MS, PA	Only difference was that at 16 months, BCT group scored higher on the mood state of vigor and quality of general sexual experience than the M group.
Fallowfield, Hall, Maguire, and Baum (1990)	115 BCT ± RT ± CT, 154 M ± CT; Not randomized (some offered choice); Presurgery, 2 weeks, 4 months, and 12 months postsurgery	PA	No differences in the incidence of anxiety and depression.

Table 1—(Continued)

Study	Participants and design[a]	Dependent variables	Results
Margolis, Goodman, and Rubin (1990)	32 BCT + RT ± CT, 22 MRM ± RC ± CT Not randomized About 49 and 38 months postsurgery	BI, MS, PA	M group felt less attractive, less sexually desirable, and more ashamed of their breasts; M group enjoyed sexual relationships less than before treatment; no group differences in psychiatric symptoms.
McArdle, Hughson, and McArdle (1990)	67 BCT ± RT ± CT, 52 M ± RT ± CT Not randomized 6, 9, and 12, months postsurgery	PA	M group tended to be higher on depression, anxiety, and insomnia.
Langer, Prohaska, Schreiner-Frech, Ringler, and Kubista (1991)	20 BCT + RT ± CT, 40 MRM ± CT, 19 MRM + EP ± CT Not randomized About 2 years postsurgery	BI, PA	No significant group differences in body image; BCT group had less illness-related stress than the other two groups; MRM group had a more unfavorable coping pattern than the other two groups.
Ganz, Schag, Lee, Polinsky, and Tan (1992)	52 BCT + RT ± CT, 57 MRM ± RT ± CT Randomized 1, 4, 7, and 13 months postsurgery	BI, GA, PA	BCT group had a better body image and fewer difficulties with clothing; no group differences in quality of life, psychosocial adjustment, or mood.
Goldberg et al. (1992)	73 BCT ± RT ± CT, 93 SM ± RT ± CT, 156 benign breast biopsy Not randomized Presurgery, 6 and 12 months postsurgery	BI, MS, PA	No group differences in body image, sexual problems, anxiety, or depression preoperatively or 6 and 12 months after surgery.

Study	Design	Measures	Results
Levy et al. (1992) (follow-up of Levy et al., 1989)	90 BCT + RT ± CT, 39 M ± CT; Not randomized; 5 days, 3 and 15 months postsurgery	PA, SA	BCT group showed tendency to be more distressed and felt less emotional support at 3 months in particular.
Lee et al. (1992)	100 BCT + RT ± CT, 97 MRM ± CT; Randomized; Presurgery, 3 and 12 months postsurgery	BI, GA, MS, PA	More in MRM group were upset about change in breast contour and stopped intercourse after treatment; no group differences in global adjustment or psychiatric morbidity.
Maraste, Brandt, Olsson, and Ryde-Brandt (1992)	79 BCT, 54 M; Not randomized; About 2 months postsurgery	PA	No group differences in anxiety, but for patients aged 50–59 morbid anxiety was higher for M group.
Omne-Pontén, Holmberg, Burns, Adami, and Bergström (1992)	37 BCT ± RT, 62 M ± RT ± CT; Not randomized; 4 and 13 months postsurgery	GA, MS, PA	There was a trend for BCT group to have superior functioning on all outcomes except sexual functioning at 4 months; less depression and better global adjustment in BCT group at 13 months.
Pozo et al. (1992)	15 BCT ± RT ± CT, 48 M ± RT ± CT; Not randomized, half of M group and all of BCT group had choice; 1 day presurgery, 10 days, 3, 6, and 12 months postsurgery	FC, GA, MS, PA, SA	Only difference was that BCT group reported greater enjoyment of their sex lives at 6 and 12 months.
Hughes (1993)	46 BCT + RT, 25 MRM; Not randomized; At time of diagnosis, and about 8 weeks postsurgery	FC, GA	No group differences in uncertainty, distress about the cancer diagnosis, or quality of life.

Table 1—(*Continued*)

Study	Participants and design[a]	Dependent variables	Results
Mock (1993)	90 BCT, 62 M, 58 M + RC (immediate), 47 M + RC (delayed) Not randomized 2 months to 2 years postsurgery	BI	No group differences in self-concept; with one body image assessment, no group differences; with another body image assessment, BCT group was better than M and the M + RC (immediate) groups.
Noguchi, Kitagawa, et al. (1993)	42 BCT + RT + CT, 48 MRM + RC (immediate) + CT Choice of treatment >1 year postsurgery	BI, FC, MS	No group differences in fear of cancer recurrence or sexual adjustment; body image and satisfaction with surgery were superior in BCT group.
Noguchi, Saito, et al. (1993)	31 BCT + RT + CT, 71 RM + CT Choice of treatment >6 months postsurgery	BI, FC, MS	Body image disturbance was a concern for 22% of RM group but for none of BCT group; no group differences in satisfaction with operative results, fear of recurrence, or sexual adjustment.
Omne-Pontén, Holmberg, and Sjödén (1994) (follow-up of Omne-Pontén et al., 1992)	26 BCT ± RT ± CT, 40 M ± RT ± CT Not randomized 6 years postsurgery	BI, GA, PA	No differences in cosmetic evaluation of surgery, but the proportion who felt multilated was marginally higher in the M group; no group differences in global adjustment, anxiety, or depression.
Schain, d'Angelo, Dunn Lichter, and Pierce (1994)	76 BCT + RT, 60 M ± RC Randomized Before randomization, 6, 12, and 24 months postsurgery	BI, FC, MS, PA, SA	At 6 months postsurgery, M group reported less control over events in their lives and more problems with sexual relations; at 6 and 12 months, M group had higher distress over their nude bodies; no group differences in social support.

Study	Treatment groups[a]	Measures	Results
Yilmazer, Aydiner, Özkan, Aslay, and Bilge (1994)	40 BCT ± RT ± CT, 40 TM ± RT ± CT Not randomized 10–48 months postsurgery	BI, SA	BCT had superior body image; no group differences in self-esteem or social support.
Schover et al. (1995)	72 BCT ± RT ± CT, 146 M + RC (immediate) ± CT Not randomized 3 months to 9.5 years postsurgery	BI, FC, GA, MS	No group differences in body image, psychosocial adjustment to illness, or satisfaction with relationships or sexual life; BCT group maintained pleasure and frequency of breast caressing during sexual activity.

Note. BCT = breast-conserving treatment; RT = radiotherapy; MRM = modified radical mastectomy; BI = body/self-image; MS = marital-sexual adjustment; PA = psychological adjustment; M = mastectomy; FC = cancer-related fears and concerns; CT = chemotherapy; SA = social adjustment; RC = breast reconstruction; RM = radical mastectomy; GA = global adjustment; SM = simple mastectomy; TM = total mastectomy; EP = expander prosthesis.

[a]Number of participants in each surgical treatment group, method of assignment to treatment, and timing of assessment(s).

(Carlsson & Hamrin, 1994; Fallowfield & Clark, 1991; Hall & Fallowfield, 1989; Kiebert et al., 1991; Schain & Fetting, 1992). The literature suffers from small sample sizes and several inconsistencies—such as variability in method of assignment to treatment, time elapsed since treatment, and definitions of quality of life (Kiebert et al., 1991; Moyer & Salovey, 1996)—thereby possibly contributing to the lack of consistent findings. These methodological features are noted in Table 1.

This review strives to clarify ambiguities in this body of research in three ways. First, meta-analytic methods are used, which can reveal patterns obscured by traditional significance testing, especially for a group of studies characterized by null or conflicting findings (Schmidt, 1992). Although meta-analytic reviews are criticized on a number of grounds, they complement traditional narrative reviews in being more systematic, explicit, and quantitative, and less likely to produce Type II errors (Rosenthal, 1990, 1991). Second, this summary includes recent studies, some larger and more sophisticated, published since this area was last reviewed. Third, this article attends to methodological factors that may influence the direction of findings. Resulting recommendations for treatment for women with breast cancer are also provided.

Research Questions

The following research questions are addressed by the meta-analysis:

1. What is the magnitude and direction of the difference (effect size, ES) in the psychosocial outcomes of breast-conserving surgical treatment versus mastectomy? To investigate conceptually distinct types of adjustment, as recommended by Durlack (1995), psychosocial outcomes were divided according to Meyerowitz's (1980) description. Separate areas of impact of breast cancer and its treatment are psychological discomfort, changes in life patterns, and fears and concerns. With these domains and the existing research as a guide, six specific types of adjustment were identified. These were (a) psychological adjustment, (b) marital–sexual adjustment, (c) social adjustment, (d) body/self-image, (e) cancer-related fears and concerns, and (f) global adjustment.

2. Do particular study features influence the ESs for these six categories of psychosocial adjustment? This study examined three characteristics of interest. The first was the method of assignment to treatment (randomized versus nonrandomized). Assigning individuals randomly to treatment or not may result in sample differences or differences in psychosocial outcome. For instance, randomization can only be ethically performed on women who have no preference (Brewin & Bradley, 1989), which limits the range of women studied. The second characteristic was the length of time since surgery (less than 12 months versus 12 months or more) because the effects of breast cancer and its treatment may differ in the long term versus the short term. Because psychological symptoms in response to breast cancer tend to attenuate by about 1 year (Schover et al., 1995) I examined outcomes before and after 12 months. The third study feature was the year the study was published. Historical changes (e.g., accrual of evidence for the efficacy of breast-conserving surgeries) might influence the findings of earlier versus later studies. Other potentially relevant variations in study features, such as presence or absence of adjuvant treatment, often differed widely among women within a particular sample, or were not precisely

documented. Thus, it was difficult to stratify investigations on these variables to examine their effects in study-level analyses. However, the possible effects of some of these variables are addressed in the Discussion.

Method

Definitions of Variables and Selection of Studies

The present analysis includes investigations that compared the psychosocial effects of breast-conserving surgical treatment (procedures that spare the breast, known by a variety of terms: local excision, wide excision, lumpectomy, partial mastectomy, tumorectomy, tylectomy, and breast conservation) with the psychosocial effects of mastectomy (surgical removal of the breast). Outcomes of interest were variables that dealt with psychological and social rather than physical or health-related effects.

Procedures for Literature Search

To identify studies, the Cumulative Index to Nursing/Allied Health, Medline, and PsychINFO (which indexes dissertations and conference proceedings as well as published articles) were searched using key terms. No language exclusions were specified. Reference sections of articles were also reviewed. Published and unpublished investigations from 1980 to October 1995 were retrieved. The search yielded 40 published articles (one non-English), 1 abstract from a scientific meeting, and 1 unpublished dissertation.

Categorization of Study Outcomes

The types of findings of investigations were sorted into six categories:

1. Psychological adjustment: This category includes measures of disturbances and feelings such as depression, anxiety, guilt, anger, and hostility. Examples include the Profile of Mood States (McNair, Lorr, & Droppleman, 1981) and the Brief Symptom Inventory (Derogatis & Melisaratos, 1983), as well as individual items.
2. Marital–sexual adjustment: This classification includes assessments of marital satisfaction and sexual functioning such as the Dyadic Adjustment Scale (Spanier, 1976) and items assessing satisfaction with one's sex life and frequency of sexual activity.
3. Social adjustment: This category encompasses one's own social functioning, such as items asking about feelings of self-consciousness in groups and expressing one's feelings, and perceptions of behavior of others within one's social network, such as social support.
4. Body/self-image: This grouping deals with measures of body image, body satisfaction, self-image, and self-esteem. Examples include the Tennessee Self Concept Scale (Roid & Fitts, 1988) and items assessing feelings of attractiveness and femininity.

5. Cancer-related fears and concerns: This category primarily involves fear of cancer recurrence and confidence in one's treatment but also includes other concerns such as worries about family members.

6. Global adjustment: This classification was included because several investigations used general measures of quality of life or compound measures that comprised several areas of adjustment in their total score. Examples include the Psychosocial Adjustment to Illness Scale (Derogatis, 1983); the Cancer Rehabilitation Evaluation System (also known as the Cancer Inventory of Problem Situations; Schag, Heinrich, Aadland, & Ganz, 1990); and the Social Adjustment Scale (Weisman, 1975), which assesses effects on one's work, social and leisure activities, family, marriage, parental role, and sexual relations.

The kappa, adjusted for chance agreement (Siegel & Castellan, 1988), for two independent raters using this classification scheme to code study outcomes was 0.95. Thus, it was deemed acceptable to use the primary rater's judgment.

Procedures for Meta-Analysis

Effect size (ES) estimates in standard deviation units were calculated using a computer software program (Schwarzer, 1989) and equations provided by Rosenthal (1991, 1994). Where possible, effect size g (Hedges & Olkin, 1985) was calculated by subtracting the mean of the score for the mastectomy group from the mean of the score for the breast-conserving surgery group and dividing by the pooled standard deviation of both groups. When group means and standard deviations were not available, summary statistics such as F, t, or p were used. When only proportions were reported, Cohen's (1988) h, a conservative estimate of ES (see Rohling, Binder, & Langhinrichsen-Rohling, 1995), was used. In a small number of instances, nonsignificant or significant findings were reported in the text of an article but no other data were provided. In the first case, an effect size of zero was assigned in order not to bias the findings toward significance; in the second case, the convention $p < .05$ was assumed, and the corresponding ES was calculated (Rosenthal, 1995; Wolf, 1990). Effect sizes derived in these ways made up 18 of the 121 individual ESs used in the analysis. Two investigations reported data in a manner that could not be converted into ESs.

Efforts were made to ensure that ESs included in the meta-analysis were independent, so that a single investigation would not disproportionately influence the results. For example, two follow-up studies reported data for participants already examined in previous studies and one investigation provided data on two separate samples. Consequently, only one ES per sample was used (Kulik & Kulik, 1989). Similarly, studies often reported more than one relevant variable for a given outcome (e.g., both depression and anxiety belong to the category psychological adjustment) or used repeated measures. In these cases, the mean ES per outcome was chosen as a composite estimate (Rosenthal & Rubin, 1986).

All g values were converted to d, an unbiased estimate of ES (Hedges & Olkin, 1985), and were combined and tested for signficance and homogeneity with a computer software program (Schwarzer, 1989). Mean ESs and mean weighted ESs, which put greater emphasis on larger studes by weighting by sample size (Hedges & Olkin, 1985; Wolf, 1986), were computed.

Results

Magnitude and Direction of ESs

Table 2 presents the mean unweighted and weighted ESs for the six categories of psychosocial outcome. (The weighted ESs here are smaller than the unweighted ESs because when unweighted ESs are greater than zero, weighted ESs correct for the "overweighting" of smaller contributing ESs; Hedges & Olkin, 1985.) The weighted ESs for psychological, marital–sexual, and social adjustment, body/self-image, and cancer-related fears and concerns were significantly different from zero and positive, indicating superior scores for patients treated with breast-conserving surgery compared with mastectomy. The weighted effect sizes are in the quite-small to small-to-medium range (Cohen, 1988).

To account for the "file drawer problem," the tendency for studies supporting the null hypothesis to remain unpublished (Rosenthal, 1979, 1991, 1995), the fail-safe N was used, where possible. This gives the number of (undiscovered) unpublished studies with ESs of zero that would reduce the overall ES below a critical value of 0.20 standard deviation units (Wolf, 1986). Because most of the ESs obtained were lower than this critical value, the fail-safe N was only meaningful for psychological adjustment and body/self-image. Their values were 2 and 41, respectively. Thus, body/self-image is the only outcome with a high tolerance for future null results. It should be noted, however, that the literature on breast-conserving treatment versus mastectomy includes several studies reporting null results for a portion (e.g., Ganz, Schag, Lee, Polinsky, & Tan, 1992; Lee et al., 1992; Meyer &

Table 2—*Psychosocial Consequences of Surgery for Breast Cancer: Numbers of Samples, Numbers of Participants, and Means and Standard Deviations for Unweighted and Weighted Effect Sizes (ESs)*

Construct	No. of samples	No. of participants	Unweighted ES		Weighted ES	
			M	SD	M	SD
Psychological adjustment	30	2,828	.238	.696	.118**	.039
Marital–sexual adjustment	23	1,860	.163	.353	.093*	.048
Social adjustment	12	796	.207	.374	.181**	.073
Body/self-image	27	2,371	.560	.512	.400*****	.043
Cancer-related fears and concerns	16	1,086	.198	.413	.161****	.063
Global adjustment	13	1,163	.082	.158	.058	.061

Note. Positive values for ESs indicate better outcomes for groups treated with breast-conserving surgery. Significance level shown only for weighted mean ES.

$*p < .05.$
$**p < .01.$
$****p < .0001.$
$*****p < .00001.$

Aspegren, 1989; Mock, 1993; Pozo et al., 1992; Schain, d'Angelo, Dunn, Lichter, & Pierce, 1994; Schover et al., 1995; Wellisch et al., 1989) or all (Fallowfield, Hall, Maguire, & Baum, 1990; Goldberg et al., 1992; Hughes, 1993; van Heeringen, van Moffaert, & de Cuypere, 1989) of the variables assessed, perhaps indicating that the file drawer problem is not very prevalent in this area of investigation.

Influence of Study Features on Psychosocial Outcomes

Many of the constructs of interest had significant tests for heterogeneity (psychological adjustment, $Q = 107.97$, $p < .00001$; social adjustment, $Q = 21.10$, $p < .05$; body/self-image, $Q = 82.08$, $p < .00001$; cancer-related fears and concerns, $Q = 28.10$, $p < .05$), indicating that variation in the effects represents systematic differences among the studies in addition to sampling error. When samples of studies are heterogeneous, examining whether particular methodological features influence study outcomes is appropriate (Durlack, 1995; Rosenthal, 1995). Tables 3 and 4 show the means and standard deviations of the ESs for each of the six psychosocial consequences by method of assigning participants to treatment (randomized versus nonrandomized) and by timing of postsurgical assessment (less than 12 months versus 12 months or more), respectively. In Table 3, the mean weighted ES (benefit for

Table 3—*Psychosocial Consequences of Surgery for Breast Cancer by Method of Assignment to Treatment: Numbers of Samples, Numbers of Participants, and Means and Standard Deviations for Unweighted and Weighted Effect Sizes (ESs)*

Construct	No. of samples	No. of participants	Unweighted ES		Weighted ES	
			M	SD	M	SD
Psychological adjustment						
Randomized	10	941	.069	.266	.060***	.066
Nonrandomized	18	1,803	.366	.865	.161	.049
Marital–sexual adjustment						
Randomized	7	616	.080	.139	.065	.081
Nonrandomized	14	1,164	.226	.434	.114	.061
Social adjustment						
Randomized	3	209	.393	.296	.334*	.140
Nonrandomized	8	457	.164	.414	.133	.088
Body/self-image						
Randomized	7	550	.627	.253	.553	.088
Nonrandomized	17	1,565	.599	.600	.351	.053
Cancer-related fears and concerns						
Randomized	6	441	.128	.268	.120	.097
Nonrandomized	10	645	.240	.489	.191	.082
Global adjustment						
Randomized	3	340	−.006	.075	−.020	.108
Nonrandomized	10	853	.108	.170	.086	.072

Note. Positive values for ESs indicate better outcomes for groups treated with breast-conserving surgery. Significance level shown only for weighted mean ES.

*$p < .05$.

***$p < .001$.

Table 4—*Psychosocial Consequences of Surgery for Breast Cancer by Length of Follow-Up: Numbers of Samples, Numbers of Participants, and Means and Standard Deviations for Unweighted and Weighted Effect Sizes (ESs)*

Construct	No. of samples	No. of participants	Unweighted ES M	Unweighted ES SD	Weighted ES M	Weighted ES SD
Psychological adjustment						
Less than 12 months	17	1,947	.061	.235	.060*****	.046
12 months or longer	19	1,890	.310	.859	.167	.048
Marital–sexual adjustment						
Less than 12 months	12	995	.174	.435	.075**	.065
12 months or longer	14	1,172	.225	.301	.155	.060
Social adjustment						
Less than 12 months	6	467	−.043	.184	−.027	.097
12 months or longer	6	395	.300	.398	.318	.108
Body/self-image						
Less than 12 months	12	906	.511	.527	.433	.068
12 months or longer	15	1,256	.522	.512	.422	.059
Cancer-related fears and concerns						
Less than 12 months	7	457	.032	.164	.052*	.097
12 months or longer	6	421	.365	.619	.254	.098
Global adjustment						
Less than 12 months	10	894	.104	.189	.069	.069
12 months or longer	8	717	.021	.126	.012	.077

Note. Positive values for ESs indicate better outcomes for groups treated with breast-conserving surgery. Significance level shown only for weighted mean ES.
*p < .05.
**p < .01.
*****p < .00001.

breast-conserving surgery) for psychological functioning was significantly higher for samples that were not randomized to treatment than for samples that were randomized. Conversely, the mean weighted ES (benefit for breast-conserving surgery) for social functioning was significantly higher for samples that were randomly assigned

Table 5—*Correlations Between Year of Study Publication and Observed Effect Size (ES)*

Construct	r	n
Psychological adjustment	.07	30
Marital–sexual adjustment	−.09	23
Social adjustment	−.27	12
Body/self-image	−.26	27
Cancer-related fears and concerns	.07	16
Global adjustment	−.05	13

Note. A positive correlation indicates that the ESs are larger for more recent studies and a negative correlation indicates that the ESs are smaller for more recent studies.

to treatment. In Table 4, the mean weighted ESs (benefit for breast-conserving surgery) for psychological and marital–sexual adjustment and cancer-related fears and concerns were significantly higher for assessments made 12 months or more after surgical treatment than for assessments less than 12 months after surgical treatment. Table 5 shows the correlations between the year that an individual study was published and its ES for each of the six psychosocial outcomes. None of the correlations were significant.

Discussion

Meta-analytic methods produced significant mean ESs, indicating benefits for breast-conserving surgical treatment for five areas of psychosocial outcome: psychological adjustment, marital–sexual adjustment, social adjustment, body/self-image, and cancer-related fears and concerns. The largest and most robust ES, showing benefits for breast-conserving surgery for body/self-image, is already a firmly established finding. However, the findings for the other four types of outcome reveal patterns that have not been observed in narrative reviews of the literature.

Psychological Adjustment

A small but significant weighted mean ES for psychological adjustment indicated benefits for breast-conserving surgery versus mastectomy. This benefit was stronger for groups not randomized to treatment. Differences may simply be harder to detect in these studies. Because only patients with no treatment preference can be randomized, differences that might occur for those who have strong feelings toward either type of treatment may be overlooked. In addition, better psychological adjustment for groups receiving breast-conserving surgery was more pronounced for assessments made 12 months or longer after treatment. During the first year postsurgery, adjuvant radiation that more often accompanies breast-conserving procedures or the combination of surgery and radiation may be a source of psychological distress (Levy et al., 1992; Steinberg et al., 1985). Thus, longer-term assessments may be more sensitive to potential advantages for breast-conserving surgery.

Although we see small benefits for breast-conserving surgery for psychological adjustment, this category includes feelings as diverse as anxiety, depression, guilt, and anger. It is possible that women treated with breast-conserving versus breast-removing surgeries may experience different levels of specific feelings. For instance, cancer itself might be associated with anxiety, whereas breast loss or disfigurement might be associated with depression (Deadman, Dewey, Owens, Lienster, & Slade, 1989). Also, women treated with different types of surgery may feel distress for different reasons. For example, in one investigation, lumpectomy patients were bothered by fatigue and their slow recovery after a small operation; on the other hand, mastectomy patients, who did not expect a swift recovery, found treatment was less difficult than anticipated (Fallowfield et al., 1986). Also, after the initial recovery ifferent sources of distress might exist depending upon type of surgical

Marital and Sexual Functioning

Breast loss or disfigurement can alter intimate and sexual relationships. An extremely small but significant weighted mean ES in favor of breast-conserving surgery was found for marital–sexual adjustment. Similar to that observed for psychological adjustment, the benefit for breast-conserving surgery was larger for groups assessed 12 months or more after treatment. Again, it may be that adjuvant radiation for conservatively treated women contributed to fatigue and loss of libido, thus disrupting sexual functioning (Schover, 1991). However, depression, anger, and fear during treatment, apart from disfigurement or adjuvant therapy's effects, may also contribute to a lack of interest in intimacy (Dean, Chetty, & Forrest, 1983; Derogatis, 1980). Thus, to the extent that psychological adjustment is superior for women treated with breast-conserving treatment, marital and sexual adjustment might benefit too.

Social Adjustment

An extremely small but significant weighted mean ES was found for social adjustment. In contrast to the observation for psychological adjustment, the benefits for breast-conserving surgery were stronger for samples that were randomized to treatment. This finding might indicate that there are benefits in terms of one's interactions with others when women have no treatment preference, have the burden of choice removed through randomization, and receive breast-conserving surgery. It is possible that women treated with breast-conserving surgery who participate in clinical trials receive more attention and support by medical personnel through involvement in a trial than they would from members of their social network itself. Social-network members may minimize the seriousness of breast-conserving surgery patients' disease because they have undergone less extensive surgery.

Body Image

The largest mean weighted ES emerging from the meta-analysis was for body/self-image. This is consistent with a number of previous findings (Kemeny et al., 1988; Lasry et al., 1987; Margolis et al., 1990; Wellisch et al., 1989; Yilmazer, Aydiner, Özkan, Aslay, & Bilge, 1994). This consistency is evident despite body image being operationalized in a range of ways: feelings about appearance and sexual desirability, shame and embarrassment about one's body, and established scales assessing body image. Because breast-conserving techniques involve less physical mutilation, such findings are not surprising.

Although some reviewers consider such results circular (Hall & Fallowfield, 1989), they may not be trivial. To the extent that body image affects psychological functioning, it is indeed relevant (Hall & Fallowfield, 1989). For instance, concerns about body disfigurement may partially mediate the adverse psychological effects of more radical surgery (S. E. Taylor et al., 1985). However, the principal advantages of breast-conserving treatment may be that it can facilitate fitting clothes, avoiding the inconvenience of a prosthesis, viewing or revealing one's nude body, or continuing a sexual relationship (Aaronson, Bartelink, van Dongen, & van Dam, 1988; Schain et al., 1983; Steinberg et al., 1985). Nevertheless, the psychological ramifications of a life-threatening disease may overshadow these smaller benefits when worries about survival supersede cosmetic concerns (Fallowfield, Baum, & Maguire, 1987; Peters-Golden, 1982; Pozo et al., 1992). In a small sample of Chinese patients, there were high levels of depression and sexual difficulties for breast cancer patients treated with mastectomy and for women with other malignancies 7 years posttreatment (Alagaratnam & Kung, 1986). The authors concluded that a diagnosis of malignancy is more worrisome than the disfigurement of mastectomy.

Cancer-Related Fears and Concerns

Much of the anxiety associated with breast cancer probably stems from fears about cancer recurrence and death because these are frequently identified psychological problems (Ganz, Schag, Polinsky, Heinrich, & Flack, 1987; Jones & Greenwood, 1994). In this investigation, a small but significant mean weighted ES indicated fewer cancer-related fears and concerns in samples treated with breast-conserving surgery. In addition, this advantage was significantly better for longer compared with shorter term assessments. The disfigurement associated with mastectomy may remind women of the threat of cancer (Aaronson et al., 1988). In contrast to this finding, in the past, researchers speculated that women treated with breast-conserving surgery might worry more about cancer returning because less of the breast had been removed. Previous research supported this belief (Fallowfield et al., 1986) or showed that women (and physicians) had doubts about the effectiveness of breast-conserving treatment (Massie & Holland, 1991; Ward, Heidrich, & Wolberg, 1989). However, more recent evidence asserts the comparable effectiveness of breast-conserving surgery (Early Breast Cancer Trialists' Collaborative Group, 1995; Jacobson et al., 1995). Such changing views have been offered to explain discrepancies in the literature, particularly between older and more recent studies (Sinsheimer & Holland, 1987); however, this trend was not observed in the present meta-analysis for any of the psychosocial outcomes.

Global Adjustment

The mean weighted ES for global adjustment was in the direction of benefits for breast-conserving surgery but was not significantly different from zero. Perhaps these general measures do not detect subtle differences between the two groups, which could be due in part to the fact that the meta-analysis used the total scores from these global measures rather than their individual subscales, which vary considerably in what they assess.

Possible Moderators of Effects of Breast-Conserving Versus More Radical Surgery

Discrepancies in the conclusions of investigations comparing breast-conserving surgery with mastectomy may be due to differences in participant or methodologic characteristics, as seen in Table 1. It was possible to examine the effects of three study-level factors: method of assignment to treatment, timing of assessment, and year of study publication.

Method of Assignment to Treatment

For some of the outcomes considered in the meta-analysis, findings differed for groups randomly versus not randomly assigned to treatment. Similarly, Levy, Herberman, Lee, Lippman, and d'Angelo (1989) observed different profiles of psychosocial adjustment for a sample that was assigned randomly to treatment compared to a sample in which treatment was negotiated. However, other reports show that participation in clinical trials per se is not associated with different levels of psychological, sexual, or social problems (Fallowfield et al., 1990).

Although random assignment controls for individual differences related to choice of surgery, it is artificial and thus may not produce generalizable results (Moyer & Salovey, 1996). Many early-stage breast cancer patients are increasingly involved in decisions made by their medical team regarding an optimal treatment strategy. More problematic is evidence that surgical principal investigators assign their patients selectively to treatment protocols, regardless of their eligibility (K. M. Taylor, Margolese, & Soskolne, 1984). Thus, women randomized to treatment may be even less representative of women with breast cancer in general. Again, the fact that it is only ethical to randomize to treatment women who indicate that they have no preference may itself contribute to the lack of differences observed (S. E. Taylor et al., 1985).

Timing of Assessment

The timing of assessment had similar effects for three outcomes. For psychological adjustment, marital–sexual adjustment, and cancer-related fears and concerns the benefit for breast-conserving surgery was significantly larger in the long term than in the short term. Although these long-term follow-ups are not extremely long (most are within a few years postsurgery), it could be argued that effects on longer-term adjustment represent more permanent and thus more important effects.

Year of Study Publication

There was no relationship found between year of study publication and the study ES for any of the psychosocial outcomes. This is surprising because several changes in the meaning and treatment of breast cancer have occurred over the period these studies were conducted (Rowland & Holland, 1989; Moyer & Salovey, 1996). However, such developments have not established either type of surgery as clearly superior. For instance, increasing assurance of the medical effectiveness of breast-conserving procedures might improve the psychosocial outcomes after this treatment, whereas wider availability of breast reconstruction might improve the outcomes after mastectomy.

As explained earlier, other potential moderating variables could not be examined at the study level. However, the following sections explore how some of these factors might affect the findings of this literature.

Level of Disfigurement in Patients Treated With Mastectomy

Breast reconstruction offers a way to improve body integrity and perhaps adjustment after mastectomy and can even result in cosmetic outcome superior to breast conservation (Cady & Stone, 1990; S. E. Taylor et al., 1985). Levels of satisfaction with body image for women who undergo reconstruction are reported to fall in between those of the women treated with mastectomy without reconstruction and those receiving breast-conserving treatment (Mock, 1993; Wellisch et al., 1989). Two investigations compared women treated with breast-conserving surgery to a group of mastectomy patients who underwent breast reconstruction. In the first sample, body image and satisfaction with surgery were superior in the breast-conserving surgery group, yet there were no group differences in sexual adjustment or fear of cancer recurrence (Noguchi, Kitagawa, et al., 1993). In the second sample, there were no group differences in body image, psychosocial adjustment to illness, or satisfaction with relationships or sexual life, although the breast conservation group maintained pleasure and frequency of breast caressing during sexual activity (Schover et al., 1995). Therefore, the inclusion of women who have had reconstruction after mastectomy in studies comparing treatments may play a role in nonsignificant findings.

Conversely, some studies included patients treated with radical mastectomy, a more mutilating procedure than the more common modified radical mastectomy. Not surprisingly, in most of these samples, compromised adjustment on some variables for mastectomy groups was more likely to be seen (Aaronson et al., 1988; Bartelink, van Dam, & van Dongen, 1985; S. E. Taylor et al., 1985; but see Noguchi, Saito, et al., 1993).

Presence or Absence of Adjuvant Treatment

The inclusion of participants with and without adjuvant treatment represents another confounding factor. Adjuvant treatment such as radiation and chemotherapy can be physically and psychologically draining because of their side effects, such as fatigue and hair loss (Kaplan, 1992; Seltzer, 1987). Treatment with chemotherapy, regardless of type of surgical treatment, is also associated with fear of cancer recurrence, possibly because it represents a sign of poorer prognosis (Lasry et al., 1987). Follow-up treatment in general may be distressing as patients repeatedly face the seriousness of their disease (Meyerowitz, 1980).

Some investigations have tried to disentangle the effects of type of surgery itself and adjuvant treatment. One study controlled for the effects of radiotherapy by assessing patients after surgery but before radiotherapy had begun (Maraste, Brandt, Olsson, & Ryde-Brandt, 1992). The results were somewhat ambiguous: A higher percentage of mastectomy patients (19%) than breast-conserving surgery patients (10%) experienced severe anxiety, but this difference was not significant. However, higher levels of anxiety were experienced by women treated with mastectomy in their fifties, as compared to women under 50 or in their sixties. This suggests that, apart from the effects of radiation therapy, there may be some benefit for breast-conserving treatment, at least in the short-term. Another investigation that included groups of patients receiving lumpectomy with and without radiation who were assessed long after adjuvant treatment had ended (up to 9 years after surgery) found few differences in distress (Lasry et al., 1987). Similarly, chemotherapy contributed to psychosocial maladjustment, sexual dysfunction, and poorer body image, regardless of type of initial surgery (Schover et al., 1995).

Opportunity to Choose Type of Surgical Treatment

Some studies reported on samples where participants (or a portion of them) chose their treatment (e.g., Fallowfield et al., 1990; Noguchi, Kitagawa, et al., 1993; Pozo et al., 1992; Steinberg et al., 1985). Allowing patients to make a decision on the basis of their own values may foster improved psychological well-being, regardless of the procedure chosen (Dean, 1988; Fallowfield et al., 1990; Maguire, 1989; Pozo et al., 1992). In addition, such control might also be an important factor promoting psychosocial adjustment, especially in the context of a disease that often makes patients feel a lost sense of control. Although pursuing treatment preferred by an individual logically appears beneficial (Morris & Ingham, 1988; Morris & Royle, 1987; Pozo et al., 1992), a separate issue is the extent to which patients desire having a choice of treatments when possible. Some investigators insist that a majority of patients appear to welcome the opportunity to be involved in treatment decisions (Ward et al., 1989). Others, however, reported that in a group of recently diagnosed breast cancer patients, 52% preferred that their surgeon decide for them (Luker, Leinster, Owens Beaver, & Degner, cited in Fallowfield, Hall, Maguire, Baum, & Hern, 1994). Decision making may be an additional burden for patients during a time of high anxiety and may result in patients feeling responsible if treatment is unsuccessful (Morris & Ingham, 1988). Regardless of the direction of influence, having a choice of treatments could affect variability in the findings.

Initial Prognosis

In studies that do not randomize patients to treatment, initial prognosis might be confounded with the type of surgery received, with participants with worse prognosis receiving more extensive surgical treatment; this could account for better psychosocial outcomes for patients treated with breast-conserving surgery. Only a few studies comparing the effect of breast-conserving surgery versus mastectomy have taken this factor into account. Levy et al. (1989, 1992) controlled for the number of lymph nodes that were positive for cancer as a measure of extent of disease. Women treated with mastectomy fared better than those treated with lumpectomy in terms of mood and perceptions of social support at the 3-month follow-up, but there were no group differences at the 15-month follow-up.

Patient Age

It is possible that younger patients may be more likely to receive breast-conserving procedures (Maunsell, Brisson, & Deschênes, 1989; Wellisch et al., 1989), or that older and younger patients have different psychosocial responses to different surgical treatments. Younger patients may react more negatively to breast removal than do older patients. Younger breast cancer patients in general may also be more distressed

(Levy et al., 1992). Maunsell et al. (1989) found that for women less than 40 years old, breast-conserving treatment was protective against psychological distress, whereas among women 50–59 years old, breast-conserving treatment was associated with more distress, and for women more than 70 years old there was no association between extent of surgery and distress. Conversely, Maraste et al. (1992) found that for women aged 50–59, those treated with breast-conserving treatment had less anxiety than those treated with mastectomy.

Strengths and Limitations of the Meta-Analysis

One strength of this analysis is that the findings probably accurately represent the available research on this topic because this analysis involved an exhaustive search of the literature and contains samples from a number of countries and cultures. Another strength is the use of weighed ESs that take into account study sample size. An important limitation, however, is that the studies on which the analysis is based include mostly self-report measures. The findings could be affected by biases introduced by self-report, whereby women who received breast-conserving surgery feel reluctant to report negative outcomes. Women treated with breast-conserving surgery sometimes feel that they should be grateful for retaining their breast and feel guilty for experiencing psychological distress (Fallowfield et al., 1987).

Clinical and Practical Implications of Study Findings

What is the meaning of the small but significant ESs found? Some procedures used in the present analysis, such as assuming an ES of zero or $p < .05$ when results were reported to be nonsignificant or significant, may have contributed to conservative overall average ES estimates. However, these made up a small proportion of the contributing ESs and probably had only a small impact. In a meta-analysis of the effectiveness of psychosocial interventions with cancer patients, Meyer and Mark (1995) found significant unweighted ESs of similar magnitude (ranging from .19 to .28). They explain that different interpretations regard the clinical significance of small ESs as either negligible or very meaningful. On one hand, effect sizes around .2 are considered "small" (Cohen, 1988), but on the other hand, even tiny effect sizes may be important in the impact they have for the individuals affected (Rosenthal, 1991), especially for a prevalent disease. For example, if an ES of .20 is expressed as the percentage of individuals scoring above the median on a given measure of adjustment, this value would be 55% for individuals treated with breast-conserving surgery compared with 45% for individuals treated with mastectomy (Rosenthal, 1994). Meyer and Mark concluded that the small ES they found should be viewed as noteworthy.

Thus, to the extent that the ESs observed in the present meta-analysis are small but solid, there is optimism for the benefits of breast-conserving surgery compared with mastectomy, particularly for body image but also for psychological adjustment, marital–sexual adjustment, social adjustment, and cancer-related fears and concerns, where the literature had before been ambiguous. To the extent that the differences between the two types of surgery are not enormous, rather than advocating one particular treatment over another, strategies such as actively matching patients to optimal treatment could be helpful. This is especially important as women begin to play a more active role in the decision-making process in early breast cancer, some by law rather than by preference. Particular areas where individual preferences may play a role in satisfaction with and adjustment to treatment include concern about body image and disfigurement, tolerance for adjuvant radiation, tolerance for future surgery, cost, beliefs about the efficacy of treatment, and the values and concerns of significant others. Therefore, despite this optimism for treatment with breast-conserving surgery, adequate preparation and support for all breast cancer patients should remain a crucial focus (Fallowfield et al., 1986; Maunsell et al., 1989; van Heeringen et al., 1989).

References

References marked with an asterisk indicate studies included in the meta-analysis.

*Aaronson, N. K., Bartelink, H., van Dongen, J. A., & van Dam, F. S. A. M. (1988). Evaluation of breast conserving therapy: Clinical, methodological and psychosocial perspective. *European Journal of Surgical Oncology, 14*, 133–140.

Alagaratnam, T. T., & Kung, N. Y. T. (1986). Psychosocial effects of mastectomy: Is it due to mastectomy or to the diagnosis of malignancy? *British Journal of Psychiatry, 149*, 296–299.

*Ashcroft, J. J., Leinster, S. J., & Slade, P. D. (1985). Breast cancer—Patient choice of treatment: Preliminary communication. *Journal of the Royal Society of Medicine, 78*, 43–46.

*Ashcroft, J. J., Leinster, S. J., & Slade, P. D. (1986). Mastectomy versus breast conservation: Psychological effects of patient choice of treatment. In M. Watson & S. Greer (Eds.), *Psychosocial issues in malignant disease* (pp. 55–71). New York: Pergamon Press.

*Baider, L., Rizel, S., & Kaplan De-Nour, A. (1986). Comparison of couples' adjustment to lumpectomy and mastectomy. *General Hospital Psychiatry, 8*, 251–257.

*Bartelink, H., van Dam, F., & van Dongen, J. (1985). Psychological effects of breast conserving therapy in comparison with radical mastectomy. *International Journal of Radiation Oncology Biology and Physics, 11*, 381–385.

*Beckman, J., Johansen, L., Richardt, C., & Blichert-Toft, M. (1983). Psychological reactions in younger women operated on for breast cancer. *Danish Medical Bulletin, 30* (Suppl. 2), 10–13.

Brewin, C. R., & Bradley, C. (1989). Patient preferences and randomised clinical trials. *British Medical Journal, 299*, 313–315.

Cady, B., & Stone, M. D. (1990). Selection of breast-preservation therapy for primary invasive breast carcinoma. *Surgical Clinics of North America, 70*, 1047–1059.

Carlsson, M., & Hamrin, E. (1994). Psychological and psychosocial aspects of breast cancer and breast cancer treatment: A literature review. *Cancer Nursing, 17*, 418–428.

Cohen, J. (1988). *Statistical power analysis for the behavioral sciences* (Rev. ed.). Hillsdale, NJ: Erlbaum.

*Cohen, R. S., Wellisch, D. K., Christensen, A., & Giuliano, A. E. (1984). Effect of mastectomy and lumpectomy on dimensions of mood, self-concept, impairment and marital satisfaction [Abstract]. *Proceedings: Annual Meeting of the American Society of Clinical Oncology, 3*, 72.

Coon, W. W. (1988). The surgeon's role in the management of the patient with breast cancer. In J. K. Harness, H. A. Oberman, A. S. Lichter, D. D. Adler, & R. L. Cody (Eds.), *Breast cancer: Collaborative management* (pp. 129–135). Chelsea, MI: Lewis Publishers.

Deadman, J. M., Dewey, M. J., Owens, R. G., Leinster, S. J., & Slade, P. D. (1989). Threat and loss in breast cancer. *Psychological Medicine, 19*, 677–681.

Dean, C. (1988). The emotional impact of mastectomy. *British Journal of Hospital Medicine, 39*, 30–32, 36, 38–39.

Dean, C., Chetty, U., & Forrest, A. P. (1983). Effects of immediate breast reconstruction on psychosocial morbidity after mastectomy. *Lancet, 1*, 459–462.

*de Haes, J. C. J. M., van Oostrom, M. A., & Welvaart, K. (1986). The effect of radical and conserving surgery on the quality of life of early breast cancer patients. *European Journal of Surgical Oncology, 12*, 337–342.

*de Haes, J. C. J. M., & Welvaart, K. (1985). Quality of life after breast cancer surgery. *Journal of Surgical Oncology, 28*, 123–125.

Derogatis, L. R. (1980). Breast and gynecologic cancers: Their unique impact on body image and sexual identity in women. In J. M. Vaeth, R. C. Blomberg, & L. Adler (Eds.), *Frontiers of radiation therapy and oncology: Vol. 14. Body image, self-esteem, and sexuality in cancer patients* (pp. 1–11). Basel, Switzerland: Karger.

Derogatis, L. R. (1983). *Psychosocial Adjustment to Illness Scale (PAIS and PAIS-SR): Administration, scoring, and procedures manual I.* Baltimore: Clinical Psychometric Research.

Derogatis, L. R. (1986). Psychology in cancer medicine: A perspective and overview. *Journal of Consulting and Clinical Psychology, 54*, 632–638.

Derogatis, L. R., & Melisaratos, N. (1983). The brief symptom inventory: An introductory report. *Psychological Medicine, 13*, 595–605.

Durlack, J. A. (1995). Understanding meta-analysis. In L. G. Grimm & P. R. Yarnold (Eds.), *Reading and understanding multivariate statistics* (pp. 319–352). Washington, DC: American Psychological Association.

Early Breast Cancer Trialists' Collaborative Group. (1995). Effects of radiotherapy and surgery in early breast cancer: An overview of the randomized trials. *New England Journal of Medicine, 333*, 1444–1455.

*Fallowfield, L. J., Baum, M., & Maguire, G. P. (1986). Effects of breast conservation on psychological morbidity associated with diagnosis and treatment of early breast cancer. *British Medical Journal, 293*, 1331–1334.

Fallowfield, L. J., Baum, M., & Maguire, G. P. (1987). Addressing the psychological needs of the conservatively treated breast cancer patient: Discussion paper. *Journal of the Royal Society of Medicine, 80*, 696–700.

Fallowfield, L. J., & Clark, A. (1991). *Breast cancer.* New York: Tavistock/Routledge.

*Fallowfield, L. J., Hall, A., Maguire, G. P., & Baum, M. (1990). Psychological outcomes of different treatment policies in women with early breast cancer outside a clinical trial. *British Medical Journal, 301*, 575–580.

Fallowfield, L. J., Hall, A., Maguire, G. P., Baum, M., & Hern, R. P. (1994). Psychological effects of being offered choice of surgery for breast cancer. *British Medical Journal, 309*, 448.

Fisher, B. (1992). Justification for lumpectomy in the treatment of breast cancer: A comment on the underutilization of that procedure. *Journal of the American Medical Women's Association, 47*, 169–173.

Fisher, B., Anderson, S., Redmond, C. K., Wolmark, N., Wickerham, D. L., & Cronin, W. M. (1995). Reanalysis and results after 12 years of follow-up in a randomized clinical trial comparing total mastectomy with lumpectomy with or without irradiation in the treatment of breast cancer. *New England Journal of Medicine, 333*, 1456–1461.

Fisher, B., Redmond, C., Poisson, R., Margolese, R., Wolmark, N., Wickerham, L., Fisher, E., Deutsch, M., Caplan, R., Pilch, Y., Slass, A., Shibata, H., Lerner, H., Terz, J., & Sidorovich, L. (1989). Eight-year results of a randomized clinical trial comparing total mastectomy with or without radiation in the treatment of breast cancer. *New England Journal of Medicine, 312*, 665–673.

*Ganz, P. A., Schag, C. A. C., Polinsky, M. L., Heinrich, R. L., & Flack, V. F. (1987). Rehabilitation needs and breast cancer: The first month after primary therapy. *Breast Cancer Research and Treatment, 10,* 243–253.

*Ganz, P. A., Schag, C. A. C., Lee, J., Polinsky, M. L., & Tan, S. (1992). Breast conservation versus mastectomy. *Cancer, 69,* 1729–1738.

*Goldberg, J. A., Scott, R. N., Davidson, P. M., Murray, G. D., Stallard, S., George, W. D., & Maguire, G. P. (1992). Psychological morbidity in the first year after breast surgery. *European Journal of Surgical Oncology, 18,* 327–331.

Hall, A., & Fallowfield, L. (1989). Psychological outcome of treatment for early breast cancer: A review. *Stress Medicine, 5,* 167–175.

Hedges, L. V., & Olkin, I. (1985). *Statistical methods for meta-analysis.* New York: Academic Press.

Henderson, I. C. (1995). Paradigmatic shifts in the management of breast cancer. *New England Journal of Medicine, 332,* 951–952.

*Holmberg, L., Omne-Pontén, M., Burns, T., Adami, H. O., & Bergström, R. (1989). Psychosocial adjustment after mastectomy and breast-conserving treatment. *Cancer, 64,* 969–974.

*Hughes, K. K. (1993). Psychosocial and functional status of breast cancer patients: The influence of diagnosis and treatment choice. *Cancer Nursing, 16,* 222–229.

Jacobson, J. A., Danforth, D. N., Cowan, K. H., D'Angelo, T., Steinberg, S. M., Pierce, L., Lippman, M. E., Lichter, A. S., Glatstein, E., & Okunieff, P. (1995). Ten-year results of a comparison of conservation with mastectomy in the treatment of stage I and II breast cancer. *New England Journal of Medicine, 332,* 907–911.

Jones, R. V. H., & Greenwood, B. (1994). Breast cancer: Causes of patients' distress identified by qualitative analysis. *British Journal of General Practice, 44,* 370–371.

Kaplan, H. S. (1992). A neglected issue: The sexual side effects of current treatments for breast cancer. *Journal of Sex and Marital Therapy, 18,* 3–19.

*Kemeny, M. M., Wellisch, D. K., & Schain, W. S. (1988). Psychosocial outcome in a randomized surgical trial for treatment of primary breast cancer. *Cancer, 62,* 1231–1237.

Kennedy, B. J. (1989). *Breast cancer.* New York: Alan R. Liss.

Kiebert, G. M., de Haes, J. C. M., & van de Velde, C. J. H. (1991). The impact of breast-conserving treatment and mastectomy on the quality of life of early-stage breast cancer patients: A review. *Journal of Clinical Oncology, 9,* 1059–1070.

Kulik, J. A., & Kulik, C.-L. C. (1989). Meta-analysis in education. *International Journal of Educational Research, 13,* 221–340.

*Langer, M., Prohaska, R., Schreiner-Frech, I., Ringler, M., & Kubista, E. (1991). Krankheitsbewältigung und Körperbild nach unterschiedlichen Operationstechniken bei Brustkrebs [Coping and body image after different operative techniques in breast cancer patients]. *Psychotherapie Psychosomatik Medizinische Psychologie, 41,* 379–384.

*Lasry, J.-C. M., Margolese, R. G., Poisson, R., Shibata, H., Fleischer, D., LaFleur, D., LeGault, S., & Taillefer, S. (1987). Depression and body image following mastectomy and lumpectomy. *Journal of Chronic Disease, 40,* 529–534.

*Lee, M. S., Love, S. B., Mitchell, J. B., Parker, E. M., Rubens, R. D., Watson, J. P., Fentiman, I. S., & Hayward, J. L. (1992). Mastectomy or conservation for early breast cancer: Psychological morbidity. *European Journal of Cancer, 28A,* 1340–1344.

*Levy, S. M., Haynes, L. T., Herberman, R. B., Lee, J., McFeely, S., & Kirkwood, J. (1992). Mastectomy versus breast conservation surgery: Mental health effects at long-term follow-up. *Health Psychology, 11,* 349–354.

*Levy, S. M., Herberman, R. B., Lee, J. K., Lippman, M. E., & d'Angelo, T. (1989). Breast conservation versus mastectomy: Distress sequelae as a function of choice. *Journal of Clinical Oncology, 7,* 367–375.

Maguire, P. M. (1989). Breast conservation versus mastectomy: Psychological considerations. *Seminars in Surgical Oncology, 5,* 137–144.

*Maraste, R., Brandt, L., Olsson, A., & Ryde-Brandt, B. (1992). Anxiety and depression in breast cancer patients at start of adjuvant radiotherapy. *Acta Oncologica, 31*, 315–320.

*Margolis, G., Goodman, R. L., & Rubin, A. (1990). Psychological effects of breast-conserving treatment and mastectomy. *Psychosomatics, 31*, 33–39.

Massie, M. J., & Holland, J. C. (1991). Psychological reactions to breast cancer in the pre- and post-surgical treatment period. *Seminars in Surgical Oncology, 7*, 320–325.

*Maunsell, E., Brisson, J., & Deschênes, L. (1989). Psychological distress after initial treatment for breast cancer: A comparison of partial and total mastectomy. *Journal of Clinical Epidemiology, 42*, 765–771.

McArdle, J. M., Hughson, A. V. M., & McArdle, C. S. (1990). Reduced psychological morbidity after breast conservation. *British Journal of Surgery, 77*, 1221–1223.

McNair, D. M., Lorr, M., & Droppleman, L. F. (1981). *Profile of Mood States manual.* San Diego, CA: Educational and Industrial Testing Service.

*Meyer, L., & Aspegren, K. (1989). Long-term psychological sequelae of mastectomy and breast conserving treatment for breast cancer. *Acta Oncologica, 28*, 13–18.

Meyer, T. J., & Mark, M. M. (1995). Effects of psychosocial interventions with adult cancer patients: A meta-analysis of randomized experiments. *Health Psychology, 14*, 101–108.

Meyerowitz, B. E. (1980). Psychological correlates of breast cancer and its treatments. *Psychological Bulletin, 87*, 108–131.

*Mock, V. (1993). Body image in women treated for breast cancer. *Nursing Research, 42*, 153–157.

Morris, J., & Ingham, R. (1988). Choice of surgery for early breast cancer: Psychosocial considerations. *Social Science and Medicine, 27*, 1257–1262.

Morris, J., & Royle, G. T. (1987). Choice of surgery for early breast cancer: Pre- and post-operative levels of clinical anxiety and depression in patients and their husbands. *British Journal of Surgery, 74*, 1017–1019.

*Moyer, A. (1995). *Quality of life following treatment for breast cancer: Breast-conserving surgery versus mastectomy.* Unpublished doctoral dissertation, Yale University, New Haven, CT.

Moyer, A., & Salovey, P. (1996). Psychosocial sequelae of breast cancer and its treatment. *Annals of Behavioral Medicine, 18*, 110–125.

*Noguchi, M., Kitagawa, H., Kinoshita, K., Earashi, M., Miyazaki, I., Tatsukuchi, S., Saito, Y., Mizukami, Y., Nonmura, A., Nakumura, S., & Michigishi, T. (1993). Psychologic and cosmetic self-assessments of breast conserving therapy compared with mastectomy and immediate breast reconstruction. *Journal of Surgical Oncology, 54*, 260–266.

*Noguchi, M., Saito, Y., Nishijima, H., Koyanagi, M., Nonomura, A., Mizukami, Y., Nakamura, S., Michigishi, T., Ohta, N., Kitagawa, H., Earashi, M., Thomas, M., & Miyazaki, I. (1993). The psychological and cosmetic aspects of breast conserving therapy compared with radical mastectomy. *Japanese Journal of Surgery, 23*, 598–602.

*Omne-Pontén, M., Holmberg, L., Burns, T., Adami, H. O., & Bergström, R. (1992). Determinants of the psycho-social outcome after operation for breast cancer: Results of a prospective comparative interview study following mastectomy and breast conservation. *European Journal of Cancer, 28A*, 1062–1067.

*Omne-Pontén, M., Holmberg, L., & Sjödén, P.-O. (1994). Psychosocial adjustment among women with breast cancer stages I and II: Six-year follow-up of consecutive patients. *Journal of Clinical Oncology, 12*, 1778–1782.

Peters-Golden, H. (1982). Breast cancer: Varied perceptions of social support in the illness experience. *Social Science and Medicine, 16*, 483–492.

*Pozo, C., Carver, C. S., Noriega, V., Harris, S. D., Robinson, D. S., Ketcham, A. S., Legaspi, A., Moffat, F. L., & Clark, K. C. (1992). Effects of mastectomy versus lumpectomy on emotional adjustment to breast cancer: A prospective study of the first year postsurgery. *Journal of Clinical Oncology, 10*, 1292–1298.

Rohling, M. L., Binder, L. M., & Langhinrichsen-Rohling, J. (1995). A meta-analytic review of the association between financial compensation and the experience and treatment of chronic pain. *Health Psychology, 14*, 537–547.

Roid, G. H., & Fitts, W. H. (1988). *Tennessee Self Concept Scale: Revised manual.* Los Angeles: Western Psychological Services.

Rosenthal, R. (1979). The "file drawer" problem and tolerance for null results. *Psychological Bulletin, 86*, 638–641.

Rosenthal, R. (1990). An evaluation of procedures and results. In K. W. Wachter & M. L. Straf (Eds.), *The future of meta-analysis* (pp. 123–133). New York: Russell Sage Foundation.

Rosenthal, R. (1991). *Meta-analytic procedures for social research* (Rev. ed.). Newbury Park, CA: Sage.

Rosenthal, R. (1994). Parametric measures of effect size. In H. Cooper & L. V. Hedges (Eds.), *Handbook of research synthesis* (pp. 231–244). New York: Russell Sage Foundation.

Rosenthal, R. (1995). Writing meta-analytic reviews. *Psychological Bulletin, 118*, 183–192.

Rosenthal, R., & Rubin, D. B. (1986). Meta-analytic procedures for combining studies with multiple effect sizes. *Psychological Bulletin, 99*, 400–406.

Rowland, J. H., & Holland, J. C. (1989). Breast cancer. In J. C. Holland & J. H. Rowland (Eds.), *Handbook of psychooncology* (pp. 188–207). New York: Oxford University Press.

*Sanger, C. K., & Reznikoff, M. A. (1981). A comparison of the psychological effects of breast-saving procedures with the modified mastectomy. *Cancer, 48*, 2341–2346.

Schag, C. C., Heinrich, R. L., Aadland, R., & Ganz, P. A. (1990). Assessing problems of cancer patients: Psychometric properties of the Cancer Inventory of Problem Situations. *Health Psychology, 9*, 83–102.

*Schain, W. S., d'Angelo, T. M., Dunn, M. E., Lichter, A. S., & Pierce, L. J. (1994). Mastectomy versus conservative surgery and radiation therapy: Psychosocial consequences. *Cancer, 73*, 1221–1228.

*Schain, W. S., Edwards, B. K., Gorrell, C. R., de Moss, E. V., Lippman, M. E., Gerber, L. H., & Lichter, A. S. (1983). Psychosocial and physical outcomes of primary breast cancer therapy. *Breast Cancer Research and Treatment, 3*, 377–383.

Schain, W. S., & Fetting, J. H. (1992). Modified radical mastectomy versus breast conservation: Psychosocial considerations. *Seminars in Oncology, 19*, 239–243.

Schmidt, F. L. (1992). What do data really mean? Research findings, meta-analysis, and cumulative knowledge in psychology. *American Psychologist, 47*, 1173–1181.

Schover, L. R. (1991). The impact of breast cancer on sexuality, body image, and intimate relationships. *CA—A Cancer Journal for Clinicians, 41*, 112–120.

*Schover, L. R., Yetman, R. J., Tuason, L. J., Meisler, E., Esselstyn, C. B., Hermann, R. E., Grundfest-Broniatowski, S., & Dowden, R. V. (1995). Partial mastectomy and breast reconstruction: A comparison of their effects on psychosocial adjustment, body image, and sexuality. *Cancer, 75*, 54–64.

Schwarzer, R. (1989). Meta-analysis Programs (Version 5.1) [Computer software]. Berlin, Germany: Author.

Seltzer, V. L. (1987). *Every woman's guide to breast cancer: Prevention, treatment, recovery.* Middlesex, England: Viking Penguin.

Siegel, S., & Castellan, N. J. (1988). *Nonparametric statistics for the behavioral sciences* (2nd ed.). New York: McGraw-Hill.

Sinsheimer, L. M., & Holland, J. C. (1987). Psychological issues in breast cancer. *Seminars in Oncology, 14*, 75–82.

Spanier, G. B. (1976). Measuring dyadic adjustment: New scales for assessing the quality of marriage and similar dyads. *Journal of Marriage and the Family, 38*, 15–28.

*Steinberg, M. D., Juliano, M. A., & Wise, L. (1985). Psychological outcome of lumpectomy versus mastectomy in the treatment of breast cancer. *American Journal of Psychiatry, 142*, 34–39.

Taylor, K. M., Margolese, R. G., & Soskolne, C. L. (1984). Physicians' reasons for not entering eligible patients in a randomized clinical trial of surgery for breast cancer. *New England Journal of Medicine, 310,* 1363–1367.

Taylor, S. E., Lichtman, R. R., Wood, J. V., Bluming, A. Z., Dosik, G. M., & Leibowitz, R. L. (1985). Illness-related and treatment-related factors in psychological adjustment to breast cancer. *Cancer, 55,* 2506–2513.

*van Heeringen, C., van Moffaert, M., & de Cuypere, G. (1989). Depression after surgery for breast cancer: Comparison of mastectomy and lumpectomy. *Psychotherapy and Psychosomatics, 51,* 175–179.

Ward, S., Heidrich, S., & Wolberg, W. (1989). Factors women take into account when deciding upon type of surgery for breast cancer. *Cancer Nursing, 12,* 344–351.

Weisman, M. M. (1975). The assessment of social adjustment. *Archives of General Psychiatry, 32,* 357–365.

*Wellisch, D. K., DiMatteo, R., Silverstein, M., Landsverk, J., Hoffman, R., Waisman, J., Handel, N., Waisman-Smith, E., & Schain, W. (1989). Psychosocial outcomes of breast cancer therapies: Lumpectomy versus mastectomy. *Psychosomatics, 30,* 365–373.

*Wolberg, W. H., Romsaas, E. P., Tanner, M. A., & Malec, J. F. (1989). Psychosexual adaptation to breast cancer surgery. *Cancer, 63,* 1645–1655.

Wolf, F. M. (1986). *Meta-analysis: Quantitative methods for research synthesis.* Newbury Park, CA: Sage.

Wolf, F. M. (1990). Methodological observations on bias. In K. W. Wachter & M. L. Straf (Eds.), *The future of meta-analysis* (pp. 139–151). New York: Russell Sage Foundation.

*Yilmazer, N., Aydiner, A., Özkan, S., Aslay, I., & Bilge, N. (1994). A comparison of body image, self-esteem and social support in total mastectomy and breast-conserving therapy in Turkish women. *Supportive Care in Cancer, 2,* 238–241.

Correction to Moyer (1997)

In the article "Psychosocial Outcomes of Breast-Conserving Surgery Versus Mastectomy: A Meta-Analytic Review" by Anne Moyer (*Health Psychology*, 1997, Vol. 16, No. 3, pp. 284–298), Table 1 contained an error, which has implications for some of the data in Table 3.

Specifically, the study by Ganz, Schag, Lee, Polinsky, and Tan (1992), listed as the third entry on the third page (p. 288) of Table 1, *Summary of Studies Comparing Psychosocial Outcomes of Breast-Conserving Surgeries Versus Those of Mastectomy*, is incorrectly described in the second column, under "Participants and design," as one that randomized patients to treatment. This study should have been described as not randomized.

As a consequence of the incorrect designation of randomization for Ganz et al.'s (1992) study, some of the data in Table 3 (p. 291) were incorrect in the published article. The data were reanalyzed on the basis of the corrected information. The magnitude of the effect sizes is not changed considerably although the previously

Table 3—*Psychosocial Consequences of Surgery for Breast Cancer by Method of Assignment to Treatment: Numbers of Samples, Numbers of Participants, and Means and Standard Deviations for Unweighted and Weighted Effect Sizes (ESs)*

Construct	No. of samples	No. of participants	Unweighted ES M	Unweighted ES SD	Weighted ES M	Weighted ES SD
Psychological adjustment						
Randomized	9	832	.083	.092	.076**	.070
Nonrandomized	19	1,912	.344	.194	.147	.048
Marital–sexual adjustment						
Randomized	7	616	.080	.139	.065	.081
Nonrandomized	14	1,164	.226	.434	.114	.061
Social adjustment						
Randomized	3	209	.393	.296	.334*	.140
Nonrandomized	8	457	.164	.414	.133	.088
Body/self-image						
Randomized	6	441	.665	.104	.593*	.099
Nonrandomized	18	1,674	.588	.138	.355	.051
Cancer-related fears and concerns						
Randomized	6	441	.128	.268	.120	.097
Nonrandomized	10	645	.240	.489	.191	.082
Global adjustment						
Randomized	2	231	.033	.033	.010	.132
Nonrandomized	11	962	.091	.052	.065	.067

Note. Positive values for ESs indicate better outcomes for groups treated with breast-conserving surgery. Significance level shown only for weighted mean ES.

*$p < .05$.

**$p < .01$.

determined .001 level of significance for the difference between randomized and nonrandomized samples for the construct of psychological adjustment reduces to .01, and the difference between randomized and nonrandomized samples for the body/self-image construct is significant at the .05 level. A corrected version of Table 3 is printed on page 287.

Part IV

Family Dynamics

Chapter 11
WHEN MOM OR DAD HAS CANCER:
Markers of Psychological Distress in Cancer Patients, Spouses, and Children

Bruce E. Compas, Nancy L. Worsham, JoAnne E. Epping-Jordan,
Kathryn E. Grant, Gina Mireault, David C. Howell,
and Vanessa L. Malcarne

The diagnosis and treatment of cancer are sources of considerable psychological stress for patients and their families. Although treatments have become increasingly effective for a wide range of cancers, the initial diagnosis still involves a threat of loss of life for many patients. Even in those cases in which the prognosis for survival is good, there may be the threat of the loss of some significant aspect of personal functioning, damage to physical appearance, or loss of physical functioning (e.g., Heinrich, Schag, & Ganz, 1984). In addition to its importance in its own right, the diagnosis of cancer represents a prototype of acute, extreme stress that confronts many families. A necessary first step in research on stressors such as cancer is to document levels of psychological distress and identify individual differences among family members in order to set the stage for subsequent research on the processes that may contribute to distress.

Cancer appears to present at least a short-term threat or crisis to patients, as reflected in increased symptoms of depression and anxiety near the time of diagnosis (e.g., Andersen, Andersen, & deProsse, 1989; Derogatis et al., 1983; Heinrich & Schag, 1987; Massie & Holland, 1987; Stanton & Snider, 1993). Distressed mood may subside for many patients in the months following diagnosis, underscoring the need to consider the length of time that has elapsed since the patient's diagnosis (Andersen et al., 1989; Northouse & Swain, 1987). Findings comparing levels of psychological distress of men and women with cancer have been mixed, with some evidence that women experience more emotional distress (e.g., Cella et al., 1987), other findings indicating that men are more distressed and their lives more disrupted by the experience (e.g., Pettingale, Burgess, & Greer, 1988), and still other studies finding no gender differences (e.g., Marks, Richardson, Graham, & Levine, 1986). Researchers have failed to control for normative differences between men and women in symptoms of psychological distress, however (e.g., Nolen-Hoeksema, 1990). Therefore, it is unclear whether differences between male and female patients

Reprinted from *Health Psychology, 13*(6), 507–515. (1994). Copyright © 1994 by the American Psychological Association. Used with permission of the author.

This research was supported by grants from the National Institute of Mental Health (MH43819) and the National Cancer Institute (P30CA22435). Its contents are solely the authors' responsibility and do not necessarily represent the official views of the National Cancer Institute. The authors are grateful to numerous individuals for their assistance in carrying out this research, including oncologists Jerome Belinson, Thomas Roland, and James Stuart; oncology nurses Elaine Owen, Susan Guillan, Debbie Potter, and Joyce Silveira; staff assistant Jeannie Bernard; research assistants Sydney Ey, Carol Kottmeier, Doug Bolton, Caroline Freidman, Cindy Gerhardt, and Pam Orosan; and undergraduate assistants Laurie Raezer and Amy Willard.

can be attributed to the diagnosis of cancer per se, above and beyond expected gender differences in the general population.

Fewer studies have investigated the impact of cancer on spouses of patients. Spouses rate cancer in their partners as a significant stressor and report a number of adverse effects of the disease on their marital relationship and daily functioning in the family (e.g., Ell, Nishimoto, Mantell, & Hamovitch, 1988; Given et al., 1993; Hannur, Gresi-Davis, Harding, & Hatfield, 1991; Lewis, Woods, Hough, & Bensley, 1989; Lichtman, Taylor, & Wood, 1987). However, the degree of psychological symptoms experienced by spouses of patients is not well documented and possible gender differences in the responses of spouses are not clear.

The psychological adjustment of children of cancer patients has been the focus of several recent studies but remains even less well understood than that of patients and spouses (e.g., Casselith et al., 1985; Lewis, Ellison, & Woods, 1985; Lewis, Hammond, & Woods, 1993; Northouse, Cracchiolo, & Appel, 1991; Siegel et al., 1992; Wellisch, Gritz, Schain, Wang, & Siau, 1991, 1992). In one of the most extensive investigations of children of cancer patients (Lewis et al., 1985; Lewis et al., 1993), parental reports indicated that children in these families experienced few behavioral or emotional problems, whereas children's self-reports indicated some negative impact on children's self-esteem and adjustment. However, data on children's adjustment were obtained several years after the parents' diagnoses. Lichtman and Taylor (1986) presented some evidence that young women are adversely affected by the diagnosis of breast cancer in their mothers, but investigations have not been conducted with other age groups or with sons and daughters of mothers and fathers with cancer.

Previous research on stress processes in cancer patients has drawn primarily on cognitive appraisal models of individual responses to stress (e.g., Lazarus & Folkman, 1984). When considering the responses of family members to cancer, however, it is necessary to include interpersonal aspects of stress (e.g., Compas & Wagner, 1991) as well as developmental differences in stress processes (e.g., Compas, Worsham, & Ey, 1992). Research on interpersonal aspects of stress has shown that women tend to be more affected than men by stress in the lives of significant others (e.g., Barnett & Baruch, 1987) and that adolescence is an important period for the emergence of these gender differences (Wagner & Compas, 1990).

On the basis of these perspectives, we examined several factors as possible markers of psychological distress in cancer patients and their family members. First, we examined both the objective characteristics of the disease (length of time since diagnosis, stage, initial prognosis, type of treatment, and functional status) and cognitive appraisals of the seriousness and stressfulness of the disease as possible correlates or markers of patients' and family members' distress. Second, we considered age, sex, and family role of family members as markers of differences in the psychological distress of patients, their spouses, and their children. We did not hypothesize specific differences in levels of psychological distress of men and women with cancer or their husbands and wives, as prior research comparing distress in men and women with cancer and comparing patients and spouses has been unclear. Furthermore, by selecting patients who have children living in the home, the present sample represents adults with cancer who are younger than typical samples of cancer patients reported in the literature (e.g., Cella et al., 1987; Derogatis et al., 1983).

We compared levels of distress among male and female preadolescent, adolescent, and young adult children whose mother or father had cancer. Psychological distress of daughters whose parents have cancer was expected to be greater than distress reported by sons, as girls have been found to perceive events affecting a member of their family as more stressful than boys (e.g., Wagner & Compas, 1990). Furthermore, the work of Lichtman and Taylor (1986) has suggested that distress may be higher in same-sex offspring of patients. Analyses of age differences in distress of children in these families were exploratory, as previous research was not sufficient to develop specific hypotheses. The association of patients' distress with the distress of spouses and children was also examined, as prior research on interpersonal stress processes in families has shown an association between the psychological distress of husbands and wives and between distress of parents and their children (e.g., Compas, Howell, Phares, Williams, & Ledoux, 1989; Given et al., 1993).

We measured psychological distress of cancer patients and their families in two ways. First, we selected symptoms of depression and anxiety as an index of generalized psychological distress of patients and family members. Second, as an index of response to a traumatic event, we used symptoms of a stress response syndrome (Horowitz, Field, & Classen, 1993) or posttraumatic stress disorder (PTSD; American Psychiatric Association, 1987) including unwanted and intrusive thoughts and emotions pertaining to the disease accompanied by efforts to avoid thoughts and reminders of it. Measures were selected to provide comparisons of levels of distress among different family members, as well as to allow for comparison of symptom levels with normative data to understand the clinical significance of these symptoms (i.e., to determine the percentage of individuals who exceed the clinical cut-offs established for each of these measures).

Method

Participants

Participants were 117 cancer patients (72% female; mean age = 41.2 years, SD = 8.2), 76 spouses (36% female; mean age = 42.0 years, SD = 9.2), 34 young-adult children (62% female; mean age = 22.9 years, SD = 3.4), 50 adolescent children (58% female; mean age = 14.6 years, SD = 2.2), and 26 preadolescent children (42% female; mean age = 7.8, SD = 1.7). All preadolescent and adolescent children lived with their parents, and young adults either lived in their parents' home or had frequent, ongoing contact with the parent diagnosed with cancer. These patients represent 75% of those eligible patients who were approached regarding the study. The number of spouses and children differed from the number of patients, as individual family members were allowed to agree or decline to participate in the study independent of the decision of the patient to participate, and families differed in number and ages of children.

Patients were diagnosed with a variety of different types of cancer including breast cancer (32%; 35 women), gynecologic cancers (21%; 23 women), brain tumors (12%; 7 men, 6 women), lung cancer (7%; 3 men, 5 women), hematologic malignancies (10%; 5 men, 6 women), gastrointestinal cancers (6%; 3 men, 3 women), testicular cancer (5%; 5 men), melanoma (4%; 4 men), and other diagnoses (5%; 3 men, 2 women). Type of diagnosis differed by sex of patient, $\chi^2(8, n = 110) = 56.90$, $p < .001$, primarily as a result of rates of breast and gynecologic cancers in the female patients. Patients were contacted for the initial data collection on average 2 months after their initial diagnosis ($M = 8.59$ weeks postdiagnosis, $SD = 5.51$). Men ($M = 8.99$ weeks) and women ($M = 8.45$ weeks) did not differ significantly in their time since diagnosis at the first data collection. We used time since diagnosis as a covariate in all analyses.

We considered the severity of patients' cancers in several ways. Stage of cancer varied with 33% Stage I, 28% Stage II, 22% Stage III, and 17% Stage IV. Men and women did not differ in stage, $\chi^2(3, n = 104) = 3.17$, ns. Initial prognosis was operationalized as patients' projected 5-year survival rates (i.e., the percentage of patients with a similar prognosis expected to be alive in 5 years) derived from the National Cancer Institute's Surveillance, Epidemiology, and End Results (SEER) program (American Cancer Society, 1992). Men ($M = 50.31\%$, $SD = 30.40$) and women ($M = 59.37\%$, $SD = 31.16$) did not differ significantly in initial prognosis. Men and women did not differ in the frequency of receiving chemotherapy (43.33% and 60.00%, respectively), radiation therapy (66.67% and 61.25%, respectively), or hormonal therapy (0% and 5% respectively). Finally, we assessed degree of functional impairment through the Eastern Cooperative Oncology Group (ECOG) performance status ratings, based on ratings of symptoms and ambulatory status abstracted from medical charts by two research assistants (interrater reliability exceeded 90%). Separate ratings for both the best and worst ECOG performance status near the time of diagnosis ranged from 0 (normal activity, asymptomatic) to 4 (patient 100% bedridden, likely terminal phase of cancer). Male and female patients did not differ significantly in either their best or worst performance status. Both ratings were highly skewed, with 96% of patients receiving a best performance status rating of 0 or 1 and 85% of patients receiving a worst performance status rating of 3. The severity of parents' diagnoses (stage, SEER ratings, performance status) and children's perceptions of the seriousness or severity of their parents' cancer did not differ among children, adolescents, and young adults who participated in the study. All children who participated in the study were aware prior to their participation in the interview that their parent had cancer.

Procedure

We recruited participants through the Medical Oncology, Radiotherapy, and Gynecologic Oncology cancer clinics of the Vermont Cancer Center, University of Vermont. A member of the medical staff contacted patients who had children either living in the home or living outside the home but in frequent contact with the family. A member of the research team obtained written consent to participate from the patient, spouse, and children over the age of 18, and written assent from children under 18 years of age. Each consenting family member participated in individual interviews of 1 to 2 hours (in person or over the telephone) and completed sets of questionnaires.

Measures

Perceptions of Severity and Stressfulness of Cancer

Perceptions of the patients' cancer were assessed for each family member during individual interviews as an index of cognitive appraisals of the cancer as a stressor (cf. Davis & Compas, 1986). In response to the question "How serious do you think the cancer is at this time," patients, spouses, and young adults rated the severity of the cancer on a 4-point Likert scale ranging from "not at all serious" to "extremely serious." Preadolescent children and adolescents were asked "How bad do you think your parent's illness is," and responded to a 4-point scale ranging from "not bad" to "very bad." In response to the question "How stressful is your experience with the cancer at this time," the stressfulness of the cancer was rated by patients, spouses, and young adults on a 4-point scale ranging from "not at all stressful" to "extremely stressful." Preadolescent children and adolescents were asked "How upsetting is your parent's illness for you right now," and provide responses ranging from "not upsetting" to "extremely upsetting."

Anxiety/Depression Symptoms

Because there is no measure of symptoms of anxiety/depression that is appropriate for use across the age range of participants, we selected age-appropriate measures for preadolescents, adolescents, young adults, patients, and spouses. Preadolescents (6–10 years old) completed the Children's Depression Inventory (CDI; Kovacs, 1980) and the Revised-Children's Manifest Anxiety Scale (R-CMAS; Reynolds & Richmond, 1978); adolescents (11–18 years old) completed the Youth Self-Report (YSR; Achenbach, 1991); and patients, spouses, and young adults completed the Brief Symptom Inventory (BSI; Derogatis & Spencer, 1982).[1]

The CDI is a 27-item self-report measure of symptoms of depression over the previous 2 weeks.[2] The CDI has good internal consistency, distinguishes children with general emotional distress from nondistressed children, and corresponds well

---

[1]There is considerable correspondence in item content across the measures of anxiety and depression symptoms used for adults (BSI), adolescents (YSR), and children (CDI and R-CMAS). Six items are common to the measures for all three age groups (sad or dysphoric affect, loneliness, worthlessness, suicidal ideation, nervousness, and fearfulness). Of the 12 items on the BSI Depression and Anxiety scales, 6 were on both the adolescent and child measures, 5 others appeared on at least one other age group measure, and 1 item appeared only on the BSI (spells of terror or panic). Of the 16 items on the Anxious and Depressed Syndrome of the YSR, 6 appeared on the adult and child measures, 6 appeared on at least one other age group measure, and 4 appeared only on the YSR (fears own impulses, needs to be perfect, suspicious, and tries to harm self). Because the CDI and R-CMAS contain many more items than either of the subscales for anxiety or depression on the BSI and YSR, more items appeared only on the child measures than on the adult and adolescent measures. Seven of the 27 items on the CDI appeared on the adult and adolescent measures (loneliness was reflected in 2 items), 6 items appeared on at least one other age group measure, and 14 items appeared only on the CDI. Of the 28 anxiety symptom items on the R-CMAS, 3 appeared on the adult and adolescent measures, 5 appeared on at least one other measure, and 20 items only on the R-CMAS.

[2]The CDI, R-CMAS, YSR, and BSI ask for reports of symptoms over different periods of time. To retain the standard administration of these scales and to allow for comparisons with normative data, these different time frames were retained for this study.

with self-report measures of self-concept (e.g., Saylor, Finch, Spirito, & Bennett, 1984). Norms for the CDI were drawn from a nonreferred sample of 1,463 children (Finch, Saylor, & Edwards, 1985).

The R-CMAS is a 37-item self-report questionnaire (28 anxiety items and 9 Lie scale items) of the presence or absence of a variety of anxiety-related symptoms in the previous 2 weeks. *Yes*-responses on the anxiety items are summed to yield a total anxiety score, and responses to the Lie scale items are summed to provide an index of socially desirable responses. The R-CMAS has acceptable internal consistency and test–retest reliability, and correlates with other measures of children's anxiety (e.g., Finch & Rogers, 1984). Norms for the R-CMAS were drawn from a sample of 329 nonreferred children (Reynolds & Richmond, 1978). In the present sample the CDI and R-CMAS were moderately correlated, $r = .50$, $p = .003$.

The YSR is a checklist of 102 behavior problem items rated by the respondent as *not true, somewhat or sometimes true,* or *very true or often true* during the past 6 months. Test–retest reliability over 1 week is excellent, and validity has been established through differentiation of referred and nonreferred youth (Achenbach, 1991). Normative data are available for the YSR in the revised 1991 profiles based on a nationally representative sample of 1,315 nonreferred youth. We used the Anxious/Depressed syndrome that includes 16 symptoms of anxiety and depression in the present analyses.

The BSI (Derogatis & Spencer, 1982) is a self-report inventory of 53 items describing a variety of emotional and somatic complaints. Test–retest and internal consistency reliabilities are adequate (Derogatis & Spencer, 1982). We focused on the Depression (6 items) and Anxiety (6 items) scales for the present analyses. Separate community (nonpatient) norms for men and women ($N = 974$) were used to generate T scores (Derogatis & Spencer, 1982). The Anxiety and Depression scales of the BSI were significantly correlated ($p < .001$) for patients ($r = .64$), spouses ($r = .71$), and young adults ($r = .67$).

Raw symptom scores on the BSI, YSR, CDI, and R-CMAS were transformed into T scores ($M = 50$, $SD = 10$) based on separate normative data for men and women available on each scale. Differences that are found as a function of gender and age are therefore more readily interpreted as related to the impact of the cancer. A T score of 63 (90th percentile) was used to identify scores in the clinical range on each measure. Because separate anxiety and depression scores are generated for the BSI, CDI, and R-CMAS, a mean T score calculated across symptoms of anxiety and depression reflecting negative affect was created for patients, spouses, and young adults on the BSI and for children on the CDI and R-CMAS (no such transformation was needed on the YSR because a combined anxiety/depression score is generated). The BSI, YSR, CDI, and R-CMAS do not allow for determination of diagnoses of clinical depression or anxiety disorders. However, these measures reflect symptoms of depression and anxiety or negative affect at the syndromal level that include fear, anxiety, sadness, and guilt (e.g., Compas, Ey, & Grant, 1993; Watson & Clark, 1984).

Stress Response Symptoms

Symptoms of a stress-response syndrome were measured in terms of the degree of avoidance and intrusive thoughts and emotions on the 15-item Impact of Event Scale

(IES; Horowitz, Wilner, & Alvarez, 1979).[3] Eight items assess avoidance (e.g., "I try to remove it from my memory") and 7 items assess intrusive thoughts and emotions (e.g., "I have waves of strong feelings about it"). Patients and spouses responded to the full 15-item scale; young adults, adolescents, and children responded to a shorter set of 8 randomly selected items (5 avoidance items and 3 intrusion items) to shorten their interviews. Participants indicated the frequency of each item with respect to their experience with the cancer in the past 7 days. The IES has been used as an index of stress-response syndrome and PTSD symptoms in cancer patients in previous studies (Horowitz et al., 1993). Internal consistency for the present sample was $\alpha = .80$ for patients, .85 for spouses, .69 for young adults, .67 for adolescents, and .49 for preadolescent children. The low reliability for children indicates that their scores must be interpreted cautiously.

Results

Correlations of Psychological Distress With Disease Variables

Stage of cancer, SEER 5-year survival ratings of the patients' cancers, time since the patients' diagnosis, patients' best and worst ECOG performance status ratings, and perceptions of the seriousness and stressfulness of their cancer were correlated with symptoms of anxiety/depression and stress response syndrome symptoms on the IES for all family members (see Table 1). In general, disease characteristics were not related to symptoms of anxiety/depression or to total stress-response syndrome symptoms on the IES. Stage of patients' cancer was related only to spouses' IES scores, and the SEER projected 5-year survival rate was related to patients', spouses', and adolescents' IES scores. For each of these correlations, a worse prognosis was related to greater distress. Measures of psychological distress and perceptions of the seriousness and stressfulness of the cancer were also generally uncorrelated with the length of time since the patients' diagnosis. The measures of psychological distress were moderately to strongly correlated with perceptions of the seriousness and stressfulness of the patients' cancer. Stress response syndrome symptoms were more consistently associated with disease characteristics and cognitive appraisals than were symptoms of anxiety/depression.

Correlations of Patients' Distress With Family Members' Distress

Patients' combined mean anxiety/depression symptom scores were significantly related to spouses' mean anxiety/depression symptoms ($r = .32$) but not related to anxiety/depression for young adults, adolescents, or children. Patients' scores on the

---

[3]The IES provides an approximation of the diagnostic criteria for PTSD in the revised third edition of the *Diagnostic and Statistical Manual of Mental Disorders* (American Psychiatric Association, 1987). Specifically, Criterion A (presence of a stressor outside the range of usual experience), Criterion B (presence of intrusive thoughts and emotions related to the stress), and Criterion C (efforts to avoid stimuli associated with the stressor) are reflected in the IES. Criterion D (persistent symptoms of increased arousal) and Criterion E (duration of at least one month) are not represented in the IES. Therefore, we have chosen to refer to the IES as an index of a stress response syndrome (Horowitz et al., 1993) rather than as an index of PTSD symptoms per se.

Table 1—*Correlations of Anxiety/Depression Symptoms and Stress Response Symptoms on the IES*

| | | Measurement | | | | | |
| | | SEER 5-Year survival rate | ECOG worst | ECOG best | Time since diagnosis | Perceived serious | Perceived stress |
Characteristic	Stage						
Patients							
Anxiety/depression	−.08	−.08	.11	.03	−.18	.14	.41***
IES	.14	−.17*	.02	−.09	.06	.27**	.56***
Spouses							
Anxiety/depression	−.02	−.14	.11	.02	−.11	.25*	.15
IES	.31**	−.43***	.11	−.04	.05	.55***	.47***
Young adults							
Anxiety/depression	−.01	−.08	−.32	.26	−.42*	.26	.09
IES	.14	−.10	−.10	−.25	−.25	.32*	.68***
Adolescents							
Anxiety/depression	−.03	−.01	.00	−.07	−.15	.03	.31*
IES	.20	−.36**	−.02	−.01	.04	.36**	.63***
Children							
Anxiety/depression	−.25	.09	—	.41*	.22	.09	.34
IES	−.20	−.02	—	.27	−.12	.23	.36

Note. The correlation between worst ECOG performance status and children's anxiety/depression and IES symptoms was indeterminant, as there was no variance in performance status for the parents of the 27 children for whom these data were available. IES = Impact of Event Scale; SEER = National Cancer Institute Surveillance, Epidemiology, and End Results prognosis; ECOG worst = Eastern Cooperative Oncology Group worst performance status rating; ECOG best = Eastern Cooperative Oncology Group best performance status rating.

$*p < .05.$
$**p < .01.$
$***p < .001.$

IES were not related to IES scores for spouses or any of the age groups of children. Thus, family members' symptoms of distress were relatively independent of the level of distress reported by patients.

Patients' and Spouses' Symptoms of Psychological Distress

Perceived seriousness of the cancer varied as a function of the interaction of sex and family role, $F(4, 180) = 5.38$, $p = .022$. Wives of patients perceived the cancer as more serious ($M = 2.97$) than either husbands whose wives were ill ($M = 2.47$), male patients ($M = 2.56$), or female patients ($M = 2.31$). Perceived stressfulness of the cancer varied as a function of sex of patient, $F(4, 180) = 4.72$, $p = .044$, and family role, $F(4, 180) = 5.75$, $p = .026$. Women ($M = 3.36$) perceived their experience with cancer as more stressful than men did ($M = 3.01$), and spouses ($M = 3.38$) perceived the cancer as more stressful than patients did ($M = 2.99$).

Means of the combined T scores for symptoms of anxiety/depression reported by patients and spouses on the BSI and for total symptoms on the IES are presented in Table 2. These scores correspond to moderate levels of anxiety/depression symptoms, with the means approximately one-half standard deviation above the normative mean. The total scores on the IES are higher than those reported in a previous study of recently diagnosed cancer patients (Horowitz, 1982), $t(160) = 9.87$, $p < .001$, indicating moderate levels of stress-response syndrome scores. We conducted two-way analyses of covariance (ANCOVAs) with sex and family role (patient vs. spouse) as the independent variables, time since diagnosis as the covariate, and T scores for anxiety/depression and total stress response syndrome symptoms as the dependent variables. Because scores for patients and their spouses cannot be assumed to be independent, family role was treated as a repeated measure. Neither the main effects, the covariate, or the interactions were significant in the ANCOVA for anxiety/depression. There were no significant effects for sex or family role or their interaction in the ANCOVA for stress-response symptoms on the IES. We conducted additional analyses with the Avoidance and Intrusion scales of the IES as separate dependent variables; we found no significant effects for sex, family role, or their interaction.

Analyses of the numbers of male and female patients in the clinical range on the BSI were conducted separately for anxiety and depression symptoms. Eight male patients (36%) and 16 female patients (21%) had T scores of above 63 on anxiety near time of diagnosis. These proportions are greater than the percentage of patients (10%) expected to exceed the cutoff by chance for men, $\chi^2(1, N = 22) = 16.99$, $p < .001$, and for women, $\chi^2(1, N = 74) = 11.10$, $p < .01$. Analyses of the Depression scale revealed that more male patients ($N = 7$, 32%) and more female patients ($n = 17$, 23%) were in the clinical range than was expected, $\chi^2(1, n = 22) = 11.64$, $p < .001$, and $\chi^2(1, n = 74) = 13.84$, $p < .01$, respectively.

On the Anxiety scale, more male ($n = 14$, 35%) and female ($n = 9$, 35%) spouses were in the clinical range on anxiety symptoms than would be expected, $\chi^2(1, N = 40) = 27.78$, $p < .001$, and $\chi^2(1, N = 26) = 17.50$, $p < .001$, respectively. The distribution for husbands and wives did not differ from one another. Analyses of the Depression scale indicated that more male spouses ($n = 9$, 23%), $\chi^2(1, N = 40) = 6.94$, $p < .01$, and more female spouses (23%) were in the clinical range than would be expected by chance, $\chi^2(1, N = 26) = 4.94$, $p < .05$.

Table 2—*Cancer Patients' and Spouses' Symptoms of Anxiety/Depression and Stress Response Symptoms on the IES*

	Women		Men	
	M	SD	M	SD
Anxiety/depression symptoms				
Patients	54.26	9.80	56.00	7.60
Spouses	54.41	10.76	54.81	10.70
IES				
Patients	31.79	7.50	29.92	8.28
Spouses	31.36	9.11	28.35	8.42

Note. IES = Impact of Event Scale.

Young Adults', Adolescents', and Children's Symptoms
of Psychological Distress

The means for symptoms of anxiety/depression from the age-appropriate measures and total stress-response symptoms on the IES for young adults, adolescents, and children whose parents had cancer are presented in Table 3. The ANCOVA for symptoms of anxiety/depression revealed a significant main effect for age, $F(2, 82) = 10.57$, $p < .001$, and a borderline significant interaction of age and sex, $F(2, 82) = 2.84$, $p = .068$ (no other main or interaction effects were significant). With regard to the main effect for age, children's mean anxiety/depression T score ($M = 45.06$) was significantly lower ($p < .05$, Newman-Keuls test) than the mean T scores for adolescents ($M = 56.93$) or young adults ($M = 56.26$). Because of the effect for age and the borderline interaction of age and sex, we examined simple effects by conducting separate 2 (sex of patient) × 2 (sex of child) ANCOVAs for each age group. There were no effects for sex of patient or child for preadolescent children. For adolescents, there was a significant effect for sex of the adolescent, $F(1, 39) = 11.74$, $p = .001$, and an interaction of sex of adolescent and sex of patient, $F(1, 39) = 5.80$, $p = .02$. Specifically, adolescent girls ($M = 60.44$) reported higher symptoms of anxiety/depression than boys ($M = 51.35$), and girls whose mothers had cancer reported more symptoms than all other groups of adolescents.[4] Finally, for young adults whose parents had cancer, there were no significant main effects or interactions.

The ANCOVA for stress-response symptoms on the IES revealed a significant main effect for age, $F(1, 94) = 3.11$, $p = .049$; an interaction of age and patient sex, $F(1, 94) = 4.44$, $p = .014$; and an interaction of sex of respondent and sex of patient, $F(1, 94) = 4.67$, $p = .033$ (no other main or interaction effects were significant). A Newman–Keuls test showed that the main effect for age was the result of higher IES scores for children ($M = 17.91$) than adolescents ($M = 14.56$) and young adults ($M = 11.82$); the latter two groups did not differ. The interaction of sex of respondent and sex of patient resulted from higher IES scores for sons whose fathers were ill ($M = 14.46$) and daughters whose mothers were ill ($M = 16.34$) than sons of ill mothers ($M = 11.72$) or daughters of ill fathers ($M = 13.67$). Because of the significant differences as a function of age and the interaction of age and patient sex, we conducted separate 2 × 2 ANCOVAS for each age group. There were no effects for preadolescent children. For adolescents, there was a significant main effect for sex of adolescent, $F(1, 45) = 5.24$, $p = .027$, and a significant interaction of sex of patient and sex of adolescent, $F(1, 45) = 8.61$, $p = .005$. Adolescent girls reported more symptoms on the IES ($M = 15.68$) than adolescent boys ($M = 11.91$). Furthermore, adolescent girls whose mothers had cancer reported more stress-related symptoms on the IES than girls whose fathers were ill or boys whose fathers or mothers were ill. The ANCOVA for young adults revealed a main effect for patient sex, $F(1, 29)$

---

[4]The greater distress of adolescent girls whose mothers were ill may have been attributable to a subgroup of girls whose mothers had sex-linked cancers (breast or gynecologic cancers), as these girls may have felt more threatened by the perception that they were personally at risk for cancer. To test this possibility we compared girls whose mothers had a sex-linked cancer ($n = 10$) with those with mothers whose cancer was not sex linked. These groups did not differ on anxiety or depression symptoms ($M = 64.7$ vs. $M = 61.6$, respectively; $t = 0.59$, ns) or on stress response syndrome symptoms ($M = 17.0$ vs. $M = 17.2$, respectively; $t = 0.04$, ns). Thus, the increased distress of adolescent girls whose mothers had cancer was not attributable to the presence of a sex-linked cancer.

Table 3—*Young Adults', Adolescents', and Children's Symptoms of Anxiety/Depression and Stress Response Symptoms on the IES*

| | Patient mother | | | | Patient father | | | |
| | Male | | Female | | Male | | Female | |
	M	*SD*	*M*	*SD*	*M*	*SD*	*M*	*SD*
Anxiety/depression								
Young adults	57.60	10.91	56.93	10.10	56.75	10.96	52.00	10.86
Adolescents	50.20	0.63	63.88	10.70	53.00	4.80	55.45	6.31
Children	46.90	6.13	42.00	7.68	43.86	7.07	48.36	8.80
IES								
Young adults	6.89	6.88	12.37	6.34	17.67	4.73	17.33	11.50
Adolescents	10.17	3.95	19.53	6.96	12.63	3.25	12.18	5.29
Children	19.50	5.73	18.00	7.25	17.00	4.24	15.00	9.42

Note. IES = Impact of Event Scale.

$= 5.87$, $p = .022$. Young adults whose fathers were ill ($M = 17.50$) reported more symptoms on the IES than those whose mothers were ill ($M = 10.61$).

We conducted separate analyses of the numbers of male and female young adults in the clinical range on the BSI for anxiety and depression symptoms. More young adult men whose fathers had cancer ($n = 2$, 50%) and more young adult women whose mothers had cancer ($n = 6$, 43%) were in the clinical range on anxiety than expected, $\chi^2(1, N = 4) = 7.11$, $p < .01$, and $\chi^2(1, N = 16) = 16.79$, $p < .001$, respectively. The percentages of young adults in the clinical range on depression symptoms did not exceed the level expected by chance.

The number of adolescents in the clinical range on the Anxious/Depressed scale revealed that only 1 of the boys (10%) whose fathers had cancer and none of the boys whose mothers had cancer were in the clinical range. Two of the girls (6%) whose fathers had cancer were in the clinical range, and 7 of the girls (25%) whose mothers had cancer were clinically elevated on this scale. Only the proportion of girls whose mothers had cancer exceeded the expected distribution, $\chi^2(1, N = 17) = 18.36$, $p < .001$.

Examination of the numbers of children in the clinical range on the R-CMAS and the CDI indicated that this sample had low levels of distress compared with normative data for these scales. Only 2 girls and 1 boy exceeded a *T* score of 63 on the R-CMAS; none of the children exceeded a *T* score of 63 on the CDI. It is noteworthy, however, that 12 of the 34 children (35%) scored above the 90th percentile on the Lie scale on the CMAS-R, indicating that this sample tended to present themselves in a favorable or socially desirable manner, $\chi^2(1, N = 34) = 24.17$, $p < .001$.

Discussion

Cancer patients, their spouses, and their children are confronted with considerable stress at the time of diagnosis. This stress was reflected in the present sample in the symptoms of anxiety/depression and levels of intrusive thoughts and avoidance associated with a stress-response syndrome reported by patients and family members. The present findings indicate that patients and their spouses are relatively similar in the levels of distress that they report. The levels of psychological symptoms in this sample of children differed, however, as a function of whether a mother or father had cancer and the individual's age and sex. Distress was strikingly high among adolescent girls whose mothers were diagnosed with cancer.

A first step in understanding the levels of distress in cancer patients and their families is to examine the relationship between distress and objective characteristics of the patients' disease. It is noteworthy that objective data reflecting the severity of patients' cancers were for the most part only moderately related to levels of anxiety/depression symptoms in this sample. Only stress-response symptoms were related to poorer prognosis for patients, spouses, and adolescents; they were also related to a worse stage of cancer for spouses. Perceptions of the seriousness and stressfulness of the patient's cancer were related to both indices of distress for patients, spouses, young adults, and adolescents, although these associations were more consistent with stress-response syndrome symptoms than with anxiety/depression symptoms.

Prior research has produced mixed results concerning the relation between disease characteristics and psychological distress in patients, with a number of studies finding an association between disease parameters and psychological distress, and others not finding an association (e.g., Cella et al., 1987; Marks et al., 1986; Pettingale et al., 1988). Psychological distress has typically been more closely related to patients' self-reports of their disease symptoms (e.g., Given et al., 1993) than to objective indices of disease severity. The independence of anxiety/depression symptoms and disease characteristics in the present sample may have resulted from several factors, including limited variance in several of the disease parameters, the use of a symptom checklist as opposed to indices of current mood used in many prior studies, the relatively young age of the patients in this sample, the assessment of psychological distress near the time of diagnosis rather than at a later point in their patients' experience with the disease, and differences among family members in their awareness of the nature of the parent's cancer. In spite of these issues, the present findings suggest that psychosocial factors may be as important as disease characteristics in understanding symptoms of depression and anxiety and stress-response syndrome symptoms in cancer patients. The data are consistent with models of stress that emphasize the role of cognitive appraisals in determining the meaning and level of threat in explaining individual differences in psychological distress (e.g., Lazarus & Folkman, 1984; Taylor, 1983). Because both cognitive appraisals and psychological distress were measured through self-reports, however, the contribution of shared method variance to these associations is unclear.

Patients' symptoms of anxiety/depression and stress-response syndrome were generally unrelated to family members' distress. With the exception of a moderate correlation between patients' and spouses' reports of anxiety/depression symptoms, the distress of spouses and children were not correlated with that of patients. These data do not suggest that families respond in a similar manner to the diagnosis of cancer in a parent, at least as it is manifested in the levels of psychological distress experienced by family members. Rather, the findings suggest that families may be best characterized by differences among members in their response to the diagnosis, with individuals' cognitive appraisals of the seriousness and stressfulness of the cancer as an important correlate of levels of distress.

Male and female patients and spouses did not differ in symptoms of anxiety/depression or stress-response syndrome. Both patients and spouses reported moderate levels of anxiety/depression and stress-response syndrome symptoms. These findings are similar to those reported by Given et al. (1993), who found that patients and caregivers (primarily spouses) did not differ in self-reported depressive symptoms and that their depressive symptoms were moderately correlated. The percentage of participants who exceeded the normative cutoff for clinical levels of symptoms of anxiety and depression was significantly greater than expected on the basis of normative data for both patients and spouses, and the mean total score on the IES was substantially higher than in a previous study of cancer patients (Horowitz et al., 1993). Thus, the diagnosis of cancer appears to be an equally significant stressor for patients and their spouses. Furthermore, the use of T scores on the BSI that were normed separately for men and women indicates that men and women in the present sample did not differ in anxiety/depression symptoms, once expected sex differences are taken into account. Thus, female patients and spouses were relatively no more distressed than males.

The data on young adult, adolescent, and preadolescent children of these patients suggest that psychological distress is influenced by their age and sex and whether their mother or father is ill. Measures of anxiety/depression symptoms provide somewhat different pictures of distress in children as compared with stress-response symptoms. Based on scores that were transformed using separate norms for each age group, anxiety/depression symptoms were higher for adolescents and young adults than for children. In contrast, total stress-response syndrome scores on the IES were greater for children than for adolescents and young adults. These data are open to two possible interpretations. First, there may be developmental differences in responses to the stress associated with a severe illness in a parent, with younger children more likely to manifest symptoms of a stress-response syndrome than symptoms of negative affect. Previous research has found that intrusive thoughts and emotions and avoidance are distinct from symptoms of generalized anxiety in children exposed to traumatic stress (Pynoos et al., 1987). This pattern may be reflected in the present sample of young children as well. Second, these seemingly contradictory findings may be the result of a response bias in the younger children. A substantial portion of young children (35%) scored above the 90th percentile on the Lie scale from the R-CMAS, indicating a tendency to try to present themselves in a socially desirable light. This may account for their relatively lower endorsement of anxiety/depression symptoms. Because the IES contained a majority of items (5 of 8) that reflected avoidance of their parents' cancer and reminders of it, children's relatively higher scores on this scale may also represent an attempt to minimize or deny the significance of their parents' disease. However, the low reliability of the children's responses on the IES indicates that these findings must be interpreted with caution. Further research on the characteristics of young children's adjustment to parents' cancer is needed.

The findings from both the anxiety/depression symptom measures and the IES indicate that adolescents' and young adults' distress varied as a function of the interaction of the sex of the ill parent and the sex of the child. Stress response syndrome symptoms on the IES were greatest for daughters whose mothers were ill and sons whose fathers were ill. The strongest effect on this measure was found for adolescent girls whose mothers were ill, as they reported the highest levels of stress-response symptoms. Similarly, adolescents' anxiety/depression symptoms differed as a function of sex of adolescent and sex of the patient, with girls whose mothers were ill again reporting the highest symptoms. These findings are consistent with reports of the concerns of daughters of women with breast cancer patients (e.g., Lichtman & Taylor, 1986; Wellisch et al., 1991, 1992), and identify adolescent girls as a highly vulnerable subgroup.

Adolescent girls may be especially vulnerable to the presence of severe disease in a parent for several reasons. Adolescents may be more cognitively aware than younger children of the meaning of the disease as a stressor for the parent with cancer and the family as a whole (cf. Compas et al., 1989). Parents may also be more willing to share information regarding the nature of their cancer with their adolescent as opposed to preadolescent children. Compared with young adults however, adolescents may be less able to cope with the threats associated with parental cancer. Adolescent girls in particular may have been faced with increased stress associated with greater caretaking responsibilities in the family, they may have perceived an increased sense of personal vulnerability to cancer for themselves, or they may have been coping in maladaptive ways. These hypotheses warrant further investigation.

The clinical significance of these findings is evident in the greater than expected proportions of patients and family members in the clinical range for anxiety and depression symptoms. Approximately one third of male patients, male and female spouses, young adult women whose mothers had cancer, and adolescent girls whose mothers had cancer reported significant levels of distress. Although these scores cannot be interpreted as reflective of diagnostic levels of depression or anxiety, they indicate that the impact of cancer on patients and their families is meaningful and may warrant interventions in the form of short-term support services. Clinicians will need to attend to symptoms characteristic of anxiety and depression, as well as those associated with PTSD.

Factors that further elucidate these differences in vulnerability to distress in cancer patients and their families will be important in developing intervention programs targeting those family members in greatest need of psychological support. The present data, combined with those from prior studies, establish that cancer is a marker of risk for patients and their families. Moreover, the diagnosis of cancer in a parent offers an important model for studying stress and adaptation in families exposed to conditions of extreme, acute stress. The processes and mechanisms through which the stress of cancer exacts a toll, including ongoing stress with the family and maladaptive coping responses, now need to be examined.

References

Achenbach, T. M. (1991). *Manual for the Youth Self-Report and 1991 profile*. Burlington: University of Vermont, Department of Psychiatry.

American Cancer Society. (1992). *Cancer facts and figures—1992*. Atlanta, GA: Author.

American Psychiatric Association. (1987). *Diagnostic and statistical manual of mental disorders* (3rd ed., rev.). Washington, DC: Author.

Andersen, B. L., Andersen, B., & deProsse, C. (1989). Controlled prospective longitudinal study of women with cancer: II. Psychological outcomes. *Journal of Consulting and Clinical Psychology, 57*, 692–697.

Barnett, R. C., & Baruch, G. K. (1987). Social roles, gender, and psychological distress. In R. C. Barnett, L. Biener, & G. K. Baruch (Eds.), *Gender and stress* (pp. 122–143). New York: Free Press.

Casselith, B. R., Lusk, E. J., Strouse, T. B., Miller, D. S., Brown, L. L., & Cross, P. A. (1985). A psychological analysis of cancer patients and their next-of-kin. *Cancer, 55*, 72–76.

Cella, D. F., Orofiamma, B., Holland, J. C., Silberfarb, P. M., Tross, S., Feldstein, M., Perry, M., Maurer, H., Comis, R., & Orav, J. (1987). The relationship of psychological distress, extent of disease, and performance status in patients with lung cancer. *Cancer, 60*, 1661–1667.

Compas, B. E., Ey, S., & Grant, K. E. (1993). Taxonomy, assessment, and diagnosis of depression during adolescence. *Psychological Bulletin, 114*, 323–344.

Compas, B. E., Howell, D. C., Phares, V., Williams, R. A., & Ledoux, N. (1989). Parent and child stress and symptoms: An integrative analysis. *Developmental Psychology, 25*, 550–559.

Compas, B. E., & Wagner, B. M. (1991). Psychosocial stress during adolescence: Intrapersonal and interpersonal processes. In M. E. Colten & S. Gore (Eds.), *Adolescent stress: Causes and consequences* (pp. 67–85). New York: Aldine de Gruyter.

Compas, B. E., Worsham, N. L., & Ey, S. (1992). Conceptual and developmental issues in children's coping with stress. In A. M. La Greca, L. J. Siegel, J. L. Wallander, & C. E. Walker (Eds.), *Stress and coping in child health* (pp. 7–24). New York: Guilford Press.

Davis, G. E., & Compas, B. E. (1986). Cognitive appraisals of major and daily stressful events during adolescence: A multidimensional scaling analysis. *Journal of Youth and Adolescence, 15*, 377–388.

Derogatis, L. R., Morrow, G. R., Fetting, J., Penman, D., Piasetsky, S., Schmale, A. M., Henrichs, M., & Carnicke, C. L. M. (1983). The prevalence of psychiatric disorders among cancer patients. *Journal of the American Medical Association, 249*, 751–757.

Derogatis, L. R., & Spencer, P. M. (1982). *Administration and procedures: BSI manual: I.* Baltimore: Clinical Psychometric Research.

Ell, K., Nishimoto, R., Mantell, J., & Hamovitch, M. (1988). Longitudinal analysis of psychological adaptation among family members of patients with cancer. *Journal of Psychosomatic Research, 32*, 429–438.

Finch, A. J., & Rogers, T. R. (1984). Self-report instruments. In T. H. Ollendick & M. Hersen (Eds.), *Child behavioral assessment: Principles and procedures* (pp. 106–123). New York: Plenum Press.

Finch, A. J., Saylor, C. F., & Edwards, G. L. (1985). Children's Depression Inventory: Sex and grade norms for normal children. *Journal of Consulting and Clinical Psychology, 53*, 424–425.

Given, C. W., Stommel, M., Given, B., Osuch, J., Kurtz, M. E., & Kurtz, J. C. (1993). The influence of cancer patients' symptoms and functional status on patients' depression and family caregivers' reactions and depression. *Health Psychology, 12*, 277–285.

Hannur, J. W., Gresi-Davis, J. G., Harding, K., & Hatfield, A. K. (1991). Effects of individual and marital variables on coping with cancer. *Journal of Psychosocial Oncology, 9*, 1–20.

Heinrich, R. L., & Schag, C. C. (1987). The psychosocial impact of cancer: Cancer patients and healthy controls. *Journal of Psychosocial Oncology, 5*, 75–91.

Heinrich, R. L., Schag, C. C. & Ganz, P. A. (1984). Living with cancer: The Cancer Inventory of Problem Situations. *Journal of Clinical Psychology, 40*, 972–980.

Horowitz, M. J. (1982). Stress response syndromes and their treatment. In L. Goldberger & S. Breznitz (Eds.), *Handbook of stress: Theoretical and clinical aspects* (pp. 711–732). New York: Free Press.

Horowitz, M. J., Field, N. P., & Classen, C. C. (1993). Stress response syndromes and their treatment. In L. Goldberger & S. Breznitz (Eds.), *Handbook of stress: Theoretical and clinical aspects* (2nd ed., pp. 757–773). New York: Free Press.

Horowitz, M., Wilner, N., & Alvarez, W. (1979). Impact of Event Scale: A measure of subjective stress. *Psychosomatic Medicine, 41*, 209–218.

Kovacs, M. (1980). Rating scales to assess depression in school-aged children. *Acta Paedopsychiatrica, 46*, 305–315.

Lazarus, R. S., & Folkman, S. (1984). *Stress, appraisal and coping.* New York: Springer.

Lewis, F. M., Ellison, E., & Woods, N. F. (1985). The impact of breast cancer on the family. *Seminars in Oncology Nursing, 1*, 206–213.

Lewis, F. M., Hammond, M. A., & Woods, N. F. (1993). The family's functioning with newly diagnosed breast cancer in the mother: The development of an exploratory model. *Journal of Behavioral Medicine, 16*, 351–370.

Lewis, F. M., Woods, N. F., Hough, E. E., & Bensley, L. S. (1989). The family's functioning with chronic illness in the mother: The spouse's perspective. *Social Science and Medicine, 29*, 1261–1269.

Lichtman, R. R., & Taylor, S. E. (1986). Close relationships and the female cancer patient. In B. L. Andersen (Ed.), *Women with cancer: Psychological perspectives* (pp. 233–256). New York: Springer.

Lichtman, R. R., Taylor, S. E., & Wood, J. V. (1987). Social support and marital adjustment after breast cancer. *Journal of Psychosocial Oncology, 5(3)*, 47–71.

Marks, G., Richardson, J. L., Graham, J. W., & Levine, A. (1986). Health locus of control and expectations of treatment efficacy in adjustment to cancer. *Journal of Personality and Social Psychology, 51*, 443–450.

Massie, M. J., & Holland, J. C. (1987). The cancer patient and pain: Psychiatric complications and their management. *Medical Clinics of North America, 71*, 243–258.

Nolen-Hoeksema, S. (1990). *Sex differences in depression.* Stanford, CA: Stanford University Press.

Northouse, L. L., Cracchiolo, A., & Appel, C. P. (1991). Psychologic consequences of breast cancer on partner and family. *Seminars in Oncology Nursing, 7*, 216–223.

Northouse, L. L., & Swain, M. A. (1987). Adjustment of patients and husbands to the initial impact of breast cancer. *Nursing Research, 36*, 221–225.

Pettingale, K. W., Burgess, C., & Greer, S. (1988). Psychological response to cancer diagnosis: I. Correlations with prognostic variables. *Journal of Psychosomatic Research, 32*, 255–261.

Pynoos, R. S., Frederick, C., Nader, K., Arroyo, W., Steinberg, A., Eth, S., Nunez, F., & Fairbanks, L. (1987). Life threat and posttraumatic stress in school-age children. *Archives of General Psychiatry, 44*, 970–1063.

Reynolds, C. R., & Richmond, B. O. (1978). What I Think and Feel: A revised measure of children's manifest anxiety. *Journal of Abnormal Child Psychology, 6*, 271–280.

Saylor, C. F., Finch, A. J., Spirito, A., & Bennett, B. (1984). The Children's Depression Inventory: A systematic evaluation of psychometric properties. *Journal of Consulting and Clinical Psychology, 52*, 955–967.

Siegel, K., Mesagno, F. P., Karus, D., Christ, G., Banks, K., & Moynihan, R. (1992). Psychosocial adjustment of children with a terminally ill parent. *Journal of the American Academy of Child and Adolescent Psychiatry, 31*, 327–333.

Stanton, A. L., & Snider, P. R. (1993). Coping with a breast cancer diagnosis: A prospective study. *Health Psychology, 12*, 16–23.

Taylor, S. E. (1983). Adjustment to threatening events: A theory of cognitive adaptation. *American Psychologist, 38*, 1161–1173.

Wagner, B. M., & Compas, B. E. (1990). Gender, instrumentality, and expressivity: Moderators of the relation between stress and psychological symptoms during adolescence. *American Journal of Community Psychology, 18*, 383–406.

Watson, D., & Clarke, L. A. (1984). Negative affectivity: The disposition to experience aversive emotional states. *Psychological Bulletin, 96*, 465–490.

Wellisch, D. K., Gritz, E. R., Schain, W., Wang, H., & Saiu, J. (1991). Psychological functioning of daughters of breast cancer patients: Part I. Daughters and comparison subjects. *Psychosomatics, 32*, 324–336.

Wellisch, D. K., Gritz, E. R., Schain, W., Wang, H., & Saiu, J. (1992). Psychological functioning of daughters of breast cancer patients: Part II. Characterizing the distressed daughter of the breast cancer patient. *Psychosomatics, 33*, 169–179.

Chapter 12
YOUNG ADOLESCENT CANCER SURVIVORS AND THEIR PARENTS:
Adjustment, Learning Problems, and Gender

Anne E. Kazak, Dimitri Christakis, Melissa Alderfer, and Mary Jo Coiro

As survival rates increase for children with cancer, the psychological sequelae of having had cancer as a young child are only beginning to be understood. The largest body of psychological literature in this field has addressed the important neuropsychological effects of cranial irradiation on intelligence. These effects are seen as linear in nature (i.e., cranial irradiation causes cognitive impairment). Given the many factors that can mediate adaptation to childhood cancer, its long-term impact is best appreciated by more contextual and systemic research.

In this article, we present data from a study of psychological sequelae of treatment with particular attention to the impact of treatment on family and educational systems. Included are data on social adjustment and distress, family environments, support systems, and hopelessness from 10–15-year-old cancer survivors and their parents at two points in time. In addition, the practical implications of treatment for these children, many of whom are coping with learning problems subsequent to their treatment regimens, were examined.

Childhood Cancer Survival

There are many gaps in the understanding of the psychological impact of childhood cancer treatment experiences. Using general outcome measures, researchers of long-term survivors of childhood cancer have indicated adequate overall psychosocial adjustment (Brown et al., 1992; Fritz, Williams, & Amylon, 1988; Greenberg, Kazak, & Meadows, 1989; Kazak & Meadows, 1989; Spirito et al., 1990; Teta et al., 1986). However, the data fail to provide a sense of the impact of cancer survival on family members or an appreciation for factors that may enhance risk or provide buffering effects.

Declines in intellectual ability, secondary to cranial irradiation at the dose of 24 Gy, are well-established pediatric cancer sequelae (cf. Madan-Swain & Brown, 1991). Many survivors of childhood leukemia, including those who received 18 Gy, have cognitive and academic difficulties over time (Eiser, 1991; Mulhern, Fairclough, & Ochs, 1991; Peckham, Meadows, Bartel, & Marrero, 1988). They often receive special education service and additional assistance in postsecondary education and training programs. The significance of this, and the meaning of long-term learning

Reprinted from *Journal of Family Psychology, 8*(1), 74–84. (1994). Copyright © 1994 by the American Psychological Association. Used with permission of the author.

This research was supported by a grant from the University of Pennsylvania Research Foundation. The authors wish to thank Michael Manolas for his assistance in chart review.

difficulties directly related to their cancer treatments, are important contextual aspects of these young survivors' lives that warrant further investigation.

With a median age of diagnosis for acute lymphocyte leukemia (ALL) of 3–4 years (Sather, 1986), many children are very young at diagnosis. Although there is empirical evidence that even some of the youngest children have vivid recollections of their disease and treatments many years later (Kazak et al., 1992), it is also clear that their understanding of the disease and of their risk for relapse evolves over time. The most prominent feature of former patients and their parents is their anxiety related to memories of the treatment experience, fear of relapse, and potential future sequelae.

Methodological Concerns in Family Health Research

A common, although disputed, assumption is that families with a child with a chronic health problem will have a higher incidence of psychopathology than will similar families without an ill child. Studies involving heterogeneous groups of children have provided evidence that chronically ill children are at increased risk of psycho-pathology (Cadman, Boyle, Szatmari, & Offord, 1987). Other studies have documented a range of coping factors (Quitner, Glueckauf, & Jackson, 1990; Walker, Ortiz-Valdes, & Newbrough, 1989; Wallander, Varni, Babani, Banis, & Wilcox, 1989) and have shown strengths as well as vulnerabilities in these families (Kazak & Marvin, 1984).

A recurrent problem in this literature on the families of chronically ill children has been the inclusion of children who are from a wide range in age. Statistically controlling for age does not overcome the problems that are created when important developmental issues are neglected. In this study, we limited our sample to young adolescents and preadolescents who were 10–15-year-olds and who had cancer when they were young children, and their parents. This age group was chosen because of the prominent parallel processes that occur during this period: Adolescents are differentiating from their family while becoming more independent and their peer group is becoming of increasing importance to them.

Both these issues seem particularly salient for children who were seriously ill while young. With adolescence comes an increased understanding of cancer and the threats that it posed and still poses. Moreover, adolescence is a time of heightened sensitivity to perceived differences in appearance, capabilities, or personal history. At this stage of survivors' lives, their risks of infertility, risks of late relapse or secondary malignancies, and possible academic limitations have a great impact.

The use of control groups in research in this field is controversial. There is a growing body of literature on families with ill children that has shown no differences between families with and without affected children. The resultant failure to reject the null hypothesis is both theoretically and methodologically troublesome. Although it is encouraging to document adaptive functioning in families despite the chronic strains of childhood illness, the need to better understand and characterize the impact these strains have on children and their families remains. It is likely that the types of differences seen are not indicative of psychopathology, but are related to more subtle aspects of adjustment and coping. Indded, the use of comparison or control groups may be altogether inappropriate because they fail to control (or contain) the critical elements in coping with childhood chronic illness (Kazak & Nachman, 1991).

The Present Study

This study is an extension of an earlier project (Kazak & Meadows, 1989) in which we found generally normative levels of psychological functioning in 10–15-year-old long-term survivors and showed that the presence of learning problems is a psychosocial risk factor for these adolescents and their families. In this article, we present data from young adolescents who have survived childhood cancer and their parents and look at their social adjustment and distress, family environment, support systems, anxiety, and hopelessness at two points in time. This design provided a short-term longitudinal approach, which examined the nature of change and stability over a year's time. It also represents one piece of a larger longitudinal study.

Variables were chosen to reflect individual and family functioning that were consistent with previous research on families of children with special health-care needs. Self-report measures of adolescent behavior, anxiety, hopelessness, social support, and family cohesion and adaptability provided data on the adolescents' views of their individual, social, and family functioning. Hopelessness was included as an alternative to depression, as it examines ways in which the future is viewed. Because of the ongoing threat to life that is inherent in survival (cf. Koocher & O'Malley, 1981), perceptions of one's future (depressive thinking) may be a more meaningful construct than is clinical depression to gain an understanding of the ways in which long-term survivors function. Although it is an important factor, gender has generally been overlooked as a variable in studies of long-term survivors. We included it as a way of further understanding the social context of adolescent long-term survivors and its impact on adjustment. Parental report variables included parents' individual distress, family functioning, and perceptions of their child's behavioral adjustment.

Specifically, we hypothesized that overall levels of adjustment for young adolescent survivors and their parents would be within normal limits for well-validated instruments. We expected to find a significant group of survivors who experience symptomatology consistent with anxiety of a distressing magnitude. It was also expected that a subset of parents of long-term survivors would experience significant psychological distress. We hypothesized that those survivors who received special education services would have poorer overall adjustment. Gender was introduced as an exploratory variable because it has not been systemically addressed in previous research on long-term survivors of childhood cancer.

Method

Subjects

Tumor registry records at the Children's Hospital of Philadelphia were used to identify survivors of childhood cancer for a prospective study of psychological adjustment. Subjects were between the ages of 10 and 15 years when they entered the study and had been off treatment and free of disease for at least 5 years.[1] Most were diagnosed and treated for cancer while they were preschoolers.

Prospective data collection began in 1987 with a sample of 10–15-year-old survivors of ALL, acute myelomonocytic leukemia (AML), and non-Hodgkin's lymphoma and their parents. Most (87%) had survived ALL; there were only minor variations in the treatments received. All of the patients had completed 2–3 years of oral, intravenous, and intrathecal chemotherapy. In 1989, the sample was increased to include more families whose children met the same inclusion criteria but were long-term survivors of a wider range of types of cancer (38% were diagnosed with ALL, 18% with Wilms' tumor, and 15% with non-Hodgkin's lymphoma) and had received a broader range of therapies. Five of the participants had relapsed but had been off treatment and free of disease for at least 5 years since their recurrence. With respect to radiation, 30.1% of the sample did not receive radiation, 39.7% had 18 Gy, 15.1% had 24 Gy; and 15.1% received other, noncranial irradiation. For this article, we report data from two collection points: the point at which the sample was increased in 1989 and one year later.

Procedure

A letter describing the study was sent in 1987 to all 65 eligible families. Because of the length of time since treatment, some shrinkage of the potential sample was inevitable because of patients who could not be reached: 18 (27.6%) of the letters were returned to us with no forwarding address, and we were unable to locate more recent phone numbers or addresses for these patients. The 47 families who were contacted successfully became our sample. In 1989, 53 more families were contacted. From this group, 12 (22.6%) could not be located. The remaining 41 families were added to the original sample, yielding a potential sample of 88. These 88 families were mailed self-report questionnaires, with self-addressed, stamped return envelopes. Written consent was obtained from parents and children with the questionnaire packet. The study was approved by the hospital's Institutional Review Board.

Participation rates for the two data points were 74 (84.1%) for Time 1 and 59 (67.0%) for Time 2. Chi-square analyses were performed to test for differences between those survivors who participated and those who did not with respect to data available from the tumor registry (i.e., age, age at diagnosis, sex, cranial radiation therapy, medical late effects of treatment, socioeconomic status, and educational placement). There were no significant differences between those who participated and those who did not on these variables.

Basic demographic data were collected at the time of each family's first participation. Data on school grade, special education placement, and whether the child had changed or was about to change schools were collected every spring. Diagnosis, treatment, physical effects of treatment, and pubertal status were collected from on-

---

[1]To study the process of transition to adolescence, 10–15 year olds were included in the study. Although 10 year olds might more aptly be termed preadolescents, they were included to capture those patients who would have early pubescence. In light of indications that younger children now participate in behaviors once associated solely with older adolescents (e.g., dating, sex, and drug and alcohol abuse), we felt that it was important to err on the side of overinclusion rather than to omit those younger patients who were experiencing adolescent biological changes and social pressures.

cology records. The following dependent measures were obtained at each data collection point.[2]

Measures for Adolescents

The Family Adaptation and Cohesion Evaluation Scales—Version III (FACES–III)

FACES–III is a 20 item self-report scale based on the Circumplex Model of Marital and Family Systems (Olson, Portner, & Bell, 1982). The model is based on the importance of cohesiveness and adaptability in family functioning. Four levels of cohesion (disengaged, separated, connected, and enmeshed) and four levels of adaptability (rigid, structured, flexible, and chaotic) are posited. Alpha reliabilities reported in the FACES–III manual range from .58 to .77 (Olson, Portner, & Lavee, 1985). The scales are useful in differentiating functional and dysfunctional families (Garbarino, Sebes, & Schellenbach, 1984; Rodick, Henggeler, & Hanson, 1986) and are a valuable tool for identifying parent–child dyads that may develop destructive interaction patterns during adolescence (Garbarino et al., 1984). FACES–III was normed on a large, national sample that provides an adequate base for generalization from the present sample. Recent research indicated that data interpretation should be linear, rather than curvilinear (Olson, 1991).

The Self-Perception Profile for Adolescents

This scale (Harter, 1986) is a self-report measure assessing perceptions of competence and self-worth with nine subscales: Scholastic Competence, Social Acceptance, Athletic Competence, Physical Appearance, Job Competence, Romantic Appeal, Conduct–Morality, Close Friendship, and Global Self-Worth. The scale is an extension of earlier work on young children and has alpha reliabilities ranging from .85 to .95.

The Social Support Rating Scale (SSRS)

The SSRS (Cauce, 1986; Cauce, Felner, & Primavera, 1982) was modified slightly to include 17 sources of social support on three factors (family, friends, and school/ other adults). Adolescents indicated the extent to which persons provided emotional support and caring, help, and guidance and the extent to which each person may have upset them on a 5-point Likert-type scale. They also indicated the extent to which they are satisfied with the emotional support and help they receive and the extent to which they are the sort of person who seeks help on a 7-point Likert-type scale. Each subscale consists of items loading 0.5 or above and each has an eigen-

---

[2]All the measures chosen have reading levels that are appropriate for 10–15 year olds. Some of the data was missing because of the occasional difficulty that subjects experienced in reading the materials. The adolescents were strongly encouraged to complete the measures independent of parental supervision.

value greater than or equal to 1.0. The scale factors have internal consistency coefficients (Cronbach's alpha) exceeding .75. Normative data are provided only for total scores; because the scale was modified, comparisons with the normative data are not valid. The SSRS is one of the few social support scales for children and adolescents and is unique in its examination of separate sources of support. Subscales were shown to correlate significantly with ratings of self-competence (Cauce, Hannan, & Sargeant, 1987).

The State-Trait Anxiety Inventory for Children (STAIC)

The STAIC (Spielberger, 1973) provides self-report ratings on a total of 40 items assessing anxiety at a particular moment in time (state) and in general (trait). The STAIC is well normed and validated, particularly with respect to factors affecting school achievement.

The Hopelessness Scale for Children (HSC)

The HSC (Kazdin, Rodgers, & Colbus, 1986) is a 17 item true–false measure of hopelessness, or negative expectations about the future. The strong psychometric properties of the HSC have been supported, including the ability to discriminate between normal and depressed adolescents (Spirito, Williams, Stark, & Hart, 1988).

The Children's Social Desirability Questionnaire (CSD)

The CSD (Crandall, Crandall, & Katkovsky, 1965) is a scale developed to assess the extent to which children are responding in a socially acceptable manner. The original scale was developed and validated on a sample of 956 students in Grades 3 through 12 and has been used in other research on adolescents (Shirk, 1987). Shorter versions of the CSD have also been used (Eisenberg, Cialdini, McCreath, & Shell, 1987). A measure of social desirability was introduced in this study for two reasons. First, the extent to which respondents answer in a socially desirable manner, which is often presumed to be a less honest manner, plagues all studies based on self-report. Second, social desirability may be affecting the responses of cancer survivors because they may feel that it is important to appear to be without problems or they may want to impress adults.

Measures for Parents

The Langner Symptom Checklist (LSC)

The LSC (Langner, 1962) is a 22-item scale that assesses symptoms of anxiety and depression. The LSC has been established as a good measure of general mental health and is used widely in assessing adjustment and demoralization (Billings & Moos, 1984; Dohrenwend, Shrout, Egri, & Mendelson, 1980) and in studies of families with chronically ill and disabled children (Kazak, 1987; Kazak, Reber, & Snitzer, 1988).

The Child Behavior Checklist (CBCL)

The CBCL (Achenbach & Edelbrock, 1978) is a widely used, 113-item, self-report questionnaire that assesses childhood and adolescent psychopathology. Four scales have been identified through factor analysis: internalizing, externalizing, behavior problems, and social competence. Median test–retest reliability is .89, with evidence that the scale differentiates between disturbed and nondisturbed children (Achenbach & Edelbrock, 1983). The scale has been used widely in studies of children with chronic illness and of children with cancer (cf. Mulhern, Wasserman, Friedman, & Fairclough, 1989).

FACES–III

The FACES–III measure was also given to parents and is described above.

Results

Because of the multiple comparisons made, we used one criterion ($p < .01$) for statistical significance with another ($p < .05$) for statistical trends.

Sample Description

The mean age of the cancer survivors at the beginning of the study was 12.3 years with a mean age at diagnosis of 3.7 years. Of the participants, 66% had been diagnosed with ALL, 8% with non-Hodgkin's lymphoma, and 8% with Wilms' tumor. Other cancers, each of which appeared in no more than 3 subjects, were sarcomas, rhabdomyosarcomas, AML, osteosarcomas, Hodgkin's disease, retinoblastomas, t-cell lymphomas, and neuroblastomas. The mean length of time since diagnosis was 96.20 months ($SD = 29.54$), with the mean length of time since treatment ended being 70.80 months ($SD = 27.30$).

More than three quarters of the sample were White, including 2 who had Asian mothers and 1 who had an Asian father. Mean parental age was in the late 30s and early 40s, with 40% having completed high school, 43% being college educated, and 18% having some postgraduate education. Median income was $35,000. Approximately one quarter ($N = 27$) were identified by their parents as receiving special services in school related to learning problems.

Chi-square analysis and t tests were performed to test for differences between the initial and expanded samples with respect to age, age at diagnosis, sex, educational placement, and family demographic variables. The groups differed in terms of their sex composition: Of the initial group 60% were male adolescents, whereas of the follow-up group, 60% were female adolescents. The groups did not differ with respect to family background variables.

Adolescent Variables

Scores on measures of adolescent adjustment at Times 1 and 2 were generally within normal limits (Table 1).

Scores on FACES–III show that these adolescents rated their families within the separated (cohesion) and structured (adaptability) ranges that are developmentally appropriate and consistent with FACES–III norms. The Harter scores were generally consistent with normative values, although several significant gender differences were found. Male adolescents rated themselves higher on physical appearance than did female adolescents at Time 1, $t(60) = 2.68$, $p < .01$, with a similar trend found at Time 2 $t(48) = 2.39$, $p < .05$. Male adolescents perceived their athletic competence higher than did female adolescents at Time 2, $t(60) = 3.2$, $p < .01$, with a similar trend for Time 1, $t(60) = 2.29$, $p < .05$. Male adolescents also perceived their scholastic competence at Time 2 higher than did female adolescents, $t(50) = 2.60$, $p < .01$.

Social support from family was rated consistently higher than was support from friends and school staff. Normative data are not available on the SRSS because of modifications made for this sample. The sample means for hopelessness fall below the norms provided for the normative (nonpsychiatric) sample ($p < .05$); 73% (Time 1) and 70% (Time 2) of the sample are in the range of low hopelessness. Those with a score in the high hopelessness range are a subset of the sample: 6% at Time 1 and 8% at Time 2.

For female adolescents, state and trait anxiety mean scores and frequency distributions were comparable to normative values. However, for male adolescents, sample scores were significantly lower than were the norms ($p < .001$). On trait anxiety, male adolescents scored significantly lower than did female adolescents (whose scores were comparable to norms) at Time 1, $t(70) = 4.89$, $p < .0001$, and Time 2, $t(52) = 3.68$, $p < .001$.

Examination of correlations between the CSD and the adolescent dependent measures revealed several significant relationships between the tendency for subjects to want to look good and the outcome measures (Table 2). Social desirability correlated significantly and inversely with anxiety measured by the STAIC. Of the Harter scales, the only consistent significant correlation was with Conduct and Morality. For social support, the primary association was between social desirability and a reporting of being upset in relationships with family and friends. There were no gender differences in social desirability scores.

Overall there was little change over the year between Time 1 and Time 2. Less social support was reported from parents, with respect to emotional support, $F(2, 44) = 11.32$, $p < .001$, and help and guidance, $F(2, 44) = 3.66$, $p < .05$. Similarly, less support was reported from teachers and other adults at school, particularly for emotional support, $F(2, 43) = 4.71$, $p < .01$.

Parental Variables

Mothers' and fathers' reports of their adolescent cancer survivor's behavior on the CBCL are consistent with normative values (Table 3). CBCL scores were examined to determine the percentage of former patients whose scores were outside one stan-

Table 1—*Means and Standard Deviations for Adolescent Variables at Times 1 and 2*

Measure/variable	Time 1 (n = 74)		Time 2 (n = 59)		Norms	
	M	SD	M	SD	M	SD
FACES–III						
Cohesion	35.2	6.5	33.8	7.0	37.1	6.1
Adaptability	23.3	6.4	22.0	5.1	24.3	4.8
Harter scale						
Female adolescents						
Scholastic competence	2.8	0.6	3.0	0.7	2.9	—
Social acceptance	3.1	0.7	3.1	0.8	3.0	—
Athletic competence	2.5	0.8	2.4	0.8	2.9	—
Physical appearance	2.5	0.7	2.5	0.7	2.9	—
Job competence	3.2	0.5	3.2	0.5	3.2	—
Romantic appeal	2.6	0.8	2.7	0.8	2.5	—
Conduct–morality	2.8	0.6	3.1	0.6	3.2	—
Close friendship	3.4	0.8	3.4	0.6	3.2	—
Global self-worth	3.1	0.7	3.2	0.7	3.1	—
Male adolescents						
Scholastic competence	3.1	0.7	3.3	0.6	2.7	—
Social acceptance	3.2	0.5	3.3	0.7	3.1	—
Athletic competence	2.9	0.8	3.0	0.6	2.7	—
Physical appearance	2.9	0.7	3.0	0.6	2.9	—
Job competence	3.4	0.6	3.4	0.4	3.0	—
Romantic appeal	2.8	0.5	2.8	0.9	2.5	—
Conduct–morality	3.1	0.4	3.2	0.4	3.4	—
Close friendship	3.1	0.5	3.4	0.5	3.4	—
Global self-worth	3.3	0.5	3.4	0.5	3.0	—
SSRS[a]						
Family						
Emotional	4.0	0.6	3.8	0.7	—	—
Help	4.0	0.6	3.8	0.7	—	—
Upset	2.4	0.9	2.5	0.7	—	—
Friends						
Emotional	3.6	0.9	3.4	0.8	—	—
Help	3.5	0.9	3.3	0.8	—	—
Upset	2.3	0.8	2.7	0.7	—	—
School						
Emotional	3.2	1.0	2.8	1.0	—	—
Help	3.2	1.0	3.0	1.0	—	—
Upset	2.1	0.8	2.3	0.7	—	—
STAIC						
Female adolescents						
State	30.5	6.0	30.7	6.6	31.8	5.8
Trait	37.9	6.8	37.8	7.2	37.3	6.0
Male adolescents						
State	28.4	5.5	30.7	6.6	30.6	5.6
Trait	30.4**	6.2	30.3**	7.7	37.3	6.7

Table continues

Table 1—(*Continued*)

	Time 1 (n = 74)		Time 2 (n = 59)		Norms	
Measure/variable	*M*	*SD*	*M*	*SD*	*M*	*SD*
HSC					3.7	3.1
Female adolescents	3.4	2.6	3.7	2.6	—	—
Male adolescents	2.2*ʻ	2.0	2.3*	1.4	—	—
CSD[a]	4.8	3.0	4.3	2.7	—	—

Note. FACES–III = Family Adaptation and Cohesion Evaluation Scales—Version III; Harter scale = Self-Perception Profile for Adolescents; SSRS = Social Support Rating Scale; STAIC = State–Trait Anxiety Inventory for Children; HSC = Hopelessness Scale for Children; CSD = Children's Social Desirability Questionnaire. Dashes indicate not applicable.

[a]Direct comparisons with normative data could not be made because of the minor modifications to the SSRS and the CSD.

*p < .05.

**p < .001.

dard deviation from the T score. This ranged from 25.4% to 48.1% across mothers' and fathers' reports at both data points. The highest percentage of extreme scores was found on the internalizing dimension, with data showing a skew toward higher levels of internalizing behaviors reported by parents.

Parental reports of their own symptoms indicative of psychological distress on the LSC are also consistent with norms and previous studies of parents of handicapped and chronically ill children (Kazak & Marvin, 1984; Kazak et al., 1988). A score of greater than 3 is considered predictive of seeking help for psychological distress, with a score above 6 being indicative of significant psychological distress. Between 20% and 30% of parents had scores above 3 at the two data points, and between 8.8% and 10.0% fell within the psychologically distressed range. On FACES–III, parental reports of cohesion are within the separated and adaptability (structured) ranges that are consistent with the norms and with the ratings provided by the adolescents.

Adolescents With Learning Difficulties

In general, those survivors with identified learning problems who were receiving some special services in school scored lower on several Harter scales. Those survivors in special education reported significantly lower scores on Scholastic Competence, $t(60) = 5.27$, $p < .001$, with similar trends seen for Physical Appearance, $t(60) = 3.05$, $p < .05$, Romantic Appeal, $t(60) = 2.21$, $p < .05$, and Athletic Competence, $t(59) = 2.50$, $p < .05$. They also reported significantly higher levels of trait anxiety, $t(58) = 3.46$, $p < .001$, and their parents reported them on the CBCL as having significantly lower levels of social competence, $t(60) = 2.73$, $p < .005$. Trends were found for higher levels of emotional support, $t(60) = 2.42$, $p < .05$, help and guidance, $t(60) = 2.42$, $p < .05$, as well as for higher levels of upset from teachers

Table 2—*Correlations Between Social Desirability and Adolescent Variables at Times 1 and 2*

	Social desirability	
Measure/variable	Time 1	Time 2
FACES–III		
Cohesion	.19	.28*
Adaptability	.14	.01
Harter scale		
Scholastic competence	−.03	.16
Social acceptance	.08	.04
Athletic competence	−.11	−.04
Physical appearance	.23	.41**
Job competence	.49**	.34
Romantic appeal	.11	.30
Conduct–morality	.38**	.41**
Close friendship	.30	.33
Global self-worth	.17	.34*
SSRS		
Family		
Emotional	.16	.20
Help	.24*	.34**
Upset	−.53****	−.31*
Friends		
Emotional	.03	−.10
Help	.07	−.10
Upset	−.27*	−.13
School		
Emotional	.05	.04
Help	.02	.14
Upset	−.15	.00
STAIC		
State	−.33**	−.33*
Trait	−.34***	−.36**
HSC	−.13	−.23

Note. FACES–III = Family Adaptation and Cohesion Evaluation Scales—Version III; Harter scale = Self-Perception Profiles for Adolescents; SSRS = Social Support Rating Scale; STAIC = State–Trait Anxiety Inventory for Children; HSC = Hopelessness Scale for Children.

    *$p < .05$.
    **$p < .01$.
    ***$p < .001$.
    ****$p < .0001$.

and other school personnel, $t(60) = 2.19$, $p < .05$, than were found for those survivors without learning difficulties. Interestingly, those survivors in special education reported lower levels of satisfaction with the help and guidance they receive, $t(60) = 3.07$, $p < .005$. There were no differences in the number of male and female ado-

Table 3—*Means and Standard Deviations in Parent Variables at Times 1 and 2*

Measure/variable	Time 1		Time 2		Norms	
	M	*SD*	*M*	*SD*	*M*	*SD*
Mothers (*n* = 71)						
FACES–III						
Cohesion	37.6	5.5	35.9	5.7	37.1	6.1
Adaptability	22.1	5.4	21.5	5.4	24.3	4.8
LSC	2.9	2.5	2.8	2.8	2.6	2.7
CBCL						
Internalizing	54.2	9.7	53.3	10.7	50.0	10.0
Externalizing	51.7	9.7	51.0	10.0	50.0	10.0
Behavior problems	54.5	10.7	53.2	11.8	50.0	10.0
Social competence	46.8	11.5	46.5	9.8	50.0	10.0
Fathers (*n* = 58)						
FACES–III						
Cohesion	36.7	6.4	35.0	6.2	37.1	6.1
Adaptability	22.8	5.2	21.6	5.7	24.3	4.8
LSC	2.4	2.9	2.2	3.2	2.6	2.7
CBCL						
Internalizing	52.5	10.4	51.3	9.3	50.0	10.0
Externalizing	50.0	9.4	49.0	9.0	50.0	10.0
Behavior problems	51.7	11.6	51.7	11.6	50.0	10.0
Social competence	46.1	10.7	42.9	9.2	50.0	10.0

Note. FACES–III = Family Adaptation and Cohesion Evaluation Scales—Version III; LSC = Langer Symptom Checklist; CBCL = Child Behavior Checklist.

lescents receiving special education services and no interaction effects between gender and special education placement.

Discussion

Our data lend confirmation to the body of research that has indicated that most survivors of childhood cancer do well in terms of general psychological outcome. This study has also provided information about the psychological adjustment of a much less-studied group, the parents of survivors. As predicted, these adolescents scored near normative levels with respect to family functioning, social support, and perceived self-competence. Their parents also showed levels of psychological distress, family functioning, and perceptions of their adolescent children that are consistent with norms for the instruments used. Nonetheless, the subgroup that was found of patients and their parents with increased levels of distress suggests the importance of ongoing research to understand the psychological impact of treatment for both the child and family. An interesting contribution of these data concerns the role of learning problems and gender in terms of understanding issues related to survival.

Although the risk for cognitive impairment and learning problems in childhood cancer survivors has been apparent for some time, the impact of a child having long-term learning difficulties on social and family functioning is less well understood. In our study, those long-term survivors receiving special education services rated themselves lower across a variety of dimensions on the Harter scales, had higher levels of anxiety, and were perceived as having more behavioral difficulties by their parents. They also received higher levels of social support and tended to have lower social desirability scores. The data support the idea that those long-term survivors with learning problems are at higher risk than are those without learning problems. This is consistent with research that has indicated that damage to the central nervous system is a key predictor of chronic adjustment difficulties in children with other handicapping conditions (Breslau, 1985). The higher levels of social support that they receive do not necessarily buffer them from psychological distress, but may reflect differences in the social relationships of children with cancer and the ways in which they are perceived by peers and teachers (Noll, Bukowski, Rogosch, LeRoy, & Kulkarni, 1990). This is clearly a complex issue and warrants future investigation to understand the relationship between learning problems and adjustment in children with and without cancer. For example, children with even mild reading disabilities have been shown to have significant impairments in their self-concept, with parental perceptions and evaluations of their child uncorrelated (Casey, Levy, Brown, & Brooks-Gunn, 1992).

Male adolescent cancer survivors in our sample scored very low on measures of anxiety and hopelessness and were below both normative values and female adolescents' scores in this sample. This result is similar to other studies of childhood cancer survivors, where an unexpected low level of depression has been found (Greenberg et al., 1989; Worchel et al., 1988). These curious results have been interpreted as being a sign of denial or as truly being a low level of depression. Clinically, these data are bothersome and inconsistent with general studies of psychological risk in children with chronic health problems (Cadman et al., 1987).

Our data suggest that gender may play a role in explaining this finding, in that male adolescents reported significantly lower levels of anxiety and hopelessness than did female adolescents, and scored below the norms on these variables. Male adolescents also tended to feel better about themselves in several domains on the Harter scales. Among the interesting questions that need to be addressed in future research are the possible developmental differences between male and female adolescents, differences in the ways that male and female childhood cancer survivors may be treated and socialized, or differences in the effects that their childhood cancer experiences had on their development and memories.

It is becoming increasingly important to understand the mechanisms that either project or endanger the growing numbers of pediatric cancer survivors. Doing so requires focusing not only on the individual survivors, but also on the systems (families, schools, hospitals, and clinics) with which these children interact. Research is needed that will follow these patients over time, be sensitive to school and gender effects, and develop measures that examine specific parameters affected by the nature of their cancer and its course. The data in this study provide information on individual adjustment, family functioning, and social support in 10–15-year-old adolescents and their parents, while explaining the importance that school placement and gender may play in psychological outcome for this population.

There are two potential problems with the methods used that warrant discussion. The first is that 27.6% of the first set of eligible patients and 22.6% of the second were lost to follow-up. Although it is disappointing that nearly one quarter of potential subjects could not be located, we chose to exclude them from our sample and believe that no significant skew resulted from this. All of these missing patients are medically cured and have no reason to maintain contact with the hospital or to provide a forwarding address. Consequently, we infer that they were no different from the population that ultimately served as our sample, except perhaps that they moved more recently. For purposes of long-term follow-up, more aggressive record keeping may be necessary to maintain contact with former patients and their families, some of whom inevitably will relocate over the course of many years.

The second concern in research of this type is its reliance on self-report measures. The unsupervised administration of the measures in this project could lead to an underreporting of problems because subjects may have sought to convince either themselves or others that they were better adjusted than they actually were. However, except in occasions where subjects might need help to understand the instructions, it is difficult to conceive of a scenario where professional supervision would lead to a decreased reporting of problems. Therefore, these data probably do represent a valid description of the minimal scope of the problem.

Continued research on long-term survivors of childhood cancer is needed to clarify some issues outlined in this article. Gender is an attribute of an individual but is very much affected by the influence of family, society, and culture. Although previously unexplored in this population, gender may help explain the long-term implications of childhood cancer survival. The presence of learning problems is a reality for many long-term survivors of childhood cancer and their parents. Further research is needed to understand the ways that school and family systems interact over time and how children and families can be prepared for the academic, emotional, family, and social implications of these long-term sequelae. Interventions for this population, including, potentially, school-based programs, can be guided by the results of this future research.

References

Achenbach, T., & Edelbrock, C. (1978). The classification of childhood psychopathology: A review and analysis of empirical efforts. *Psychological Bulletin, 85,* 1275–1301.

Achenbach, T., & Edelbrock, C. (1983). *Manual for the Child Behavior Checklist and Revised Child Behavior Profile*. Burlington: University of Vermont, Department of Psychiatry.

Billings, A., & Moos, R. (1984). Coping, stress, and social resources among adults with unipolar depression. *Journal of Personality and Social Psychology, 96,* 877–891.

Breslau, N. (1985). Psychiatric disorder in children with disabilities. *Journal of the American Academy of Child Psychiatry, 24,* 87–94.

Brown, R., Kaslow, N., Hazzard, A., Madan-Swain, A., Sexson, S., Lambert, R., & Baldwin, K. (1992). Psychiatric and family functioning in children with leukemia and their parents. *Journal of the American Academy of Child and Adolescent Psychiatry, 31,* 495–502.

Cadman, D., Boyle, M., Szatmari, P., & Offord, D. (1987). Chronic illness, disabilities and mental and social well-being: Findings of the Ontario Child Health Study. *Pediatrics, 79,* 805–813.

Casey, R., Levy, S., Brown, K., & Brooks-Gunn, J. (1992). Impaired emotional health in children with mild reading disability. *Developmental and Behavorial Pediatrics, 13,* 256–260.

Cauce, A. (1986). Social networks and social competence: Exploring the effects of early adolescent friendships. *American Journal of Community Psychology, 14,* 607–628.

Cauce, A., Felner, R., & Primavera, J. (1982). Social support in high risk adolescents: Structural components and adaptive impact. *American Journal of Community Psychology, 10,* 417–428.

Cauce, A., Hannan, K., & Sargeant, M. (1987). *Negative events, social support, and locus of control in adolescence: Continutions to well-being.* Paper presented at the 95th Annual Convention of the American Psychological Association, New York, NY.

Crandall, V., Crandall, V., & Katkovsky, W. (1965). A children's social desirability questionnaire. *Journal of Counseling Psychology, 29,* 27–36.

Dohrenwend, B., Shrout, P., Egri, G., & Mendelson, F. (1980). Nonspecific psychological distress and other dimensions of psychopathology. *Archives of General Psychiatry, 37,* 1229–1238.

Eisenberg, N., Cialdini, R., McCreath, H., & Shell, R. (1987). Consistency-based compliance: When and how do children become vulnerable? *Journal of Personality and Social Psychology, 52,* 1174–1181.

Eiser, C. (1991). Cognitive deficits in children treated for leukemia. *Archives of Disease in Childhood, 66,* 164–168.

Fritz, G., Williams, J., & Amylon, M. (1988). After treatment ends: Psychosocial sequelae in pediatric cancer survivors. *American Journal of Orthopsychiatry, 58,* 552–561.

Garbarino, J., Sebes, J., & Schellenbach, C. (1984). Families at risk for destructive parent–child relations in adolescence. *Child Development, 55,* 174–183.

Greenberg, H., Kazak, A., & Meadows, A. (1989). Psychological adjustment in 8 to 16 year old cancer survivors and their parents. *Journal of Pediatrics, 114,* 488–493.

Harter, S. (1986). *Self-Perception Profile for Adolescents.* Denver, CO: University of Denver, Department of Psychology.

Kazak, A. (1987). Families with disabled children: Stress and social networks in three samples. *Journal of Abnormal Child Psychology, 15,* 137–146.

Kazak, A., & Marvin, R. (1984). Differences, difficulties, and adaptation: Stress and social networks in families with a handicapped child. *Family Relations, 33,* 67–77.

Kazak, A., & Meadows, A. (1989). Families of young adolescents who have survived cancer: Social–emotional adjustment, adaptability, and social support. *Journal of Pediatric Psychology, 14,* 175–191.

Kazak, A., & Nachman, G. (1991). Family research on childhood chronic illness: Pediatric oncology as an example. *Journal of Family Psychology, 4,* 462–483.

Kazak, A., Reber, M., & Snitzer, L. (1988). Childhood chronic disease and family functioning: A study of phenylketonuria. *Pediatrics, 81,* 224–230.

Kazak, A., Stuber, M., Torchinsky, M., Houskamp, B., Christakis, D., & Kasiraj, J. (1992, August). *Post traumatic stress in childhood cancer survivors and their parents.* Poster presented at the 100th Annual Convention of the American Psychological Association, Washington, DC.

Kazdin, A., Rodgers, A., & Colbus, D. (1986). The Hopelessness Scale for Children: Psychometric characteristics and concurrent validity. *Journal of Consulting and Clinical Psychology, 54,* 241–245.

Koocher, G., & O'Malley, J. (1981). *The Damocles Syndrome,* New York: McGraw-Hill.

Langner, T. (1962). A 22-item screening score of psychiatric symptoms indicating impairment. *Journal of Health and Human Behavior, 3,* 269–276.

Madan-Swain, A., & Brown, R. (1991). Cognitive and psychosocial sequelae for children with acute lymphocytic leukemia and their families. *Clinical Psychology Review, 11,* 267–294.

Mulhern, R., Fairclough, D., & Ochs, J. (1991). A prospective comparison of neuropsychologic performance of children surviving leukemia who received 18 Gy, 24 Gy, or no cranial irradiation. *Journal of Clinical Oncology, 9,* 1348–1356.

Mulhern, R., Wasserman, A., Friedman, A., & Fairclough, D. (1989). Social competence and behavioral adjustment of children who are long-term survivors of cancer. *Pediatrics, 83,* 18–25.

Noll, R., Bukowski, W., Rogosch, F., LeRoy, S., & Kulkarni, R. (1990). Social interactions between children with cancer and their peers: Teacher ratings. *Journal of Pediatric Psychology, 15,* 43–56.

Olson, D. (1991). Commentary: Three dimensional (3-D) Circumplex Model and revised scoring of FACESIII. *Family Process, 30,* 74–79.

Olson, D., Portner, J., & Bell, R. (1982). Family Adaptability and Cohesion Evaluation Scales. In D. Olson, H. McCubbin, H. Barnes, A. Lavsen, M. Muxen, & M. Wilson (Eds.), *Family inventories: Inventories used in a national survey of families across the family life cycle.* St. Paul: University of Minnesota, Department of Family Social Science.

Olson, D., Portner, J., & Lavee, Y. (1985). *FACESIII.* St. Paul: University of Minnesota, Department of Family Social Science.

Peckham, V., Meadows, A., Bartel, N., & Marrero, O. (1988). Educational late effects in long-term survivors of childhood ALL. *Pediatrics, 81,* 127–133.

Quitner, A., Glueckauf, R., & Jackson, D. (1990). Chronic parenting stress: Moderating versus mediating effects of social support. *Journal of Personality and Social Psychology, 59,* 1266–1278.

Rodick, J., Henggeler, S., & Hanson, C. (1986). An evaluation of the Family Adaptability and Cohesion Evaluation Sales and the Circumplex Model. *Journal of Abnormal Child Psychology, 14,* 77–87.

Sather, H. (1986). Age at diagnosis in childhood acute lymphoblastic leukemia. *Medical and Pediatric Oncology, 14,* 166–172.

Shirk, S. (1987). Self-doubt in late childhood and early adolescence. *Journal of Youth and Adolescence, 16,* 59–68.

Spielberger, C. (1973). *The State–Trait Anxiety Inventory for Children.* Palo Alto, CA: Consulting Psychologists Press.

Spirito, A., Stark, L., Cobiella, C., Drigan, R., Androkites, A., & Hewitt, K. (1990). Social adjustment of children successfully treated for cancer. *Journal of Pediatric Psychology, 15,* 359–371.

Spirito, A., Williams, C., Stark, L., & Hart, K. (1988). The Hopelessness Scale for Children: Psychometric properties with normal and emotionally disturbed adolescents. *Journal of Abnormal Child Psychology, 16,* 445–458.

Teta, M., Po, M., Kasl, S., Meigs, J., Myers, M., & Mulvihill, J. (1986). Psychosocial consequences of childhood and adolescent cancer survival. *Journal of Chronic Diseases, 39,* 751–759.

Walker, L., Ortiz-Valdes, J., & Newbrough, J. (1989). The role of maternal employment and depression in the psychological adjustment of chronically ill, mentally retarded, and healthy children. *Journal of Pediatric Psychology, 14,* 357–370.

Wallander, J., Varni, J., Babani, L., Banis, H., & Wilcox, K. (1989). Family resources as resistance factors for psychological maladjustment in chronically ill and handicapped children. *Journal of Pediatric Psychology, 14,* 157–174.

Worchel, F., Nolan, B., Willson, V., Purser, J., Copeland, D., & Pfefferbaum, B. (1988). Assessment of depression in children with cancer. *Journal of Pediatric Psychology, 13,* 101–112.

Chapter 13
INVOLVING PARENTS IN CANCER RISK REDUCTION:
A Program for Hispanic American Families

Marian L. Fitzgibbon, Melinda R. Stolley, Mary E. Avellone,
Sharon Sugerman, and Noel Chavez

Dietary habits have been implicated in the etiology of cancer of the colon, stomach, pancreas, and breast (Steinmetz, Kushi, Bostick, Folsom, & Potter, 1994). Although controversy exists as to the precise role of diet in cancer prevention, there is little doubt that a prudent approach to dietary intake may help reduce the risk of cancer morbidity and mortality.

Differing estimates of the contribution of diet to cancer have emerged. Wynder and Gori (1977) estimated that as many as 40% of cases of cancer were associated with diet, while Doll and Peto (1981) suggested that a range of 20–90% of cancer deaths were related to diet. The National Academy of Sciences has asserted that most cancers are related to dietary intake (National Research Council, 1989). Specifically, in countries where fat intake is 20% or less of total caloric intake, the rates of both breast and colon cancer are lower than in the United States (Prentice & Sheppard, 1990; Rose, Boyar, & Wynder, 1986). In the United States, the average fat intake is 34% of total calories (McDowell et al., 1994).

Similarly, cancer rates are lower in countries where complex carbohydrates contribute to the majority of calories (Liu et al., 1979; Phillip, 1975) and total dietary fiber is more than double that of the United States (i.e., 25–30 g vs. 13–15 g per day; Carroll, Abraham, & Dresser, 1983; National Research Council, 1989). Studies have shown a protective effect of fiber from vegetables, especially green vegetables (Hu et al., 1991), and fruits and grains (Giovannucci, Stampfer, Colditz, Rimm, & Willett, 1992). Decreases in stomach cancer have been documented in populations with increased intake of fruits and vegetables (Miller et al., 1994). Studies in the United States and China have shown fruit and vegetable consumption to have a protective effect against oral and pharynx cancers (McLaughlin et al., 1988; Zheng et al., 1992).

Comparisons of genetically similar populations residing in the United States and non-Western countries have revealed higher cancer rates in the United States. Data show that second- and third-generation Japanese women born on the U.S. mainland have breast cancer rates comparable to those of U.S. women and higher than those of Japanese women born and living in Japan (Muir, Waterhouse, Mack, Powell, & Whelan, 1987; Shimuzu et al., 1991). In addition, an increased rate of colon cancer

Reprinted from *Health Psychology, 15*(6), 413–422. (1996). Copyright © 1996 by the American Psychological Association. Used with permission of the author.

This study was funded by Grant CCP04-93 from the American Cancer Society, Illinois Division, Inc. The authors wish to thank the staff of COMMONs education program, Joy Brown for her assistance in conducting the intervention, Kristin Flynn for developing the curriculum, and Vicky Singh and Lisa Blackman for technical assistance. The authors also would like to thank Erlinda Binghay for her involvement in the project.

in Puerto Ricans has been associated with increased length of stay on the U.S. mainland (Mallin & Anderson, 1988).

Hispanics are the fastest growing ethnic minority in the United States. Between 1993 and 2000, there will be a 24.2% increase in the U.S. Hispanic population and only a 3.1% increase in non-Hispanic Whites (U.S. Bureau of the Census, 1990). Unfortunately, 25% of Mexican Americans and 38% of Puerto Ricans live below the poverty level (Mendoza et al., 1991). Moreover, in Hispanic Americans, health problems occur disproportionately more frequently among those of lower socioeconomic and education levels (Hazuda, Stern, Gaskill, Haffner, & Gardner, 1983). Poverty is a risk factor for cancer. Cancer incidence increases and survival rate decreases as income declines (U.S. Dept. of Health and Human Services, 1991; Millon-Underwood, 1992). The development of culturally appropriate prevention strategies to reduce morbidity and mortality associated with cancer in this rapidly growing population has considerable public health implications.

Health-compromising behaviors, such as poor nutritional habits, begin during childhood (Voors, Sklov, Wolf, Hunter, & Berenson, 1982). During the formative years, the family has a large influence in shaping and maintaining the eating habits and food preferences of its members (Annest, Sing, Biron, & Mongeau, 1979; Hertzler & Vaughan, 1979). Similarities have been shown between family members regarding behavioral correlates of health risk factors, such as eating habits (Patterson, Rupp, Sallis, Atkins, & Nader, 1988), exercise habits (Sallis, Patterson, Buono, Atkins, & Nader, 1988), and smoking behavior (Hunter, Baugh, Webber, Sklov, & Berenson, 1982). Adult family members provide the initial learning environment and serve as role models for their children.

Dietary interventions aimed at families, such as home-based correspondence programs, have been successful with more affluent non-Hispanic White populations. Perry et al. (1988) showed short-term reductions in total fat and saturated fat consumption and increased complex carbohydrate consumption. However, follow-up revealed that these changes were not maintained (Perry et al., 1988), Hearn et al. (1992) found that factors related to socioeconomic status influenced participation in a home-based health promotion program. Specifically, there was lower participation among those with lower occupational and educational status. The potential limitations of home-based programs underscore the growing need to tailor interventions to different ethnic and socioeconomic groups. In a community-based, culturally specific intervention for African American, inner-city mothers and daughters, positive changes were reported for eating behavior, nutrition knowledge, and attitudes toward healthy eating (Fitzgibbon, Stolley, & Kirschenbaum, 1995). Similarly, the San Diego Family Health Project required weekly family participation of Hispanic and non-Hispanic White families and found improvement in families' eating habits that were maintained 1 year after completion of the intervention (Nader, Sallis, & Rupp, 1986).

In this article, we report the results of a study in which we compared the efficacy of a 12-week, family-based intervention with a no treatment control. Our overall goal in the study was to examine the effects of a family-based, culture-specific dietary intervention intended to reduce cancer risk among low-literacy, low-income Hispanics. Specifically, we had four aims: (a) to reduce fat intake, (b) to increase fiber intake, (c) to increase nutrition knowledge, and (d) to increase parental support for healthy eating. We hypothesized that (a) families who were randomized to a 12-week active intervention would reduce fat and increase fiber significantly more than would families randomized to a literature-only control group, (b) treatment families' nutrition knowledge would increase significantly more than would control families' nutrition knowledge, and (c) treatment mothers would increase their parental support significantly more than would control mothers.

Method

Participants

We recruited the families (38 mothers with a total of 17 sons and 31 daughters) in the study from a literacy training program in a largely Hispanic community of Chicago. The program serves primarily low-income, minority women. Potential subjects who were self-admitted alcoholics or consumed more than two alcoholic drinks per day were excluded. For a family to be eligible for the study, the children had to be ages 7–12 and both the mother and the children had to be willing and able to attend 12 weekly 1-hr classes and complete an assessment that included a health screening and a series of questionnaires prior to and post intervention. Each family received $5.00 each week they attended the program. In addition, the mothers received $20.00 and the children $10.00 each time they completed an assessment. The inability to read or speak English or Spanish did not make a subject ineligible. All classes and materials were presented in both English and Spanish, and questionnaires were read to subjects who could not read in whichever language they felt most comfortable hearing.

We used a back-translation approach (Marin & Marin, 1991). That is, one independent translator translated from English to Spanish, and a second independent translator translated from Spanish back into English. We then compared the two versions in the original language (English) to identify inconsistencies and loss or change of meaning.

Procedure

When mothers expressed an interest in the program and were eligible for the study, we grouped them and all their eligible children as a family and randomized them to the active-intervention condition or the literature-only control condition. Families in both conditions participated in a preintervention assessment before randomization. During this assessment, baseline information was collected on weight, height, blood pressure, eating behavior, nutrition knowledge, physical activity, and parental support and role modeling. To help reduce socially desirable responses, we did not inform the data collectors and interventionists of the study hypotheses.

The Curriculum

After the initial assessment, the active-intervention group was exposed to a 12-week, culture-specific, cancer prevention curriculum that encouraged adoption of a low-fat, high-fiber diet. In developing the curriculum, we relied heavily on information gathered in a needs assessment conducted earlier in the year with a similar population

(Fitzgibbon, Stolley, Avellone, Sugerman, & Chavez, 1996). We incorporated several of the most salient points derived from the needs assessment. First, we made the curriculum activity based and not solely didactic. Many mothers had limited nutrition knowledge but were interested in changing both their own and their children's dietary habits. They expressed interest in learning how to adapt traditional recipes and in experimenting with recipes in the classes. We were also sensitive to the differences in ethnic foods between Mexican Americans and Puerto Ricans.

Second, the curriculum accommodated both English and Spanish speakers. We gave all participants the choice of attending a Spanish class with Spanish-written materials or an English class with English-written materials. In this way, we were able to include families who were not yet fluent or comfortable with the English language, without excluding families who preferred English.

Third, we offered the curriculum in a familiar location, the site of a literacy training program that all participants regularly attended. Given that many participants did not speak fluent English, the fact that they could participate in the study at a place they knew and felt safe in was probably instrumental in the low attrition rate of the study (36 of 38 families completed the curriculum).

Fourth, the curriculum focused on the incorporation of ethnic foods that could be purchased at local ethnic markets. Many older mothers stated that they and their spouses wished to eat traditional Latin foods.

Fifth, we specifically addressed issues related to children's resistance to eating healthy foods, for example, making lower fat foods more enticing for them.

We encouraged dialogue between the mothers and children in the active-intervention condition throughout the program. Each week, several mothers and their children met in small groups (Spanish or English speaking) to discuss a "concept of the week," after which they participated in various activities designed to reinforce the information. The concepts were as follows:

Session 1: Concept: Cancer and diet: Introduction to fat. Amounts of fat in food.

Session 2: Concept: Cancer and diet: Introduction to fiber. Amounts of fiber in food.

Session 3: Concept: Reading labels, units of measurement. Serving sizes.

Session 4: Concept: Go foods, foods that make you go—grain-based foods.

Session 5: Concept: Glow foods—plant foods.

Session 6: Concept: Grow foods—meat and dairy products.

Session 7: Concept: Holiday meal planning.

Session 8: Concept: The importance of exercise.

Session 9: Concept: Meal planning, menus, and recipes.

Session 10: Concept: Food preparation—group meal.

Session 11: Concept: Review of the foregoing and the Food Guide Pyramid.

The control group received standard pamphlets on health behaviors and nutrition, with no accompanying classes. We distributed these pamphlets on a weekly basis to the mothers' mailboxes at the literacy training program and also sent copies to their homes.

Measures

We assessed participants before the intervention and 1 week after the end of the intervention. Demographic information obtained included age, marital status, employment, education, and socioeconomic status. To further describe our sample, we collected information on height, weight, percent overweight, blood pressure, level of acculturation, and physical activity.

Demographic and Physiological Variables

Height and weight. Height and weight were measured by trained research assistants after the participant's shoes and heavy outer clothing were removed. We used a standard medical balance-beam scale and height bar. Scales were calibrated to zero at the beginning of each assessment.

Percent overweight. We calculated percent overweight for the mothers, using as the ideal weight the median for a medium frame listed in the Metropolitan Life Insurance Company's 1983 height–weight tables. We used Tanner height–weight charts for the children (Tanner, Goldstein, & Whitehouse, 1970). Maternal obesity was defined as weight equal to or greater than 120% of ideal body weight. Percent overweight for children was calculated using the 50th percentile weight for height as the ideal body weight.

Body mass index. We calculated body mass index as weight (kilograms)/height (meters)^2 for adults and children.

Acculturation. We measured the extent of the mothers' and children's acculturation using a scale developed by Marin and Marin (1991). It contains four items that address language used at home, with friends, when reading and speaking, and when thinking. Correlations between this scale and other measures of acculturation have been high (rs = .69–.76).

Behaviorable Variables

Physical activity. We measured physical activity with a single yes/no question that provides valid information about who is participating in regular exercise: "Do you currently participate in any regular activity or program (either on your own or in a formal class) designed to improve or maintain your physical fitness?" (Schectman, Barzilai, Rost, & Fisher, 1991). The response to this question has been significantly associated, after age adjustment, with body mass index and oxygen capacity in both sexes and with high-density lipoprotein level in women.

We chose our measures to enable us to examine our four study aims. Our first two goals were to assess reduction in fat intake and increased fiber consumption. We also wished to assess increases in nutrition knowledge and parental support of healthy eating behavior.

Mothers' eating behaviors. We measured the mothers' dietary intake with the Food Behavior Checklist (FBC; Kristal et al., 1990) and the Quick Check for Fat (QCF; Schaefer, Selzer, Rosenfield, Danrell, & Blankenhorn, 1992). The FBC is a simplified, structured 24-hr dietary recall. It was specifically designed to evaluate group-level behavior change in community nutrition interventions without imposing the burden and expense of having nutrition professionals collect and code multiple food records or recalls. The FBC was developed to be used with ethnically diverse populations and refined with focus groups that included Hispanics (Kristal et al.,

1990). It was recently used to evaluate changes in fruit, vegetable, and fiber intake in a California population that was 23% Mexican Americans (DiSogra, Abrams, & Hudes, 1994). On the FBC, respondents indicate whether they ate a specific list of foods in the previous 24-hr period (e.g., salad). On the basis of the findings of our needs assessment (Fitzgibbon et al., 1996), we added as vegetable examples specific Latin American/Caribbean root vegetables and squashes not named on the original instrument (ñame, yautia, malanga, calabaza, and chayote). We also added a Hispanic-specific fat source, avocado/guacamole, immediately after the butter/margarine item. We used this instrument to assess intake of fiber, fruits, and vegetables.

The QCF is a computer-assisted, focused food frequency that characterizes an individual's typical dietary intake of fat, saturated fat, and dietary cholesterol. Respondents are first asked how often they eat each of 46 different foods, with response options ranging from *every day* to *less than once a month or never*. Next, a picture of an average serving of each food is displayed, and respondents are asked to identify the portion of the food they typically eat, ranging from half of the serving shown to 4 times the serving (item dependent). The QCDIET software program (Nutrition Scientific, 1995) estimates fat intake by assigning standard nutrient values to the average size for each item and the multiplying those values by the frequency and number of portions eaten.

Children's eating behaviors. To assess the children's dietary intake, we used a Food Frequency Questionnaire (FFQ; Resnicow et al., 1992). The FFQ was developed to identify the foods most commonly eaten by school-age children taking part in the Know Your Body health intervention program. The 37-item dietary assessment for Grades 1–3 is pictorial. Frequency choices are *almost never, sometimes,* and *almost always.* The 87-item instrument for Grades 4–6 is written. It uses a 5-point Likert scale, with choices *never* to *daily*. For both age groups, high- and low-fat foods as well as a variety of fruits and vegetables that are high in fiber and low in fat are listed. Group means were compared before and after intervention regarding the frequency of and changes in these foods.

The FFQ had been used extensively to evaluate change in eating behavior with ethnically diverse and inner-city populations, including one that was 60% Hispanic (Resnicow et al., 1992). It was designed to be self-administered by persons reading at the level of Grades 4–6. An open-ended question at the end of the instrument allows participants to identify other important foods not included on the list.

Mothers' and children's nutrition knowledge. The National Adolescent Student Health Survey (NASHS; Portnoy & Christensen, 1989) was developed to accrue data on the knowledge, attitudes, and self-reported practices of 8th and 10th graders in eight health areas, including nutrition. The NASHS pays particular attention to behaviors relevant to the risks of cancer. Questions and questionnaire administration for the NASHS were pilot-tested extensively with young people of diverse ethnic backgrounds. The Nutrition Knowledge Questionnaire (NKQ) includes 10 multiple-choice questions covering such topics as dietary fat, fiber, and vitamin content and their health effects. We changed a word on one question on the NKQ to accommodate the reading level of our participants.

Parental support and role modeling. This self-report measure consists of 10 questions on the frequency with which the respondent performs supportive or modeling behaviors for healthy eating (e.g., "How often do you check food labels?''). This questionnaire is part of the survey used in the Child and Adolescent Trial for

Cardiovascular Health being conducted with more than 400 parents (Hearn et al., 1992).

Results

After providing descriptive characteristics of the population, we present baseline differences between the treatment and control groups. We then analyze differences pretreatment and posttreatment between the treatment and control groups. Finally, we examine the relationship between children's and mothers' eating behaviors.

Descriptive Characteristics

All 38 families were Hispanic (21 Puerto Rican, 11 Mexican American, 3 Central American, and 3 other). Chicago has the fifth largest Hispanic population in the United States (U.S. Bureau of the Census, 1993). However, unlike many cities with large Hispanic populations (e.g., Los Angeles, Tampa, and New York), Chicago's Hispanic population is ethnically diverse: 65% is Mexican American, 22.6% Puerto Rican, and 12.4% other Latin American countries (U.S. Bureau of the Census, 1990). Given the diversity of the Chicago Hispanic community, we were unable to recruit an ethnically homogeneous sample. Eighty-four percent of the mothers in the present study were not born on the U.S. mainland or were born in Puerto Rico or in countries other than the United States. The majority (76%) were on public assistance. More than 90% of the mothers reported having difficulty paying for basic living needs. More than half (53%) of the mothers did not have a high school education. Fifty percent were obese according to the Metropolitan Life Insurance Company (1983) tables. This is similar to a recent national estimate that 46.7% of Mexican Americans are obese (Kuczmarski, Flegal, Campbell, & Johnson, 1994). Sixty-four percent thought that being overweight was very harmful to one's health. Seventy-nine percent of the mothers said they did not exercise regularly.

Baseline Differences Between the Treatment and Control Groups

There were no significant differences between treatment and control mothers or children on any demographic variables. In addition, there were no significant differences on dependent variables for the children. For the mothers, there were no differences on dependent variables, except for diastolic blood pressure, $t(42) = 2.24$, $p < .03$; resisting relapse, $t(18) = 3.65$, $p < .002$; and FBC fruits and vegetables, $t(34) = 2.92$, $p < .006$. Demographic data for the treatment and control mothers and children are presented in Tables 1 and 2, respectively.

After the pretreatment assessment, all participants were randomly assigned to the treatment or control group regardless of their language preference (Spanish or English). However, we found that mothers who preferred English were better educated ($M = 10.3$ years, $SD = 2.7$ years) than those who preferred Spanish ($M = 7.6$ years, $SD = 4.4$ years), $t(33) = 1.87$, $p < .07$, but this difference was not significant. Further, mothers who completed the program had more children than those who dropped out, $t(33) = 9.10$, $p < .05$. Only 2 families did not complete the program.

Table 1—*Demographic Profile of Mothers*

Variable	M	SD
Age (years)	35.0	6.60
Weight (kg)	70.1	14.30
Body mass index (kg/m^2)	28.7	5.40
Education (years)	9.1	3.99
Socioeconomic status	16.3	7.50
Acculturation	3.3	.69
% calories from fat	36.0	6.10
Income (%)		
Less than $5,000	52.6	
$5,000–$11,999	28.9	
$12,000–$15,999	2.6	
$16,000–$24,999	15.8	
Marital status (%)		
Married	21.1	
Separated or divorced	57.4	
Single	28.9	
Widowed	2.6	
Preferred language (%)		
English	58.0	
Spanish	43.0	

There were no other differences between mothers who completed the 12 wk program and those who dropped out.

Pretreatment to Posttreatment Changes on Main Study Variables

To assess treatment effects, we performed a 2 (treatment vs. control) × 2 (pretreatment vs. posttreatment) repeated measures multivariate analysis of variance (MANOVA) and follow-up univariate analyses of variance (ANOVAs) on the behavioral variables for mothers (percent of total calories eaten from fat and saturated fat as measured by the QCF; fiber, fruit, and vegetable intake as measured by the FBC; and parental support). Behavioral variables for children included intake of fruit, vegetables, sweets, high-fat dairy, high-fat meat, heart-unhealthy snack foods, and heart-healthy grain foods as measured by the FFQ. We conducted separate ANOVAs on

Table 2—*Demographic Profile of Children*

Variable	M	SD
Age (years)	9.0	2.0
Weight (kg)	39.2	15.3
Body mass index (kg/m^2)	20.0	5.0
Education (years)	4.2	2.0
Acculturation	3.4	1.1

nutrition knowledge and blood pressure. To examine changes in activity level from pretreatment to posttreatment, we constructed two separate contingency tables for the treatment and control groups. We also examined the correlations between attendance and the dependent variables at posttreatment. We conducted analyses separately for mothers and children.

Mothers

The repeated measures MANOVA on the pretreatment and posttreatment fat, saturated fat, and parental support variables indicated a significant effect of group, Wilks's lambda = .77, $F(3, 32) = 3.1$, $p < .05$, and a significant effect of time, Wilks's lambda = .62, $F(3, 32) = 6.4$, $p < .01$, but no Group $\times$ Time interaction. Follow-up ANOVAs of the group effect showed significant effects of percent fat intake, $F(1, 34) = 6.8$, $p < .05$; percent saturated fat intake, $F(1, 34) = 3.8$, $p < .05$; and parental support, $F(1, 34) = 4.9$, $p < .05$. Follow-up ANOVAs of the time effect showed an overall increase from pretreatment to posttreatment for parental support, $F(1, 34) = 13.9$, $p < .001$. Examination of the means showed that treatment mothers reduced their mean percent fat and saturated fat intake from 34% to 29%, whereas the control group's mean percent fat intake remained the same at posttreatment as it had been at pretreatment (36%). The relatively small sample size makes it more difficult to see a significant effect even when the means are in the expected direction. Means and standard deviations for the behavioral variables are presented in Table 3.

When we correlated the percentage of calories from fat and saturated fat and parental support and role modeling for healthy eating with program attendance, we found that the more sessions the mothers attended, the lower their percent fat intake at posttreatment ($r = -.53$, $p < .05$). There was a positive correlation between attendance and parental support and role modeling ($r = .60$, $p < .005$). The correlation between saturated fat and attendance showed a trend toward significance ($r = -.41$, $p < .08$).

From the mothers' scores on the FBC, we determined changes in fiber intake and fruit and vegetable intake. We found main effects of group, Wilks's lambda = .81, $F(2, 31) = 3.6$, $p < .05$, and time, Wilks's lambda = .80, $F(2, 31) = 4.4$, $p < .05$.

Table 3—*Mothers' Scores on Behavioral Variables Before and After Treatment*

| Variable | Treatment ($n = 18$) | | | | Control ($n = 18$) | | | | |
| | Baseline | | Post-treatment | | Baseline | | Post-treatment | | |
	M	SD	M	SD	M	SD	M	SD	$F(3, 32)$
% calories from fat	34.3	6.20	29.3	8.50	36.3	5.50	36.7	6.10	4.20
% calories from saturated fat	12.2	2.60	11.2	4.00	12.9	2.20	13.6	3.10	2.40
Fiber intake	0.7	0.87	1.0	0.73	0.3	0.49	0.8	0.81	0.14
Fruit and vegetable intake	2.0	1.30	2.6	1.20	0.9	1.00	1.5	1.00	0.82
Parental support and role modeling	21.2	8.70	28.3	7.10	17.6	8.30	21.3	9.40	1.30

Follow-up ANOVAs of the group effect showed increased fruit intake, $F(1, 32)$, $p <$ .01, but no increase in fiber. The time effect showed increases in fiber, $F(1, 32) = 4.8$, $p < .05$, and fruit and vegetables, $F(1, 32) = 4.6$, $p < .05$, from pretreatment to posttreatment. When we correlated fiber intake and fruit and vegetable intake with program attendance, we found that the more sessions mothers attended, the greater their fiber intake at posttreatment ($r = .59$, $p < .005$). The correlation between attendance and fruit and vegetable intake showed a trend toward significance ($r = .45$, $p < .06$). Percent overweight was negatively associated with fruit and vegetable intake ($r = -.55$, $p < .05$) but was not associated with fiber intake. We also found that parental support and role modeling were positively associated with fiber intake ($r = .71$, $p < .005$) and fruit and vegetable intake ($r = .60$, $p < .005$).

In the treatment group, the percentage of mothers who reported some exercise rose from 25% before treatment to 56% after treatment ($p < .05$). In the control group, the change from pretreatment to posttreatment was not significant. Physical activity was positively associated with parental support and role modeling ($r = .55$, $p < .05$).

The mothers' nutrition knowledge was not significantly affected by group, time, or the interaction of the two. However, examination of the means showed that the treatment group did improve their level of knowledge, albeit not significantly, whereas the control group's knowledge remained at the same level after treatment as it had been before treatment (see Table 5). Nutrition knowledge was associated with increased attendance ($r = .74$, $p < .005$), increased fruit and vegetable intake ($r = .44$, $p < .01$), and increased fiber intake ($r = .33$, $p < .01$).

Results for blood pressure showed no main effect of group or an interaction effect. There was a main effect for time, however, Wilks's lambda = .47, $F(4, 28) = 7.7$, $p < .001$. Follow-up ANOVAs showed reductions from pretreatment to posttreatment for systolic blood pressure, $F(1, 29) = 6.2$, $p < .05$, and diastolic blood pressure, $F(1, 29) = 20.9$, $p < .001$.

Children

For the older children, the repeated measures MANOVA on the pretreatment and posttreatment food behavior variables indicated no main effect of group or a Group × Time interaction effect. However, there was a main effect of time, Wilks's lambda = .70, $F(7, 12) = 4.1$, $p < .05$. Follow-up ANOVAs of the time effect showed a significant increase from pretreatment to posttreatment for fruit consumption, a decrease in meat consumption, an increase in dairy foods, a decrease in sweets, and a decrease in heart-unhealthy food. However, when we combined the data for the older and younger children, we found no significant effect of group, time, or the interaction of the two. The data for older children are presented in Table 4.

For children's blood pressure, there was no significant effect of group or a Group × Time interaction, but there was a significant effect of time. Systolic blood pressure increased from pretreatment to posttreatment, Wilks's lambda = .72, $F(2, 40) = 7.7$, $p < .01$.

For the children's nutrition knowledge, there was a significant effect of time, $F(1, 44) = 4.1$, $p < .05$, and a Group × Time interaction, $F(1, 44) = 5.6$, $p < .05$. There was no main effect of group. There was also a positive correlation between

Table 4—*Older (Grades 4–6) Children's Scores on Behavioral Variables Before and After Treatment*

| | Treatment (n = 9) | | | | Control (n = 11) | | | | |
| | Baseline | | Post-treatment | | Baseline | | Post-treatment | | |
Variable	M	SD	M	SD	M	SD	M	SD	$F(2, 31)$
Fruits	2.7	0.96	2.6	0.86	2.5	0.60	2.5	0.80	0.06
Vegetables	2.1	0.63	2.0	0.50	1.7	0.48	1.7	0.63	1.50
Meat	2.6	0.64	2.1	0.79	2.4	0.47	2.4	0.53	0.46
Dairy	2.4	0.60	2.5	0.66	2.6	0.66	2.4	0.49	0.03
Sweets	3.0	1.00	2.8	1.00	2.9	0.96	2.5	0.55	1.80
Heart-healthy food	2.6	0.76	2.2	0.86	2.1	0.52	2.2	0.52	0.40
Heart-unhealthy food	3.6	1.00	2.8	1.00	3.5	0.77	2.9	0.93	0.13

attendance and children's nutrition knowledge ($r = .29$, $p < .05$). Means and standard deviations for the mothers' and children's dependent variables are presented in Table 5.

Correlations Between Mothers and Children at Posttreatment

Children's improved nutrition knowledge was associated with a lower fat intake in their mothers. It was also positively associated with parental support and role modeling ($r = .60$, $p < .001$). Increased parental support and role modeling by the mothers were also associated with children's increased consumption of heart-healthy food ($r = .38$, $p = .05$), increased consumption of fruit ($r = .31$, $p < .05$), and increased consumption of vegetables ($r = .31$, $p < .05$) at posttreatment. Mothers' intake of vegetables was positively associated with children's intake of vegetables ($r = .31$, $p < .05$). Correlations for selected study variables are presented in Table 6.

Table 5—*Mothers' and Children's Nutrition Knowledge Scores Before and After Treatment*

| | Baseline | | After treatment | |
Group	M	SD	M	SD
Mothers				
Treatment (n = 18)	4.4	1.2	4.6	1.2
Control (n = 17)	3.8	1.3	3.8	1.3
Children				
Treatment (n = 27)	3.3	2.0	4.6	2.2
Control (n = 19)	3.4	1.5	3.4	1.6

Note. Time, $F(1, 44) = 4.1$, $p < .05$; Group $\times$ Time, $F(1, 44) = 5.6$, $p < .05$.

Table 6—*Correlations Between Selected Study Variables After Treatment*

Variable	1	2	3	4	5	6	7	8	9	10
1. Mothers' nutritional knowledge	—	-.21	.33*	.24	.25	.53***	.72***	.74***	.43***	.04
2. Mothers' fat intake (FBC)	-.21	—	-.03	-.06	-.45***	-.24	-.40*	-.43*	-.12	.25
3. Mothers' fiber intake (FBC)	.33*	-.03	—	.87***	.11	.71***	.58***	.59***	.21	-.05
4. Mothers' fruit and vegetable intake (FBC)	.24	-.06	.87***	—	.17	.60***	.43*	.46*	.05	-.04
5. Children's nutritional knowledge	.25	-.45***	.11	.17	—	.28	.21	.25	.29	-.27
6. Parental support	.53***	-.24	.71***	.60***	.28	—	.63***	.60***	.38**	-.03
7. Children's attendance of program	.72***	-.40*	.58***	.43*	.21	.63***	—	.99***	.32	-.16
8. Mothers' attendance of program	.74***	-.43*	.59***	.46*	.25	.60***	.99***	—	.29	-.22
9. Children's intake of heart-healthy food (FFQ)	.43***	-.12	.21	.05	.29	.38**	.32	.29	—	.23
10. Children's intake of heart-unhealthy food (FFQ)	.04	.25	-.05	-.04	-.27	-.03	-.16	-.22	.23	—

Note. FBC = Food Behavior Checklist; FFQ = Food Frequency Questionnaire.

*p < .05.
**p < .005.
***p < .0005.

Discussion

Our findings support previous data showing the importance of family involvement in making dietary changes (Patterson et al., 1988). Interestingly, similar to the results of other dietary intervention studies, the mothers in the present study made behavior changes without showing concomitant increases in knowledge (Vega et al., 1987). It is important to note that the behavioral effects were seen in both the treatment and control groups. The control group received pamphlets that presented health-related information and this may have been particularly effective for these highly motivated women attending a literacy training program. In addition, probable contact between the treatment and control groups was an inherent problem with this project. Given that this study demonstrates the feasibility of this type of intervention, future studies with sufficient resources and accessibility to multiple sites can address the problem of contamination more fully. There also may have been some contact between treatment and control children. However, the control children were not part of the literacy program and had no consistent contact with the children in the treatment group.

The increase in the children's knowledge is encouraging given recent data that indicate that Hispanic American children have limited nutrition knowledge (Olvira-Ezzell, Power, Cousins, Guerra, & Trujillo, 1994). Although knowledge and behavior are not necessarily linked, it may be that these children's limited nutrition knowledge is related to increased prevalence of obesity, diabetes, and other health risk factors (Basch, Shea, & Zybert, 1992; Kumanyika et al., 1990; Murphy, Castillo, Martorell, & Mendoza, 1990). Unfortunately, the increase in nutrition knowledge we observed in the children in the present study was not seen in the mothers. We speculate that the measure we used to assess nutrition knowledge contained more items referring to food commonly consumed by Anglo American populations than items referring to traditional Hispanic food. These foods were common to the children's diets but were less frequently eaten by the mothers, who tended to eat more traditional foods. During the intervention, a significant issue for many mothers was that they had to cook two types of meals: one for themselves and their spouse and another using more Americanized foods for their children. Given that we did see a change in the mothers' food intake, we conclude that although we were able to have an impact on the foods they regularly ate, this did not generalize to didactic knowledge about foods with which they were less familiar.

It is also noteworthy that attendance affected the behavior and knowledge of both children and adults. Other family studies have not shown a relationship between attendance and behavior change (e.g., Nader et al., 1986). In our sample, children who attended more sessions learned more about nutrition. Mothers who attended more sessions reported larger reductions in fat intake and reported increases in physical activity; fruit, vegetable, and fiber intake; and support for their children's healthy eating. This study provides more data to suggest that health promotion programs should use the family as the unit of intervention (Baranowski & Nader, 1985). Parental support and role modeling clearly played a role in effecting positive dietary changes in the children.

The methodological limitations of the present study require that caution be used in interpreting and extending these results. First, all the data were obtained by self-report. The accuracy of self-report data, particularly dietary behavior, has been questioned (Klesges, Eck, & Ray, 1995). In addition, response problems such as extreme

responses, acquiescent responses, and socially desirable responses have been documented in Hispanic samples in proportions higher than those reported for non-
Hispanic Whites (e.g., Hui & Triandis, 1989). Hui and Triandis (1989) reported that
Hispanics tended to use extreme responses, such as *always true*, rather than more
moderate responses, such as *sometimes true*. Acquiescent responding is the tendency
of participants to agree with a statement, regardless of its content. Ross and Mirowsky (1984) found that among Hispanics, acquiescent responses were more likely
to be given by men, older individuals, and persons of low socioeconomic status.
They also found that Hispanics tended to answer in ways they perceived to be correct,
regardless of their behavior or experience of the question content. These types of
responses among low-income Hispanics can be interpreted as the deferential responding of persons of lower socioeconomic status (Ross & Mirowsky, 1984). Alternatively, Marin and Marin (1991) have suggested that the concept of *simpatia* (Triandis,
Marin, Lisansky, & Betancourt, 1984) among Hispanics, meaning the preference for
politeness and deference rather than confrontation, plays a large role in socially
desirable responses.

However, the reliability of the present results is enhanced by the fact that some
children's dietary data correlated with their mother's dietary data ($r = .31$, $p < .05$),
even though they answered their questionnaires separately. This may mean that both
mothers and the children were answering in a socially desirable way, but it may also
reflect actual correlations between their eating habits (Patterson et al., 1988). Parent–
child correlations have been found for intake of carbohydrates, fats, and calories.
Correlations have ranged from .15 to .30 for parent–child pairs (Laskarzewski et al.,
1980; Patterson et al., 1998). Patterson et al. (1988) found that among Anglos, mothers' and fathers' dietary habits were significantly correlated with younger children's
dietary habits but not those of older children. However, among Mexican Americans,
family members tended to have similar dietary habits for fat and sodium intake.

A second limitation of the present data is generalizability. The women involved
in this program were attending a literacy training program and so may not be representative of all low-income Hispanic women. In addition, their expressed interest
in nutrition may have made them more likely candidates for dietary change. Generalizability could be increased only through continued empirical investigation with
Hispanics in other areas of the country and of different socioeconomic status. The
participants in our sample were relatively homogenous in age and education, but
they were not ethnically homogenous. Given the heterogeneity of the Hispanic population in Chicago, we were unable to recruit only one ethnic subgroup. The sample
is representative of the literacy training program and the part of the city from which
it was recruited. Chicago is unlike other large American cities (e.g., New York and
Los Angeles) that have a dominant Hispanic subgroup. In addition, because the
sample did not include any adult male participants, the dietary behavior of Hispanic
men cannot be inferred.

A third limitation is that our findings are less than clean-cut because the control
group received an intervention, albeit a less intensive one. Ideally, the control group
should have received no intervention or a delayed intervention.

A fourth limitation is the lack of follow-up data. Maintenance of positive dietary
changes over a period of at least 1 year would bode well for these types of culture-
specific, community-based, family interventions.

A fifth limitation is the relatively small sample size. Because we were able to document changes in this small sample with little power, we would most likely show more robust changes with a larger sample.

These limitations notwithstanding, the present study documents that positive dietary changes can be effected by a 12-week, culture-specific community intervention. Parental support appears to be a critical component associated with positive changes in both mothers and children. We documented changes in both the treatment and control mothers and children. Clearly, more work is needed in this area to determine the appropriate dose–response relationship for optimal behavioral change among low-income Hispanic Americans.

References

Annest, J., Sing, C., Biron, P., & Mongeau, J. (1979). Familial aggregation of blood pressure and weight in adoptive families. *American Journal of Epidemiology, 110,* 479–491.

Baranowski, T., & Nader, P. R. (1985). Family involvement in health behavior change programs. In D. C. Turk & R. D. Kerns (Eds.), *Health, illness, and families* (pp. 81–107). New York: Wiley.

Basch, C. E., Shea, S., & Zybert, P. (1992). Food sources, dietary behavior, and the saturated fat intake of Latino children. *American Journal of Public Health, 82,* 810–815.

Carroll, M. D., Abraham, S., & Dresser, C. M. (1983). Dietary intake source data: United States, 1976–80. *Vital & Health Statistics–Series 11: Data from the National Health Survey, 11*(231), 1–483.

DiSogra, L., Abrams, D., & Hudes, M. (1994). Low prevalence of healthful dietary behaviors in a California agricultural county: Emphasis on White and Mexican-American adults. *Journal of the American Dietetic Association, 94,* 544–554.

Doll, R., & Peto, R. (1981). The causes of cancer: Quantitative estimates of avoidable risks of cancer in the United States today. *Journal of the National Cancer Institute, 66,* 1191–1308.

Fitzgibbon, M. L., Stolley, M. R., Avellone, M. E., Sugerman, S. B., & Chavez, N. (1996). *Involving parents in cancer risk reduction: A needs assessment.* Unpublished manuscript.

Fitzgibbon, M. L., Stolley, M. R., & Kirschenbaum, D. S. (1995). Obesity prevention in African-American pre-adolescent girls: A pilot study. *Journal of Nutrition Education, 27,* 93–97.

Giovannucci, E., Stampfer, M. J., Colditz, G., Rimm, E. B., & Willett, W. C. (1992). Relationship of diet to risk of colorectal adenoma in men. *Journal of the National Cancer Institute, 84,* 91–98.

Hazuda, H. P., Stern, M. P., Gaskill, S. P., Haffner, S. M., & Gardner, L. (1983). Ethnic differences in health knowledge and behaviors related to the prevention and treatment of coronary heart disease. *American Journal of Epidemiology, 117,* 717–728.

Hearn, M., Bigelow, C., Nader, P., Stone, E., Johnson, C., Parcel, G., Perry, C., & Luepker, R. (1992). Involving families in cardiovascular health promotion: The CATCH feasibility study. *Journal of Health Education, 23,* 22–31.

Hertzler, A., & Vaughan, C. (1979). The relationship of family structure and interaction to nutrition. *Journal of the American Dietetic Association, 74,* 23–27.

Hu, J., Liu, Y., Yu, Y., Zhao, T. A., Liu, S. D., & Wang, Q. (1991). Diet and cancer of the colon and rectum: A case-control study in China. *International Journal of Epidemiology, 20,* 362–367.

Hui, C. H., & Triandis, H. C. (1989). Effects of culture and response format on extreme response style. *Journal of Cross Cultural Psychology, 20,* 296–309.

Hunter, S., Baugh, J., Webber, L., Sklov, M., & Berenson, G. (1982). Social learning effects on trial and adoption of cigarettes smoking in children: The Bogalusa Heart Study. *Preventive Medicine, 11,* 29–42.

Klesges, R. C., Eck, L. H., & Ray, J. W. (1995). Who underreports dietary intake in a dietary recall? Evidence from the Second National Health and Nutrition Examination Survey. *Journal of Consulting and Clinical Psychology, 63,* 438–444.

Kristal, A. R., Abrams, B. F., Thornquist, M. D., DiSogra, L., Croyle, R. T., Shattuck, A. L., & Henry, H. J. (1990). Development and validation of a food use checklist for evaluation of community nutrition interventions. *American Journal of Public Health, 80,* 1318–1322.

Kuczmarski, R. J., Flegal, K. M., Campbell, S. M., & Johnson, C. L. (1994). Increasing prevalence of overweight among US adults: The National Health and Nutrition Survey. *Journal of the American Medical Association, 272,* 205–211.

Kumanyika, S. K., Huffman, S. L., Bradshaw, M. E., Waller, H., Ross, A., Serdula, M., & Paige, D. (1990). Stature and weight status of children in an urban kindergarten population. *Pediatrics, 85,* 783–790.

Laskarzewski, P., Morrison, J. A., Khoury, P., Kelly, K., Glatfelter, L., Larsen, R., & Glueck, C. J. (1980). Parent–child nutrient intake relationships in school children ages 6 to 19: The Princeton School District Study. *American Journal of Clinical Nutrition, 33,* 2350–2355.

Liu, K., Stamler, J., Moss, D., Garside, D., Parkey, V., & Soltero, I. (1979). Dietary cholesterol, fat, and fibre, and colon cancer mortality: An analysis of international data. *Lancet, 2,* 782–785.

Mallin, K., & Anderson, D. (1988). Cancer mortality in Illinois Mexican and Puerto Rican immigrants. *International Journal of Cancer, 41,* 670–676.

Marin, G., & Marin, B. V. (1991). *Research with Hispanic populations.* Newbury Park, CA: Sage.

McDowell, M. S., Briefel, R. R., Alaimoka, K., Bischof, A. M., Caughman, C. A., Carroll, M., Loria, C. M., & Johnson, C. L. (1994). *Energy and macronutrient intakes of persons ages 2 months and over in the United States: Third National Health and Nutrition Examination Survey, Phase 1, 1988–1991. Advance data from vital and health statistics* (No. 255). Hyattsville, MD: National Center for Health Statistics.

McLaughlin, J. K., Gridley, G., Block, G., Winn, D., Preston-Martin, S., Schoenberg, J., Greenberg, R., Sternhagen, A., Austin, D., Ershow, A., Blot, W., & Fraumeni, J. (1988). Dietary factors in oral and pharyngeal cancer. *Journal of the National Cancer Institute, 80,* 1237–1243.

Mendoza, F. S., Ventura, S. J., Valdez, A. B., Castillo, R. O., Salvidar, L. E., Baisden, K., & Martorell, R. (1991). Selected measures of health status for Mexican-American, mainland Puerto Rican, and Cuban-American children. *Journal of the American Medical Association, 265,* 227–232.

Metropolitan Life Insurance Company. (1983). Metropolitan height and weight tables. *Statistical Bulletin, 64,* 3–8.

Miller, A. B., Berrino, F., Hill, M., Pietinen, P., Riboli, E., & Wahrendorf, J. (1994). Diet in the aetiology of cancer: A review. *European Journal of Cancer, 2,* 207–220.

Millon-Underwood, S. (1992). *Cancer and the poor: Focusing the challenge.* Atlanta, GA: American Cancer Society.

Muir, C., Waterhouse, J., Mack, T., Powell, J., & Whelan, S. (Eds.). (1987). *Patterns of cancer incidence in five continents* (Vol. 5). Lyons, France: International Agency for Research on Cancer.

Murphy, S. P., Castillo, R. O., Martorell, R., & Mendoza, F. S. (1990). An evaluation of food group intakes by Mexican-American children. *Journal of the American Dietetic Association, 90,* 388–393.

Nader, P. R., Sallis, J. F., & Rupp, J. (1986). The Family Health Project: Reaching families through the school. *Journal of School Health, 56,* 227–231.

National Research Council. (1989). *Diet, nutrition, and cancer: Report of the Committee on Diet, Nutrition and Cancer, Assembly of Life Sciences.* Washington, DC: National Academy Press.

Nutrition Scientific. (1995). Quick Check for Diet Progress [Computer software]. South Pasadena, CA: Author.

Olvira-Ezzell, N., Power, T. G., Cousins, J. H., Guerra, A. M., & Trujillo, M. (1994). The development of health knowledge in low-income Mexican-American children. *Child Development, 65,* 416–427.

Patterson, T. L., Rupp, J. W., Sallis, J. F., Atkins, C. J., & Nader, P. (1988). Aggregation of dietary calories, fats, and sodium in Mexican-American and Anglo families. *American Journal of Preventive Medicine, 4,* 75–82.

Perry, C. L., Luepker, R. V., Murray, D. M., Hearn, M., Halper, A., Dudovitz, B., Maile, M., & Smyth, M. (1988). Parental involvement with children's health promotion: A one-year follow-up of the Minnesota Home Team. *Health Education Quarterly, 16,* 171–180.

Phillip, R. L. (1975). Role of life stress and dietary habits in risk of cancer among Seventh Day Adventists. *Cancer Research, 35,* 3515–3522.

Portnoy, B., & Christenson, C. M. (1989). Cancer knowledge and related practices: Results from the National Adolescent Health Survey. *Journal of School Health, 59,* 218–224.

Prentice, R. L., & Sheppard, L. (1990). Dietary fat and cancer: Consistency of the epidemiologic data, and disease prevention that may follow from a practical reduction in fat consumption. *Cancer Causes and Control, 1,* 81–97.

Resnicow, K., Cohn, L., Reinhardt, J., Cross, D., Futterman, R., Kirschner, E., Wynder, E., & Allegrante, J. (1992). A three year evaluation of the Know Your Body Program in inner city schoolchildren. *Health Education Quarterly, 19,* 1–17.

Rose, D. P., Boyar, A. P., & Wynder, E. L. (1986). International comparisons of mortality rates for cancer of the breast, ovary, prostate, and colon, and per capita food consumption. *Cancer, 58,* 2363.

Ross, C. E., & Mirowsky, J. (1984). Socially desirable response and acquiescence in a cross-cultural survey of mental health. *Journal of Health and Social Behavior, 25,* 189–197.

Sallis, J., Patterson, T., Buono, M., Atkins, C., & Nader, P. (1988). Aggregation of physical activity habits in Mexican-American and Anglo families. *Journal of Behavioral Medicine, 11,* 31–41.

Schaefer, D., Selzer, R. H., Rosenfield, F., Danrell, C., & Blankenhorn, D. H. (1992). Quick Check for Fat: A bar coded food frequency analysis to accompany blood cholesterol screening. *Nutrition Metabolism and Cardiovascular Disease, 2,* 174–177.

Schectman, K. B., Barzilai, B., Rost, K., & Fisher, E. B. (1991). Measuring physical activity with a single question. *American Journal of Public Health, 81,* 771–773.

Shimuzu, H., Ross, R. K., Bernstein, L., Yatani, R., Henderson, B. E., & Mack, T. M. (1991). Cancer of the prostate and breast among Japanese and White immigrants in Los Angeles County. *British Journal of Cancer, 63,* 963–966.

Steinmetz, K. A., Kushi, L., Bostick, R., Folsom, A., & Potter, J. (1994). Vegetables, fruit, and colon cancer in the Iowa Women's Health Study. *American Journal of Epidemiology, 139,* 1–15.

Tanner, J., Goldstein, H., & Whitehouse, R. (1970). Standards for children's height at ages 2–9 allowing for height for parents. *Archives of Disease in Children, 45,* 755–762.

Triandis, H. C., Marin, G., Lisansky, J., & Betancourt, H. (1984). Simpatia as a cultural script of Hispanics. *Journal of Personality and Social Psychology, 47,* 1363–1375.

U.S. Bureau of the Census. (1990). *Summary of social, economic, and housing characteristics. U.S. income and poverty status in 1989–1990* (Publication No. CPH–5–1). Washington, DC: U.S. Government Printing Office.

U.S. Bureau of the Census. (1993). *Current population reports: Hispanic Americans today.* (Publication No. P23-183. Washington, DC: U.S. Government Printing Office.

U.S. Department of Health and Human Services. (1991). *Healthy people 2000: National health promotion and disease prevention objectives* (DHHS Publication No. PHS 91-50212). Washington, DC: U.S. Government Printing Office.

Vega, W. A., Sallis, J. F., Patterson, T., Rupp, J., Atkins, C., & Nader, P. R. (1987). Assessing knowledge of cardiovascular health-related diet and exercise behaviors in Anglo and Mexican-Americans. *Preventive Medicine, 16,* 696–709.

Voors, A. W., Sklov, N. C., Wolf, T. M., Hunter, S. M., & Berenson, G. S. (1982). Cardiovascular risk factors in children and coronary-related behavior. In T. J. Coates, A. L. Peterson, & C. L. Perry (Eds.), *Promoting adolescent health: A dialogue on research and practice* (pp. 281–304). New York, NY: Academic Press.

Wynder, E. L., & Gori, G. B. (1977). Contribution of the environment to cancer: An epidemiologic exercise. *Journal of the National Cancer Institute, 58,* 825–832.

Zheng, W., Blot, W. J., Shu, X.-O., Diamond, E. L., Gao, Y., Ji, B. T., & Faumeni, J. F., Jr. (1992). Risk factors for oral and pharyngeal cancer in Shanghai, with emphasis on diet. *Cancer Epidemiology, Biomarkers and Prevention, 1,* 441–448.

Part V

Disease Course

Chapter 14
PREDICTORS OF CANCER PROGRESSION IN YOUNG ADULT MEN AND WOMEN:
Avoidance, Intrusive Thoughts, and Psychological Symptoms

JoAnne E. Epping-Jordan, Bruce E. Compas, and David C. Howell

This year over one million Americans will be diagnosed with cancer. Of this group, approximately 450,000 will be alive in 5 years (American Cancer Society, 1992). Whereas initital disease severity is likely to influence course of cancer and ultimate survival most prominently, it is widely suggested and debated that secondary psychological factors also affect cancer progression. Overcoming cancer through mind over body has been promoted by the media and authors of popular books (e.g., Cousins, 1989; Siegel, 1986). However, health research has lagged behind in this line of inquiry. Available empirical evidence describing the relationship between psychological factors and disease progression in cancer patients is mixed (for a review, see Levenson & Bemis, 1990) and generalizations from this research are complicated by the use of varied designs and the measurement of different variables across studies.

Investigators looking at the relationship between psychological factors and cancer progression can be guided by emerging models of psychological stress, emotions, and disease (for reviews see Andersen, Kiecolt-Glaser, & Glaser, 1994; Herbert & Cohen, 1993; O'Leary, 1990; Weisse, 1992). A premise of these models is that exposure to acute or chronic psychological stress triggers emotional, cognitive, behavioral, and biological processes that lead to increased vulnerability to disease. Disruptions in the body's immune system are hypothesized to be an important pathway through which psychological factors affect health (O'Leary, 1990). Intense affect may alter the immune system's level of functioning, resulting in increased susceptibility to disease (Herbert & Cohen, 1993). Psychological factors such as stress may also affect health by disrupting certain health practices such as adherence and compliance (Andersen et al., 1994; Cohen & Williamson, 1991).

Several studies have found no relationship between psychological factors and cancer progression (e.g., Buddeberg et al., 1991; Cassileth, Lusk, Miller, Brown, & Miller, 1985; Jamison, Burish, & Wallston, 1987; Richardson, Zarnegar, Bisno, & Levine, 1990). For example, Cassileth et al. (1985) prospectively studied psychosocial predictors of survival in cancer patients with advanced disease. Independent

Reprinted from *Health Psychology, 13*(6), 539–547. (1994). Copyright © 1994 by the American Psychological Association. Used with permission of the author.

This research was supported by grants from the National Institute of Mental Health (MH43819) and the National Cancer Institute (P30CA22435). Its contents are solely the authors' responsibility and do not necessarily represent the official views of the National Cancer Institute. The authors are grateful to numerous individuals for their assistance in carrying out this research, including oncologists Jerome Belinson, Thomas Roland, and James Stuart; oncology nurses Elaine Owen, Susan Guillan, Debbie Potter, and Joyce Silveira; staff assistant Jeannie Bernard; research assistants Sydney Ey, Carol Kottmeier, Nancy Worsham, Doug Bolton, Caroline Freidman, Kathy Grant, Gina Mireault, Pam Orosan, and Cindy Gerhardt; Amy Willard, Laurie Raezer, and Vanessa Malcarne.

variables, measured within 4 weeks of diagnosis, included patients' social ties and marital history, job satisfaction, general life satisfaction, and degree of hopelessness and helplessness. Analyses indicated that these social and psychological factors, individually or in combination, did not predict the length of survival or time until relapse. Jamison et al. (1987) conducted a comparable study by measuring self-esteem, hostility, and symptoms of depression and anxiety in breast cancer patients. Similar to Cassileth et al. (1985), they found nonsignificant results when comparing these psychological variables between short-term and long-term survival groups. Both research groups concluded that in cases of advanced cancer, the inherent biology of the disease alone determines the prognosis, overriding the potentially mitigating influence of these psychological factors.

Other studies, however, have shown a significant relationship between psychological factors and progression of cancer (e.g., Derogatis, Abeloff, & Melisaratos, 1979; Levy, Herberman, Maluish, Schlien, & Lippman, 1985; Levy, Lee, Bagley, & Lippman, 1988; Rogentine et al., 1979; Spiegel, Bloom, Kraemer, & Gottheil, 1989). The majority of evidence suggests that efforts to suppress dysphoric feelings (e.g., Derogatis et al., 1979; Levy et al., 1985) and other forms of cognitive and behavioral avoidance of the cancer and of associated negative emotions are associated with shorter disease-free survival. Avoidant coping efforts are defined as active cognitive or behavioral attempts to escape or minimize the significance of the cancer but do not include efforts that center on positive reappraisal. Cancer patients who report that they need to make large adjustments to cope with their cancer—which may reflect low levels of avoidance—have significantly higher survival rates 1 year post diagnosis than those who respond with a low rating of perceived adjustment (Rogentine et al., 1979). One notable exception to these findings has been reported by Greer and colleagues (Greer, 1991; Greer, Morris, & Pettingale, 1979; Greer, Morris, Pettingale, & Haybittle, 1990), who found that breast cancer patients displaying either a fighting spirit or denial/positive avoidance were most likely to survive their diseases. That is, both avoidance and more active, confrontive forms of coping were associated with better disease outcomes. It is noteworthy, however, that avoidance in this sample was characterized as "positive avoidance" and included patients' efforts to put the disease behind them and get on with their lives (Greer, 1991).

Studies of psychological interventions that assist patients in coping with their disease have also shown evidence of an association of psychological variables with cancer progression. Psychological interventions aimed at expression of feelings and active coping with cancer have been associated with immunological changes and longer survival. For example, Spiegel et al. (1989) prospectively studied the effects of support groups on survival time in metastatic breast cancer patients. Results revealed that, although treatment and control groups did not differ significantly in initial severity of cancer or prognosis, treatment group members lived significantly longer than controls (on average, nearly 18 months longer). The authors speculated that supportive group environments might have increased survival time by providing outlets for the identification and expression of feelings. Fawzy and colleagues (Fawzy et al., 1993; Fawzy, Cousins, et al., 1990; Fawzy, Kemeny, et al., 1990) conducted a 6-week structured intervention designed to teach malignant melanoma patients stress management and active coping skills. At the conclusion of the intervention, they found that the treatment group, when compared with a control group, showed significantly lower levels of depressive symptoms, fatigue, confusion, and total mood disturbance and higher levels of vigor. In addition, immunological analyses revealed that the treatment group had significantly more large-granular lymphocytes and natural killer cells, both of which have been hypothesized to have antiviral and antitumor functions (Kiecolt-Glaser & Glaser, 1992). A 6-year follow-up of these patients indicated that survival was significantly enhanced by participation in the intervention (more patients were alive), although changes in immune function did not fully account for survival differences (Fawzy et al., 1993).

In summary, the majority of these studies suggest that minimization and avoidance of thoughts and feelings about one's cancer may be related to poorer disease outcomes, whether avoidance occurs spontaneously or in association with random assignment to control groups in psychological intervention studies. It is noteworthy, however, that none of these studies has directly measured self-reported avoidance. Rather, most have focused on self-reported mood and psychological symptoms as predictors of cancer progression (e.g., Cassileth et al., 1985; Derogatis et al., 1979; Jamison et al., 1987), resulting in mixed findings. Considering the reviewed literature, we believe that it is important to investigate avoidance directly.

In considering avoidance as a possible predictor of cancer progression, an important correlate of avoidance emerges as another potentially significant factor: the presence of intrusive thoughts and emotions. These are defined as unwanted images and strong waves of feelings in response to and associated with a specific stressor (Zilberg, Weiss, & Horowitz, 1982). Intrusive thoughts can be conceptualized as a stimulus for avoidance, which would cause patients to try avoiding unwanted thoughts and emotions. Alternatively, intrusive thoughts may be a result of unsuccessful avoidance efforts; individuals who attempt unsuccessfully to avoid negative thoughts and feelings about their disease are likely to report high levels of intrusive thoughts on an ongoing basis.

Significant relationships between intrusive thoughts and physiological functioning have been demonstrated in generally healthy individuals (Antoni et al., 1990; Davidson & Baum, 1986; Workman & LaVia, 1987) but have not yet been examined with regard to cancer progression. Previous studies have associated intrusive thoughts with markers of stress-related arousal processes such as higher systolic blood pressure (Davidson & Baum, 1986), increased levels of norepinephrine (Davidson & Baum, 1986) and cortisol (Antoni et al., 1990; Davidson & Baum, 1986), and decreased T-lymphocyte polyclonal proliferation (Workman & LaVia, 1987). Because no studies on cancer have yet examined intrusive thoughts as a variable associated with disease progression, the relationship between avoidance, intrusive thoughts, and course of cancer remains unclear. However, these prior studies with noncancer patients (Antoni et al., 1990; Davidson & Baum, 1986; Workman & LaVia, 1987) suggest that high levels of intrusive thoughts may be a marker of emotional arousal and associated dysfunctional physiological processes along with the use of avoidant coping.

In summary, cognitive and behavioral avoidance of one's cancer and its associated negative emotions, coupled with high levels of intrusive or unwanted thoughts and feelings, are strong candidates as predictors of cancer progression. Taken together, high levels of avoidance and intrusive thoughts and emotions are viewed as hallmark characteristics of a generalized stress-response syndrome (Horowitz, Field, & Classen, 1993) and are core symptoms of post-traumatic stress disorder (PTSD; American Psychiatric Association, 1987). The research cited in the previous paragraph (e.g., Antoni et al., 1990; Davidson & Baum, 1986) suggests that avoidance and intrusive thoughts may be more sensitive indices of cognitive/affective and physiological responses to the stress associated with cancer diagnosis and treatment than are measures of generalized psychological distress. Therefore, avoidance and intrusive thoughts may be stronger predictors of adverse physiological outcomes than are generalized symptoms of distress. From the perspective of cognitive–behavioral models of health and illness (e.g., Cohen & Williamson, 1991), avoidance and intrusive thoughts might affect the course of cancer (a) by leading to increased and prolonged physiological arousal and compromised immune functioning, (b) by causing avoidance of important health maintenance or treatment-related behaviors, or (c) by both of these processes.

We designed the present study to examine whether the psychological variables of avoidance, intrusive thoughts, and psychological symptoms, measured near time of diagnosis, predict disease status 1 year postdiagnosis after controlling for initial prognosis. We examined the following hypotheses, which were based on the reviewed literature: (a) Greater levels of intrusive thoughts near time of diagnosis would significantly predict poorer disease status 1 year postdiagnosis; and (b) greater levels of avoidance near time of diagnosis would significantly predict poorer disease status 1 year post diagnosis. We also hypothesized that the psychological variables of avoidance and intrusive thoughts would be stronger predictors of the progression of cancer than would psychological symptoms. Efforts were taken to control for possible third variables that would account for an association between psychological variables and disease outcome, including patient age, the type of information shared with patients by their physicians, and the nature of the treatment they received.

Method

Participants

Participants were 66 cancer patients (80% female and 20% male; mean age = 41.4 years; SD = 8.0) drawn from a larger sample of 126 patients (72% female and 28% male) participating in a longitudinal study of family coping and adjustment with cancer. Inclusion in the present study was based on availability of disease-status data collected 1 year postdiagnosis. Because of the large geographic area from which we drew subjects, a number of participants received follow-up treatment at locations other than those from which they were originally recruited; follow-up medical data were not available from these sites. Comparisons between participants for whom 1-year follow-up data were available (N = 66) and those for whom it was unavailable (n = 60) revealed that participants did not differ from nonparticipants in initial levels of intrusive thoughts, avoidance, or psychological symptoms or with regard to initial disease prognosis, treatments received, or prognosis offered by their physician. Patients in the present study were diagnosed with a variety of different types of cancer, including the most frequent diagnoses of breast cancer (37.9%), gynecologic cancers (19.2%), hematologic malignancies (13.6%), brain tumors (9.1%), and malignant melanoma (4.5%). Because the larger study from which these participants were drawn focused on patients who had children living in their homes, subjects in the present study tended to be younger than the general cancer population, and consequently their diagnoses represent types of cancer that are more common among younger adults.

Procedure

Participants were recruited through three cancer clinics: Medical Oncology ($n = 26$, 39% of the sample), Radiotherapy ($n = 28$, 42%), and Gynecologic Oncology ($n = 12$, 18%) of the Vermont Cancer Center. Patients were approached near their time of diagnosis by a member of the medical staff (nurses, physicians' assistants, or physicians) about participating in the study. For those who were willing, a member of the research team then contacted the person and obtained written consent. The overall sample of 126 represents approximately 75% of patients who were approached regarding participation in the study. Each patient participated in individual structured interviews (in person or over the telephone) and completed written questionnaires assessing psychological variables near the time of diagnosis (mean time from diagnosis to interview = 10.1 weeks, $SD = 8.1$).

Measures

Psychological Symptoms

Psychological symptoms were measured by the Brief Symptom Inventory (BSI; Derogatis & Spencer, 1982). The BSI is a 53-item self-report questionnaire covering symptoms of psychological and physical distress experienced during the previous 7 days. Internal consistency and validity are well-established for the BSI. For this study, we used a modified version of the Global Severity Index (GSI) of the BSI, the mean of ratings for all items. For this population, several somatic items are direct side effects of chemotherapy and radiation and therefore could falsely raise GSI scores for those patients receiving aggressive treatment and potentially confound the GSI with indices of disease severity. In order to address this issue, we asked four oncology professionals, two nurses and two physicians, to indicate those items on the BSI that would be expected to be affected by standard cancer treatment such as chemotherapy and radiation. We removed those items from the GSI that at least three out of four oncology specialists had marked. Thirteen items were deleted, leaving 40 items for inclusion in the modified GSI.[1] The alpha coefficient for the modified GSI indicated good internal consistency ($\alpha = .96$). Additionally, correlational analyses between the original GSI and this modified version revealed a high association, $r(65) = .98$, $p = < .0001$. However, because the modified GSI represents a measure of psychological symptoms free from the confound of physical symptoms, we retained this modified version for predictive analyses. For purposes of comparison to the original normative sample on the BSI, we calculated normalized T scores for the

---

[1]Items deleted from the BSI to create the modified GSI were nervousness or shakiness inside, faintness or dizziness, trouble remembering things, feeling easily annoyed or irritated, poor appetite, feeling blue, nausea or upset stomach, trouble falling asleep, difficulty making decisions, hot or cold spells, numbness or tingling in parts of body, trouble concentrating, and feeling weak in parts of body.

full set of items. Patients in this sample had a mean GSI T score of 55.11 (SD = 7.88), and 12.1% scored above the clinical cutoff of $T > 63$.

Avoidance and Intrusive Thoughts

We measured avoidance and intrusive thoughts by the Impact of Event Scale (IES; Horowitz, Wilner, & Alvarez, 1979). The IES is a 15-item measurement that assesses current degree of impact experienced in response to a specific stressful event, in this case, cancer. Participants responded to the IES as part of their interviews. We asked them to indicate how frequently each item had been true with aspect to their cancer in the 7 days preceding the interview. Responses were made with 4-point scales, from *not at all true* to *often true* (scores corresponding to 0, 1, 3, and 5). There are two subscales to the IES, Avoidance (eight items, range = 0–40) and Intrusion (seven items, range = 0–35), composed of mutually exclusive items. Sample items in the Avoidance subscale include "I try to remove it from my memory," "I stay away from reminders of it," "I try not to talk about it," and "I try not to think about it." Examples of items in the Intrusion subscale include "I think about it when I don't mean to," "I have waves of strong feelings about it," "I have dreams about it," and "Pictures about it pop into my mind." Higher scores correspond to greater degree of impact. Internal consistency of the subscales was adequate in the present sample (α = .73 for Intrusion and α = .70 for Avoidance). In original validation studies (Horowitz et al., 1979), the two subscales correlated at $r(64)$ = .42 (p = < .01). In this sample, Avoidance and Intrusion were correlated at $r(64)$ = .51 (p = < .01). These correlation coefficients are small enough to infer that the scales represent relatively separate constructs but also indicate a moderate degree of covariation.

Disease Variables

We obtained data on disease variables by reviewing medical charts, and we obtained patients' reports of the prognosis they received from their oncologist from the structured interviews. A research assistant and an oncology nurse, both of whom were unaware of patients' psychological data, jointly reviewed each patient's chart. A research assistant unaware of previous findings conducted a separate review and interrater reliability was established at greater than 90%.

Initial prognosis was defined as projected 5-year survival rate. This percentage is derived from statistics that the National Cancer Institute's Surveillance, Epidemiology, and End Results (SEER) program collects (American Cancer Society, 1992) and is used to rate cancer severity at time of diagnosis. Survival rates, which can theoretically range from 1% to 99%, are based on both site and pervasiveness of cancer. Although this study followed patients to 1 year post diagnosis, we used the projected 5-year survival rate, taken directly from the SEER table, because it offers a common prognostic index for this sample of patients with heterogeneous types of cancer. Initial stage ratings I through IV—representative of tumor size and severity —were highly correlated with projected 5-year survival rate, $r(62)$ = −.80, $p < .01$.

We obtained patients' reports of the prognosis that they had been given by their physician by asking the question "Has your physician talked with you about the prognosis of your cancer? [If yes] What have you been told?'' Independent raters coded the responses as reflecting a good prognosis, uncertain prognosis, or poor prognosis. Interrater reliability of 89% agreement was achieved by two independent raters. Five (7.6%) patients reported receiving a poor prognosis, 36 (54.5%) reported receiving an uncertain prognosis, and 25 (37.5%) reported receiving a good prognosis.

An index of the number of treatments was derived by adding the total number of the following treatments that each patient received: surgery (87.9% of patients underwent surgery), hormonal therapy (4.5%), chemotherapy (60.6%), and radiation therapy (63.6%). Thus, the number of treatments could range from 0 to 4. Eight (12.1%) patients received only one form of treatment, 39 (59.1%) received two forms of treatment, 19 (28.8%) patients received three forms of treatment, and no patients received all four forms of treatment.

Disease status was measured 1 year postdiagnosis and was dichotomized into (a) no disease or (b) presence of original cancer, recurrence of cancer, or death. This outcome variable was dichotomized because of the categorical nature of disease status and the low sample size in each of the disease subcategories. Of those participants who were not disease free at 1 year, 14 had died from their cancer, 2 had their original cancer, and 2 had experienced a recurrence.

Results

Descriptive Statistics

Means and standard deviations for predictor variables measured near time of diagnosis are displayed in Table 1. The means for the Avoidance ($M = 10.4$) and Intrusion ($M = 12.5$) subscales of the IES were moderately high, greater than those of community samples but somewhat lower than a clinical sample of adults experiencing parental bereavement (Horowitz et al., 1979). Although norms are not available and therefore T scores cannot be computed for this modified version of the GSI, the mean ($M = 0.33$) indicates that, on average, patients responded somewhere between 0, *not at all*, and 1, *a little bit*, on the retained items. However, the value of the standard

Table 1—*Means and Standard Deviations of Predictor Variables*

Predictor variable	M	SD
Initial SEER prognosis	58.29	30.81
Physician's prognosis	2.30	0.61
Number of treatments	2.17	0.62
Intrusive thoughts	12.53	7.37
Avoidance	10.39	7.30
Modified GSI items	0.33	0.40

Note. SEER = Surveillance, Epidemiology, and End Results program (American Cancer Society, 1992); GSI = Global Severity Index from the Brief Symptom Inventory (Derogatis & Spencer, 1982).

deviation (SD = 0.4) in relation to the mean indicates that the distribution was positively skewed; this signifies that, as assessed by this measure, the majority of patients were subclinical and only a minority reported a high level of psychological symptoms.

Correlational Analyses

Intercorrelations for both the predictor variables measured near time of diagnosis and disease status measured 1 year post diagnosis are shown in Table 2. The three psychological predictors were moderately correlated in the range of .34 to .52. As previously noted, the correlation between the Avoidance and Intrusion subscales of the IES, $r(64)$ = .51, p < .001, is similar to the correlation in original validation study for this measure (r = .42, p < .01; Horowitz et al., 1979). Significant correlations of the Intrusion subscale with the modified GSI, $r(64)$ = .34, p < .01, and of the Avoidance subscale with the modified GSI, $r(64)$ = 0.52, p < .001, are similar to prior studies of highly stressed adults (e.g., Davidson & Baum, 1986).

Initial prognosis based on SEER data and patients' reports of the prognosis that they had received from their physician were only moderately correlated, $r(64)$ = .48, p < .001. As expected, initial prognosis based on SEER data was highly correlated with 1-year disease status, $r(64)$ = −.72, p < .001. Similarly, patients' reports of the prognosis that they had received from their physician were also correlated with 1-year disease status, $r(64)$ = −.48, p < .001. The number of treatments received was not related to either of the initial prognosis variables or with 1-year disease status. The psychological variables of Avoidance, Intrusion, and the modified GSI items were not significantly associated with initial disease prognosis. However, Avoidance was significantly correlated with disease status 1 year post diagnosis, $r(64)$ = 0.25, p < .05. Finally, age was unrelated to any of the disease parameters and was related to only one psychological variable (a negative correlation with avoidance).

Table 2—*Intercorrelations of Predictor Variables Near Diagnosis and Disease Status at 1 Year*

Predictor variable	1	2	3	4	5	6	7	8
1. Intrusive thoughts	—							
2. Avoidance	.51***	—						
3. Modified GSI	.34**	.52***	—					
4. Initial SEER prognosis	.03	−.11	.03	—				
5. Physician's prognosis	−.12	−.19	−.10	.48***	—			
6. Number of treatments	.14	.11	.03	.07	.15	—		
7. 1-Year disease status	.02	.25*	−.02	−.72***	−.48***	−.11	—	
8. Patient age	−.25*	.07	−.09	.11	.08	−.02	−.03	—

Note. GSI = Global Severity Index from the Brief Symptom Inventory (Derogatis & Spencer, 1982); SEER = Surveillance, Epidemiology, and End Results program (American Cancer Society, 1992).

p < .05.
**p* < .01.
***p* < .001.

Logistic Regression Analyses

Forty-eight patients (72.7%) were disease free 1 year post diagnosis, and 18 patients (27.3%) had their original cancers, had experienced a recurrence, or had died. The percentage of subjects who were disease free after only 1 year postdiagnosis was greater than their corresponding 5-year survival rate ($M = 58.3\%$), although this is expected when considering 1-year data with a 5-year predictor.

Because the criterion variable for this study is dichotomous (disease free vs. ill or deceased), we conducted logistic regressions to address the research questions and hypotheses in this study. Logistic regression provides the same type of analyses as linear multiple regression. That is, multiple independent variables are used to predict variance in a dependent variable. However, linear multiple regression and logistic regression use different methods to create optimal predictive models. Linear regression uses a least-squares criterion to model the predicted outcome. Logistic regression usually uses a maximum likelihood procedure to model the log of the odds ratio, where the latter is expressed as the natural log of the probability of survival divided by the probability of nonsurvival. (For further discussion of logistic regression see Darlington, 1990; Hosmer & Lemeshow, 1989).

In the first logistic regression equation we modeled the probability of survival as a function of a set of control variables composed of patient age, initial SEER prognosis, patients' reports of the prognosis they received from their physician, and the number of treatments patients' received. These variables were treated as covariates and were common to all regressions. Next, to allow direct comparisons with prior studies using a general psychological symptom index, the modified GSI scores were entered along with the control variables. We then added the measure of avoidance to the model, followed in the final analysis by the measure of intrusive thoughts.

In the first regression, age and medically related control variables were used to predict disease status at 1 year. The results of this analysis are shown in Table 3. The overall equation provided a significant fit with the data, $\chi^2(4, N = 66) = 42.67$, $p < .001$. As expected, the SEER 5-year survival estimate was a strong predictor of 1-year survival status, although neither age, the patients' reports of the prognosis they had received from the physician, or the number of treatments received accounted for any significant variance in the outcome.

Adding the modified GSI—a global measure of psychological distress—to the model did not lead to a significant improvement in fit. The test for this model produced $\chi^2(5, N = 66) = 42.71$. This represents a gain in chi-square of only .04 units, which is itself a chi square on 1 degree of freedom and is not significant. We chose to retain this global measure in future models, however, to maintain comparability with previous studies.

Adding the Avoidance scale of the IES produced a model with a good fit to the data, $\chi^2(6, N = 66) = 49.72$, $p < .001$, which is a significant improvement over the previous model. The test on the improved fit of the model was $\chi^2(1, N = 66) = 7.01$, $p < .025$. As can be seen in Table 3, in this model both the initial SEER 5-year prognosis and the Avoidance subscale were significant predictors. The coefficient for the avoidance measure is -0.211, which can be used to calculate an index of the difference in the odds of survival associated with a fixed difference in the avoidance score. If we take a difference in avoidance scores equal to one half of a standard deviation as being a psychologically meaningful difference, this would be associated

Table 3—*Logistic Regressions Predicting Disease Status at 1 Year From Initial Disease Parameters and Psychological Variables Near Diagnosis*

Predictor entered	β	χ^2	Probability
Control variables, $\chi^2(4, N = 66) = 42.67*$			
Intercept	−5.20	2.81	.094
Patient age	−0.01	0.04	.834
SEER prognosis	0.08	11.65	.001
Physician's prognosis	0.90	1.07	.300
Number of treatments	0.59	0.82	.365
Psychological symptoms, $\chi^2(5, N = 66) = 42.71*$			
Intercept	−5.33	2.76	.097
Patient age	−0.01	0.03	.863
SEER prognosis	0.08	11.52	.001
Physician's prognosis	0.91	1.08	.299
Number of treatments	0.56	0.71	.401
Modified GSI	0.34	0.04	.848
Avoidance and psychological symptoms, $\chi^2(6, N = 66) = 49.72*$			
Intercept	−7.27	3.11	.078
Patient age	0.05	0.46	.498
SEER prognosis	0.11	8.52	.004
Physician's prognosis	0.40	0.14	.706
Number of treatments	1.23	1.70	.192
Avoidance subscale	−0.21	5.51	.019
Modified GSI	3.19	1.73	.188
Avoidance, intrusion, and psychological symptoms, $\chi^2(7, N = 66) = 50.54*$			
Intercept	−8.54	3.89	.049
Patient age	0.60	0.84	.360
SEER prognosis	0.11	8.33	.004
Physician's prognosis	0.30	0.08	.774
Number of treatments	1.20	1.49	.222
Intrusion subscale	0.10	0.78	.378
Avoidance subscale	−0.28	4.69	.030
Modified GSI	3.49	1.87	.172
Intrusion and psychological symptoms, $\chi^2(6, N = 66) = 43.36*$			
Intercept	−5.00	2.06	.151
Patient age	−0.01	0.04	.836
SEER prognosis	0.85	11.04	.001
Physician's prognosis	0.85	0.90	.344
Number of treatments	0.73	1.03	.311
Intrusion subscale	−0.06	0.63	.427
Modified GSI	0.84	0.18	.675

Note. SEER = Surveillance, Epidemiology, and End Results program (American Cancer Society, 1992); GSI = Global Severity Index from the Brief Symptom Inventory (Derogatis & Spencer, 1982).

*$p < .001$.

with a difference of 0.488 in the odds of survival. Thus, holding all other variables constant, including initial prognosis, a patient whose avoidance score is one half of a standard deviation above that of another patient would have only approximately half the odds of being disease free at the end of 1 year.

The complete model added the Intrusion subscale of the IES to the variables in the previous model. This produced a model with $\chi^2(7, N = 66) = 50.54, p < .001$. Although this model does fit the data better than chance, it does not fit significantly better than the simpler previous model; the change was $\chi^2(1, N = 66) = 0.82, p > .10$. In addition, the initial 5-year prognosis and the Avoidance subscale remained significant predictors, but the intrusion measure did not contribute significantly.

The Intrusion and Avoidance subscales of the IES were moderately correlated ($r = .51$) and may have been competing for common variance in predicting 1-year disease status. Therefore, to determine if intrusion was a significant predictor in the absence of avoidance, we included in our final model the control variables, the modified GSI, and the Intrusion subscale of the IES as predictors. The overall model was a good fit, $\chi^2(6, N = 66) = 43.36, p < .001$. However, intrusion was not a significant predictor; initial SEER 5-year prognosis was the only significant predictor.[2]

Discussion

In the present study we used a prospective design to test psychological symptoms, avoidance, and intrusive thoughts as predictors of cancer progression over a period of 1 year. The findings indicate that avoidance, but not psychological symptoms or intrusive thoughts, predict disease status 1 year later, after controlling for initial prognosis.

In the present sample, psychological symptoms, avoidance, and intrusive thoughts were moderately intercorrelated near time of diagnosis but differentially predictive of subsequent disease status: Avoidance was the sole psychological marker of cancer progression. Prior researchers have not directly measured avoidance of one's disease or reminders of it as a predictor of cancer progression, but have focused on self-reported mood and psychological symptoms as predictors of cancer progression (e.g., Cassileth et al., 1985; Derogatis et al., 1979; Jamison et al., 1987), resulting in mixed findings. The current data extend the significance of avoidant responses by implicating their role in predicting cancer progression. These findings are consistent with the more general literature that has shown an association between avoidance and poor physical and psychological outcomes (e.g., Billings & Moos,

---

[2]A somewhat simpler analysis of the association between the Avoidance subscale of the IES and disease status at 1 year was conducted by creating groups high and low in avoidance using a median split. Thirty-four individuals were below the median (< 9), and 32 participants were above the median. A 2 × 2 chi-square analysis was used to examine the number of participants who were above and below the median on the Avoidance subscale and who were disease free versus ill or deceased at 1 year. Of the 34 who were low in avoidance, 29 were disease free and 5 were ill or deceased. Of the 32 who were high in avoidance, 19 were disease free and 13 were ill or deceased. This pattern of observed cases was significantly different from the expected distribution, $\chi^2(1, N = 66) = 5.58, p = .018$. Specifically, the expected number of individuals high in avoidance and ill or deceased was 8.7, compared with an observed frequency of 13.

1981; Holahan & Moos, 1986, 1987; Suls & Fletcher, 1985). In most of these studies, however, physical symptoms have been assessed by self-reports. The present findings establish an association between self-reported avoidance and objective measures of disease status 1 year later.

Consistent with initial hypotheses, psychological symptoms as reflected in the BSI near time of diagnosis did not predict disease status 1 year postdiagnosis. Similar results were reported by Cassileth et al. (1985) and Jamison et al. (1987), who found psychosocial symptom measures to be unrelated to cancer progression. Our findings suggest that psychological symptoms may not clearly reflect the cognitive and emotional processes that are most closely related to subsequent disease progression in cancer patients, which would account for previous studies' nonsignificant findings. The levels of psychological distress reported by patients in the present sample and in other recent studies of cancer patients (e.g., Stanton & Snider, 1993) reflect low to moderate levels of generalized distress. These symptom patterns, due to their low levels and restricted range, may not play a central role in patients' response to the stress of a cancer diagnosis and early phases of treatment. In contrast, higher levels of psychological distress, reflected by symptoms strong enough that they meet diagnostic criteria for depressive disorders, are related to compromised immune function and disease (Herbert & Cohen, 1993; Weisse, 1992). Furthermore, high levels of avoidance and intrusive thoughts and emotions may reflect a more central way in which cancer patients manifest their distress, that is, through symptoms more characteristic of PTSD.

Contrary to initial hypotheses, intrusive thoughts did not significantly predict disease status in this study. Several explanations could account for this nonsignificant finding. First, intrusive thoughts may reflect short-term levels of high distress in response to a traumatic event such as the diagnosis of cancer. Intrusive thoughts may subside over time as the original trauma is resolved (Horowitz et al., 1993), and therefore they may not be a powerful predictor of longer term physical and psychological outcomes. Second, in light of the positive association between avoidance and intrusive thoughts observed in the present sample, intrusive thoughts may play an important role as a precipitant of continued avoidance. A subgroup of cancer patients who experience high levels of intrusive thoughts and feelings about their illness may be engaging in a cycle of unsuccessful avoidance that may place them at increased risk for poorer disease outcome. The present findings suggest that avoidance of intrusive thoughts and emotions may be a better predictor of disease progression than the presence of intrusive thoughts and emotions alone. This hypothesis is plausible given the significant relationship between avoidance—which can be conceptualized as unsuccessful efforts to avoid particular thoughts and feelings—and subsequent disease progression, as well as the significant positive relationship between intrusive thoughts and avoidance.

It is noteworthy that in the present study all psychological variables were unrelated to initial prognosis. The literature is mixed with regard to the relationships between psychological distress and physical status in cancer patients. Some studies have reported significant relationships (e.g., Cassileth, Lusk, & Tenaglia, 1983; Cella et al., 1987; Taylor et al., 1985), particularly for those with more advanced forms of cancer (e.g., Pettingale, Burgess, & Greer, 1988), whereas others have found that only perceived severity of illness (e.g., Marks, Richardson, Graham, & Levine, 1986) is related to psychological distress. To make sense of these discrepant findings, it is important to consider the ways in which researchers have defined psychological distress. This variable has been operationalized as daily mood (Cella et al., 1987), symptoms of depression and anxiety (Pettingale et al., 1988), body image and satisfaction (Cassileth et al., 1983), and a factor-derived compilation of daily mood with patient- and observer-rated adjustment (Taylor et al., 1985). In the present study, we used self-report measures of generalized psychological symptoms, intrusive thoughts, and avoidance efforts spanning retrospectively 1 week from the time of response. It is possible that the present psychological indices are more stable indicators of psychological functioning and therefore less closely correlated with physical variables than daily mood measures might be.

The present study's prospective findings help in clarifying prior conflicting findings regarding the influence of psychological factors on disease progression. These findings indicate that the literature's discrepant results may have been caused by differences in psychological variables chosen for examination. Findings of previous research examining the influence of generalized psychological symptoms on cancer progression have been mainly nonsignificant (e.g., Cassileth et al., 1985; Jamison et al., 1987), whereas those studies investigating the relationship of more specific symptoms and behavior (in particular, situational adjustment and coping) on disease status have been primarily significant (e.g., Fawzy, Kemeny, et al., 1990; Rogentine et al., 1979). In support of this hypothesis, our study found that avoidance of thoughts and reminders of the cancer, but not more generalized psychological symptoms, was a predictor of cancer progression. Furthermore, it is important to note that the association between initial avoidance and later disease outcomes was not the result of such possible "third variables" or confounds as the patients' age, initial prognosis, the information communicated to patients by their physicians, or the number of treatments that they received.

The mechanisms by which avoidance might affect cancer outcome require further investigation. At least two hypotheses are worth pursuing. First, avoidance might affect immune functioning in cancer patients by contributing to continued high distress and emotional arousal. Second, avoidance might result in decreased compliance with cancer treatments, which in turn could lead to worsened disease status. The relationship of avoidance of intrusive thoughts and emotions with other aspects of patients' coping with their illness warrants further attention as well. These questions are unfortunately beyond the scope of this study.

These results offer important guidance to future work in this area. First, the findings warrant replication with a larger sample size and over a longer period of time. The present sample was limited with regard to age, sex, type of cancer, and presence of children in the home and may not be representative of cancer patients in general. Therefore, the generalizability of these results needs to be examined, as the present findings pertain primarily to relatively young married women with cancer. Second, the outcome measure, first-year disease status, is a somewhat coarse indication of physical functioning that does not reflect finer gradations of cancer progression or tumor reduction; future studies using more refined measures of disease outcome are needed. Third, the possible mechanisms that may account for the association between avoidance and disease outcome are a high priority for future research. Understanding of the long-term significance of psychological factors on cancer progression remains an important and realistic goal for research in this area. In addition to warranting continued research on the association between psychological factors and cancer progression, these findings suggest that further research on the applied implications of avoidance and cancer progression is also warranted. Enhancing patients' use of coping skills and use of social support as ways to manage or reduce avoidance of troubling thoughts and emotions may be an important target for intenventions to assist cancer patients in coping with their disease.

References

American Cancer Society. (1992). *Cancer facts and figures—1992*. Atlanta, GA: Author.

American Psychiatric Association. (1987). *Diagnostic and statistical manual of mental disorders* (3rd ed., rev.). Washington, DC: Author.

Andersen, B. L., Kiecolt-Glaser, J. K., & Glaser, R. (1994). A biobehavioral model of cancer stress and disease course. *American Psychologist, 49,* 389–404.

Antoni, M. H., August, S., LaPerriere, A., Baggett, H. L., Klimas, N., Ironson, G., Schneiderman, N., & Fletcher, M. A. (1990). Psychological and neuroendocrine measures related to functional immune changes in anticipation of HIV-1 serostatus notification. *Psychosomatic Medicine, 52,* 496–510.

Billings, A. G., & Moos, R. H. (1981). The role of coping responses and social resources in attenuating the stress of life events. *Journal of Behavioral Medicine, 4,* 139–157.

Buddeberg, C., Wolf, C., Sieber, M., Riehl-Emde, A., Bergant, A., Steiner, R., Landolt-Ritter, C., & Richter, D. (1991). Coping strategies and course of disease of breast cancer patients. *Psychotherapy and Psychosomatics, 55,* 151–157.

Cassileth, B. R., Lusk, E. J., Miller, D. S., Brown, L. L., & Miller, C. (1985). Psychosocial correlates of survival in advanced malignant disease. *New England Journal of Medicine, 312,* 1551–1555.

Cassileth, B. R., Lusk, E. J., & Tenaglia, B. S. (1983). Patients' perceptions of the cosmetic impact of melanoma resection. *Plastic and Reconstructive Surgery, 7,* 73–75.

Cella, D. F., Orofiamma, B., Holland, J. C., Silberfarb, P. M., Tross, S., Feldstein, M., Perry, M., Maurer, L. H., Comis, R., & Orav, E. J. (1987). The relationship of psychological distress, extent of disease, and performance status in patients with lung cancer. *Cancer, 60,* 1661–1667.

Cohen, S., & Williamson, G. M. (1991). Stress and infectious disease in humans. *Psychological Bulletin, 109,* 5–24.

Cousins, N. (1989). *Head first: The biology of hope.* New York: Dutton.

Darlington, R. B. (1990). *Regression and linear models.* New York: McGraw-Hill.

Davidson, L. M., & Baum, A. (1986). Chronic stress and posttraumatic stress disorders. *Journal of Consulting and Clinical Psychology, 54,* 303–308.

Derogatis, L. R., Abeloff, M. D., & Melisaratos, N. (1979). Psychological coping mechanisms and survival time in metastatic breast cancer. *Journal of the American Medical Association, 242,* 1504–1508.

Derogatis, L. R., & Spencer, P. M. (1982). *The Brief Symptom Inventory (BSI) administration, scoring and procedures manual.* Baltimore, MD: Author.

Fawzy, F. I., Cousins, N., Fawzy, N. W., Kemeny, M., Elashoff, R., & Morton, D. (1990). A structured psychiatric intervention for cancer patients: I. Changes over time in methods of coping and affective disturbance. *Archives of General Psychiatry, 47,* 720–725.

Fawzy, F. I., Fawzy, N. W., Hyun, C. S., Elashoff, R., Guthrie, D., Fahey, J. L., & Morton, D. L. (1993). Malignant melanoma: Effects of an early structured psychiatric intervention, coping, and affective state on recurrences and survival 6 years later. *Archives of General Psychiatry, 50,* 681–689.

Fawzy, F. I., Kemeny, M. E., Fawzy, N. W., Elashoff, R., Morton, D., Cousins, N., & Fahey, J. L. (1990). A structured psychiatric intervention for cancer patients: II. Changes over time in immunological measures. *Archives of General Psychiatry, 47,* 729–735.

Greer, S. (1991). Psychological response to cancer and survival. *Psychological Medicine, 21,* 43–49.

Greer, S., Morris, T., & Pettingale, K. W. (1979, October 13). Psychological response to breast cancer: Effect on outcome. *The Lancet,* 785–787.

Greer, S., Morris, T., Pettingale, K. W., & Haybittle, J. L. (1990). Psychological response to breast cancer and 15 year outcome. *The Lancet,* 49–50.

Herbert, T. B., & Cohen, S. (1993). Depression and immunity: A meta-analytic review. *Psychological Bulletin, 113,* 472–486.

Holahan, C. J., & Moos, R. H. (1986). Personality, coping and family resources in stress resistance: A longitudinal analysis. *Journal of Personality and Social Psychology, 51,* 389–395.

Holahan, C. J., & Moos, R. H. (1987). Risk, resistance, and psychological distress: A longitudinal analysis with adults and children. *Journal of Abnormal Psychology, 96,* 3–13.

Horowitz, M. J., Field, N. P., & Classen, C. C. (1993). Stress response syndromes and their treatment. In L. Goldberger & S. Breznitz (Eds.), *Handbook of stress: Theoretical and clinical aspects* (2nd ed., pp. 757–773). New York: Free Press.

Horowitz, M., Wilner, N., & Alvarez, W. (1979). Impact of event scale: A measure of subjective stress. *Psychosomatic Medicine, 41,* 209–218.

Hosmer, D. W., & Lemeshow, S. (1989). *Applied logistic regression.* New York: Wiley.

Jamison, R. N., Burish, T. G., & Wallston, K. A. (1987). Psychogenic factors in predicting survival of breast cancer patients. *Journal of Clinical Oncology, 5,* 772–786.

Kiecolt-Glaser, J. K., & Glaser, R. (1992). Psychoneuroimmunology: Can psychological interventions modulate immunity? *Journal of Consulting and Clinical Psychology, 60,* 569–575.

Levenson, J. L., & Bemis, C. (1990). The role of psychological factors in cancer onset and progression. *Psychosomatics, 32,* 124–132.

Levy, S. M., Herberman, R. B., Maluish, A. M., Schlien, B., & Lippman, M. (1985). Prognostic risk assessment in primary breast cancer by behavioral and immunological parameters. *Health Psychology, 4,* 99–113.

Levy, S. M., Lee, J., Bagley, C., & Lippman, M. (1988). Survival hazards analysis in first recurrent breast cancer patients: Seven-year follow-up. *Psychosomatic Medicine, 50,* 520–528.

Marks, G., Richardson, J. L., Graham, J. W., & Levine, A. (1986). Role of health locus of control beliefs and expectations of treatment efficacy in adjustment to cancer. *Journal of Personality and Social Psychology, 51,* 443–450.

O'Leary, A. (1990). Stress, emotion, and human immune function. *Psychological Bulletin, 108,* 363–382.

Pettingale, K. W., Burgess, C., & Greer, S. (1988). Psychological response to cancer diagnosis: I. Correlations with prognostic variables. *Journal of Psychosomatic Research, 32,* 255–261.

Richardson, J. L., Zarnegar, Z., Bisno, B., & Levine, A. (1990). Psychological status at initiation of cancer treatment and survival. *Journal of Psychosomatic Research, 34,* 189–201.

Rogentine, G. N., van Kammen, D. P., Fox, B. H., Docherty, J. P., Rosenblatt, J. E., Boyd, S. C., & Bunney, W. E. (1979). Psychological factors in the prognosis of malignant melanoma: A prospective study. *Psychosomatic Medicine, 41,* 647–655.

Siegel, B. S. (1986). *Love, medicine and miracles.* New York: Harper & Row.

Spiegel, D., Bloom, J. R., Kraemer, H. C., & Gottheil, E. (1989, October 14). Effect of psychosocial treatment on survival of patients with metastatic breast cancer. *The Lancet,* 888–891.

Stanton, A. L., & Snider, P. R. (1993). Coping with a breast cancer diagnosis: A prospective study. *Health Psychology, 12,* 16–23.

Suls, J., & Fletcher, B. (1985). The relative efficacy of avoidant and nonavoidant coping strategies: A meta-analysis. *Health Psychology, 4,* 249–288.

Taylor, S. E., Lichtman, R. R., Wood, J. V., Bluming, A. Z., Dosik, G. M., & Leibowitz, R. L. (1985). Illness-related and treatment-related factors in psychological adjustment to breast cancer. *Cancer, 55,* 2506–2513.

Weisse, C. S. (1992). Depression and immunocompetence: A review of the literature. *Psychological Bulletin, 111,* 475–489.

Workman, E. A., & LaVia, M. F. (1987). T-lymphocyte polyclonal proliferation: Effects of stress and stress response style on medical students taking national board examinations. *Clinical Immunology and Immunopathology, 43,* 308–313.

Zilberg, N. J., Weiss, D. S., & Horowitz, M. J. (1982). Impact of Event Scale: A cross-validation study and some empirical evidence supporting a conceptual model of stress response syndromes. *Journal of Consulting and Clinical Psychology, 50,* 407–414.

Chapter 15
PESSIMISM, AGE, AND CANCER MORTALITY

Richard Schulz, Jamila Bookwala, Judith E. Knapp, Michael F. Scheier, and Gail M. Williamson

Research examining the relation between psychosocial factors and the occurrence and course of cancer has yielded mixed findings. Some studies report significant associations between cancer survival and psychological factors such as personality style, depressed mood, hopelessness, social support, and anger (Colon, Callies, Popkin, & McGlave, 1991; Derogatis, Abeloff, & Melisaratos, 1979; Greer, 1991; Greer, Morris, & Pettingale, 1979; Hislop, Waxler, Coldman, Elwood, & Kan, 1987; Phillips & Smith, 1990; Phillips, Todd, & Wagner, 1993; Spiegel, Bloom, Kraemer, & Gottheil, 1989; Temoshok & Dreher, 1992), whereas others do not (Cassileth, Lusk, Miller, Brown, & Miller, 1985; Jamison, Burish, & Wallston, 1987; Morgenstern, Gellert, Walter, Ostfeld, & Siegel, 1984; Silberfarb et al., 1991; Zonderman, Costa, & McCrae, 1989). Reviewers of this literature have focused on a variety of methodological and conceptual issues that might account for these discrepant findings; however, all agree with the general conclusion that this topic is worthy of further attention (Fox, Temoshok, & Dreher, 1988; Jensen, 1991; Levenson & Bemis, 1991; Redd et al., 1991). In particular, they suggest that future research in this area concentrate on prospective studies of cancer mortality, develop more focused hypotheses regarding the role of specific psychological factors that might affect cancer mortality, and investigate underlying mechanisms that might account for the observed associations. This conclusion is further supported by a recent review of the broader literature on person variables and health carried out by Scheier and Bridges (1995).

Instead of the global omnibus psychosocial measures often used in studies of this type, we focused on two related constructs that have been frequently but not consistently linked with cancer mortality: optimism and pessimism. Researchers such as Greer and colleagues found that having a "fighting spirit," as opposed to stoic acceptance or feelings of helplessness and hopelessness, was predictive of cancer survival (Greer, 1991; Greer et al., 1979). In their study of Chinese-Americans, Phillips et al. (1993) suggested that the shortened survival of "ill-fated" individuals could be attributed to "giving up" among persons who developed cancer.

In the past, optimism and pessimism have been treated as bipolar opposites, and indeed in most contexts in which they have been studied their effects have been complementary (Carver et al., 1993; Mroczek, Spiro, Aldwin, Ozer, & Bosse, 1993; Scheier & Carver, 1985). More recent research, however, suggests that they are not simply two sides of the same coin (e.g., they can have different correlates and they tend to emerge as separate factors in factor analyses; Mroczek et al., 1993). Although this issue is not yet fully resolved, these findings have led researchers to suggest that

Reprinted from *Psychology and Aging, 11*(2), 304–309. (1996). Copyright © 1996 by the American Psychological Association. Used with permission of the author.

Preparation of this article was supported in part by grants from the National Cancer Institute (CA48635 and CA61303) and the National Institute of Mental Health (MH52247 and MH46015).

the effects of optimism and pessimism be evaluated separately as a matter of course (Scheier, Carver, & Bridges, 1994). Consequently, for purposes of the present research, we treated these constructs as distinct dimensions and examined the effects of optimism and pessimism separately in predicting survival among cancer patients.

A second factor that may contribute to the inconsistent pattern of results in psychosocial cancer research is the age-heterogeneity of populations being studied. The role of psychosocial factors and the impact of an illness like cancer may vary as a function of the individual's location in the life course (Fox, 1978; Ryff, 1991; Temoshok, 1991). The experience of cancer for an older person is likely to be substantially different from that of a younger person. Several reasons may explain these differences. First, getting a serious illness like cancer is more normative among older persons and therefore more likely to be expected. Second, older persons are likely to have greater prior experience with both acute and chronic illnesses because of their own direct experience with illness and disability or because they have observed them in friends and relatives. Finally, the threat of an illness like cancer may be lessened among older adults because the perceived losses are not as great; they have most of their lives and accomplishments behind them as opposed to ahead of them (Ryff, 1991). In general, the psychological significance of a major life event such as physical illness may vary substantially as a function of the individual's location in the life course (Heckhausen & Schulz, 1995). For an illness such as cancer, the impact on older people is likely to be blunted, and the role of psychological factors in contributing to mortality may be dampened when compared to the young (Fox, 1978). Addressing these issues would require that researchers investigate interactions between age and psychosocial variables as predictors of mortality in cancer patients. This was the strategy adopted in this study. Controlling for type and severity of cancer symptoms at baseline, we examined the independent effects of optimism and pessimism in predicting survival among younger and older patients.

Methods

Participants

Patients with recurrent or metastasized cancer ($N = 268$) were recruited consecutively from radiation therapy departments of five urban and suburban hospitals in western Pennsylvania as part of a study on the home care needs and home care utilization patterns of cancer patients. See Table 1 for descriptive information about the sample. Eligibility criteria included (a) being age 30 years or older, (b) having a diagnosis of recurrent or metastasized cancer, (c) initiating a course of outpatient radiation therapy for palliation of symptoms, (d) having a life expectancy of at least 1 year based on the judgment of medical staff, and (e) living at home. Patients enrolled in a hospice program were not eligible to participate.

Baseline interviews were conducted in most cases within 1 week of initial contact and consent. Two follow-up interviews were completed approximately 4 and 8 months later. The survey instrument took approximately 90 min to administer and focused on patient needs for and utilization of home care services as well as sociodemographic characteristics and a variety of health-related and psychosocial measures, including optimism, pessimism, depression, self-reported physical sympto-

Table 1—*Descriptive Information About the*
Patient Sample (N = 238)

Characteristic	n	%
Gender		
Male	117	49.2
Female	121	50.8
Race		
White	216	90.8
Black	22	9.2
Marital status[a]		
Single	12	5.1
Cohabiting or married	152	63.9
Widowed	45	18.9
Separated or divorced	27	11.3
Education		
High school or less	141	59.2
Trade or technical school	43	18.1
Some college	22	9.2
College graduate	19	8.0
Graduate or professional school	13	5.5
Site of cancer		
Breast	55	23.1
Lung	47	19.7
Head or neck	30	12.6
Gynecologic	21	8.8
Prostate	19	8.0
Colorectal	12	5.0
Gastrointestinal	9	3.8
Other	45	18.9

Note. Percentages do not add up to 100% because of rounding off.
[a]Because of missing data, *N* does not total 238.

matology, and site of cancer (assessed at baseline). Although survival status was not a primary endpoint of the study, mortality was ascertained at the 8-month follow-up among all individuals who remained in the study. Of the 268 persons originally recruited to the study, 30 were lost between the baseline assessment and the 8-month follow-up because of illness, refusal, or inability to locate. Because the mortality status of these 30 individuals was not ascertained at the follow-up, they were excluded from the analyses. As a group, these individuals were similar to the nonsurvivors in terms of their health status at baseline. The analyses reported in this study are based on the 238 individuals whose mortality status could be definitively ascertained at the 8-month follow-up assessment.

Measures

Dispositional optimism and pessimism were measured using the Life Orientation Test (LOT; Scheier & Carver, 1985). The LOT consists of 8 items (plus 4 filler items).

Four of the scored items are phrased in a positive manner (e.g., "In uncertain times, I usually expect the best."), and four are phrased in a negative manner (e.g., "I hardly ever expect things to go my way."). Separate subscales for optimism and pessimism can be created from the LOT by summing responses to the positively and negatively worded items, respectively. Cronbach's alpha for the optimism subscale was .72; for the pessimism subscale, it was .77. Depression was measured with the 20-item Center for Epidemiological Studies—Depression (CES–D; Radloff, 1977) scale (α = .85). Total number of symptoms was assessed by summing patient responses to the presence of 16 disease- or treatment-related symptoms that cancer patients often experience (Given, Given, & Stommel, 1994). The symptoms assessed included, among others, pain, fatigue, nausea, and bowel and bladder problems.

Results

Of the 238 patients, a total of 70 had died by the 8-month follow-up. Descriptive information about the sample is provided in Table 1. Breast cancer and lung cancer were the most prevalent forms of cancer, whereas colorectal and gastrointestinal cancers were the least common. The vast majority of study participants were White, and approximately 50% of the sample was female. Table 2 provides data for survivors and nonsurvivors separately on indicators of physical symptomatology, depression, optimism, pessimism, and age. Correlations among these variables are provided in Table 3.

We performed two separate logistic regression analyses using surviving patients and nonsurvivors at Time 3 (n = 229),[1] in order to examine the moderating role of age on the effects of an optimistic versus pessimistic life orientation (assessed at baseline) on mortality status at the 8-month follow-up. A forced-entry model was used in which mortality (coded as 0 for survivors, n = 163, and 1 for nonsurvivors, n = 66) was regressed on baseline physical health status, life orientation (optimism or pessimism), age, and the interaction between age and an optimistic or pessimistic life orientation. To control for health status at baseline, the two indicators of physical health, patient's site of cancer and reported physical symptomatology, were entered on Step 1 of the analysis. Site of cancer was coded as seven dummy variables (0 = *absence of site-specific cancer*, 1 = *presence*) based on the eight different sites of cancer (breast, lung, head/neck, gynecologic, prostate, colorectal, gastrointestinal, and other). Pessimism or optimism scores and patient's age were entered on the second step of the analysis. Finally, the interaction between optimism or pessimism and age was entered in the equation.

In the logistic regression analysis examining the effects of optimism, physical symptoms were highly predictive of mortality (p < .0001), suggesting that this variable is a good proxy indicator for severity of illness. When optimism and age were added to the regression analysis, no main effects for either variable were found; additionally, no Optimism $\times$ Age interaction effect was observed (all t values had a p > .05). In the second regression analysis focusing on the effects of pessimism, physical symptoms were again highly predictive of mortality, and although no main

---

[1]Participants with missing data on any health or psychosocial variable were excluded from the analysis.

Table 2—*Group Means on Physical Symptomatology, Psychosocial Measures, and Age Assessed at Baseline (N = 238)*

Variable	Survivors			Nonsurvivors		
	n[a]	M	SD	n[a]	M	SD
Physical symptomatology[b]	168	4.88	2.74	70	7.31	2.55
Pessimism[c]	163	5.54	3.09	66	6.50	3.53
Optimism	163	11.48	2.92	55	11.23	3.02
Depression[b]	164	8.24	8.18	66	11.86	8.55
Age	168	62.89	11.02	70	62.60	10.05

Note. Higher scores indicate greater symptomatology, higher pessimism, optimism, and depression scores.

[a]Group sizes vary because of missing data.
[b]Group means different at $p < .05$.
[c]Group means different at $p < .01$.

effects of pessimism or age on mortality status were noted, a Pessimism × Age interaction effect was obtained indicating that patients' age moderated the relation between pessimism and survival. Hence, only the results of the analyses involving pessimism are reported here (see Table 4).

On all steps of the analysis, the goodness-of-fit test statistic indicated that the data fit the model being tested (χ^2 values ranged from 217.79, $df = 217$, $p > .47$, to 220.02, $df = 220$, $p > .48$). Site of cancer and physical symptomatology, entered on Step 1, yielded a significant model chi-square value, χ^2 (8, $N = 229$) = 38.40, $p < .0001$. Total number of symptoms was the strongest predictor of mortality (Wald = 20.59, $p < .0001$). On Step 2, patients' pessimism scores and age were added to the model, resulting in a nonsignificant improvement in the model chi-square value, χ^2(2, $N = 229$) = 4.40, $p > .10$; however, neither pessimism nor age significantly predicted patient mortality at follow-up (Wald = 1.80 and 2.46, respectively, $p > .10$). Finally, the interaction between pessimism and age, entered on Step 3, produced a significant improvement in the model chi-square value, χ^2(1, $N = 229$) = 4.11, $p < .05$), and predicted mortality status at follow-up (Wald = 3.98, $p < .05$). In terms of overall

Table 3—*Intercorrelations Among Predictor and Outcome Variables (N = 238)*

Variable	1	2	3	4	5	6	7
1. Depression	—						
2. Pessimism	.39**	—					
3. Physical symptoms	.47**	.14*	—				
4. Age	−.07	.01	.09	—			
5. Optimism	−.42**	−.52**	−.14*	.09	—		
6. Married/not married	−.02	−.09	.08	−.02		—	
7. Education	−.09	−.31**	−.08	−.16*	.09	−.08	—
8. Survivor/nonsurvivor	.20**	.14*	.38*	−.01	.04	.03	−.02

*$p < .05$.
**$p < .01$.

Table 4—*Pessimism and Age as Predictors of Mortality: Hierarchical Regression Analyses (N = 238)*

Predictor	β	SE	Wald	Odds ratio
Step 1. Model χ^2(8, N = 238) = 38.40***				
Site of cancer				
Head/neck	−0.22	0.56	0.15	0.80
Gastrointestinal	−1.00	1.14	0.78	0.37
Colorectal	−0.31	0.76	0.16	0.74
Lung	0.13	0.47	0.08	1.14
Breast	−1.00	0.52	3.65	0.37
Gynecologic	−0.35	0.65	0.29	0.70
Prostate	0.08	0.65	0.02	1.09
Physical symptoms	0.29	0.06	20.59***	1.34
Step 2. Model improvement χ^2(2, N = 238) = 4.40				
Pessimism	0.07	0.05	1.80	1.07
Age	−0.33	0.21	2.46	0.72
Step 3. Model improvement χ^2(1, N = 238) = 4.11*				
Pessimism × Age	−0.12	0.06	3.98*	0.88

*$p < .05$.
***$p < .0001$.

classification, the model accurately classified the survival status at follow-up of 74.24% of the respondents.

Next, we performed follow-up analyses to examine the specific way in which age moderated the relation between pessimism and mortality status. Age was trichotomized to create three groups of roughly equivalent size representing younger cancer patients (ages 30–59, n = 83), middle-aged cancer patients (ages 60–69, n = 73), and older cancer patients (ages 70 and older, n = 82). Logistic regression analyses were conducted for the three age groups separately in which mortality status at follow-up was regressed on pessimism scores after controlling for physical health status at baseline. A strong predictive effect of pessimism on mortality status was obtained only for the youngest group (ages 30–59; Wald = 4.29, p < .05); the addition of pessimism significantly improved the fit of the model, χ^2(1, N = 80) = 4.60, p < .05. In contrast, for the two older age groups (age ranges 60–69 and > 69, respectively), pessimism scores did not significantly improve the model chi-square value, χ^2(1) < 1, *ns*, nor did they predict mortality status at follow-up (Wald < 1, *ns*).

Finally, we examined the interaction between age and pessimism on survival by plotting the mean levels of pessimism by age group and mortality status. As illustrated in Figure 1, the two older groups exhibited a relatively stable pessimistic orientation, regardless of mortality status. In contrast, in the youngest group of patients, those who had survived until follow-up were characterized by lower levels of pessimism than those who had died.

To compare the effects of depression and pessimism, we carried out a series of

Age Groups

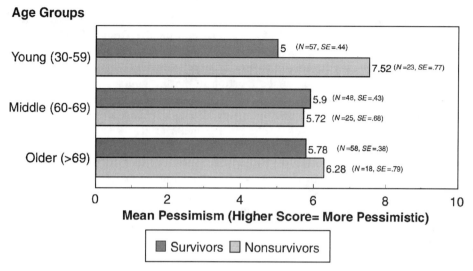

Figure 1. Mean scores for pessimism in survivors and nonsurvivors by age group.

parallel analyses examining the effects of depression. Because pessimism and depression are typically correlated ($r = .39$, in this study), we first examined whether adding depression to the analysis on pessimism and mortality would render the Age × Pessimism interaction statistically insignificant. We repeated the analysis just described, this time controlling for the effect of depression on mortality by entering depression scores in the analysis prior to pessimism, age, and their interaction. Our earlier findings remained unchanged; depression did not weaken the significant interaction effect obtained between pessimism and age, nor did it have a direct effect on mortality. Second, we examined whether age also moderated the relationship between depression and mortality. Logistic regressions similar to those using pessimism scores were performed once again. Mortality status was regressed on physical health at baseline (Step 1), depression and age (Step 2), and the interaction between depression and age (Step 3). No direct effect of depression or age on mortality was obtained, nor did we find a significant interaction between depression and patient age after physical health status had been controlled (all t values $p > .05$). These findings suggest that the effects of pessimism on the mortality status of younger cancer patients described earlier are unique to this construct.

Discussion

Our findings indicate that the endorsement of a pessimistic life orientation may function as an important risk factor for mortality among younger (ages 30–59) cancer patients. Attempts to replicate this finding with conceptually related constructs such as depression did not yield significant associations for either younger or older patients, suggesting that negative expectations about the future may contribute to mortality in unique ways.

These findings are generally consistent with other studies that show a link between psychosocial variables and cancer mortality (Colon et al., 1991; Derogatis et al., 1979; Greer, 1991; Greer et al., 1979; Hislop et al., 1987; Phillips & Smith, 1990; Phillips et al., 1993; Spiegel et al., 1989; Temoshok & Dreher, 1992), and they may help clarify why such associations are not found consistently. Our data suggest that this association may be unique to specific psychological constructs whose effects vary as a function of the individual's location in the life course.

What is unique about pessimism? First, our data are consistent with those of others showing that pessimism and optimism, although related, are not opposite ends of a single continuum (Mroczek et al., 1993; Scheier et al., 1994). Individuals may lack optimism without necessarily being pessimistic. Second, our data also show that pessimism overlaps with other psychological constructs such as depression. Pessimistic individuals report more depressive symptomatology. Despite this overlap, our findings show that there appears to be something unique about pessimism that distinguishes it from depression, a view similar to that of Temoshok and Dreher (1992), who describe depression and hopelessness as overlapping yet distinct constructs. The unique aspect of pessimism is perhaps best understood if we examine the specific items used to measure pessimism. Respondents who are highly pessimistic endorse items such as "If something can go wrong for me it will," "I hardly ever expect things to go my way," "Things never work out the way I want them to," and "I rarely count on good things happening to me." The underlying theme in all of these items is the expectation of a bleak future. Like the "ill-fated" individuals in the Phillips et al. (1993) study, the lives of pessimists appear to be predetermined as negative. Unfortunately, our data do not allow us to address the important question of mechanisms through which pessimism affects mortality. It is possible, for example, that pessimism affects behaviors such as adherence to a medical regimen, or that it directly affects the endocrine and immune systems, or both (Andersen, Kiecolt-Glaser, & Glaser, 1994).

Explaining the Age × Pessimism interaction requires that we view these data from a life-course perspective. One possible explanation is that the physiological progression of the cancer is slower among older than younger persons. Thus, our failure to find a pessimism–mortality effect among older individuals could be attributed to the relatively brief 8-month follow-up period of our study. Had we followed these patients for a longer period of time, we might have found that older persons also exhibit the pessimism–mortality effect. However, the fact that mortality rates were not significantly greater among the older group when compared with the younger group argues against this explanation.

A second possible reason for the age effect is that different age cohorts attach different meaning to the items measuring pessimism. One of the hallmarks of aging is the increased reliance on cognitive coping strategies as opposed to active primary-control strategies directed at the external environment (Heckhausen & Schulz, 1995; Schulz & Heckhausen, in press; Schulz, Heckhausen, & Locher, 1991). Under conditions of threat, cognitive coping strategies provide a rich array of options designed to maintain high levels of functioning. Individuals can adjust to anticipated losses by invoking strategies such as "defensive pessimism" (e.g., "I expect the worst"; Norem & Cantor, 1986; Norem & Illingworth, 1993). Thus, for an older person, endorsing pessimism may simply reflect a coping strategy that has become adaptive in the face of declining ability to control important life outcomes such as health. For younger persons, on the other hand, endorsing such items may reflect genuine hopelessness and despair about the future. The behavioral response engendered by these psychological states may vary by age as well. Because pessimism is more normative for older persons, it is less likely to lead to or reflect disengagement from life goals. For younger individuals, the behavioral consequences of pessimism may be considerably more negative, leading to disengagement from goals and activities that might be beneficial to survival.

A third possibility is that the psychological threat of an illness like cancer is not as great among older people when compared with the young. Cancer is more normative among older adults; that is, they are far more likely to know someone in their peer group who has experienced (and perhaps coped successfully with) cancer. In addition, older people have typically had more prior experience with illness and disability in general than have younger persons. As a result, coping with illness may become more customary, and the role of some psychological factors such as pessimism may be dampened.

Although the available data do not allow us to choose among these various explanations, they help make the point that the relation between cancer mortality and psychosocial factors is more complex than existing research suggests. Researchers pursuing this area in the future should consider several related issues. It is important to focus on the role of specific psychological constructs as opposed to diffuse, global measures that incorporate a wide array of psychological phenomena. The greater the specificity of psychological constructs, the easier it will be to identify mechanisms that account for observed effects. The search for mechanisms that link psychological states to physiological outcomes should continue to receive high priority. Finally, it is important to keep in mind that both physiology and psychology change in predictable ways with age. As a result, psychological processes may vary dramatically as a function of where the person is located in the life course.

References

Andersen, B. L., Kiecolt-Glaser, J. K., & Glaser, R. (1994). A biobehavioral model of cancer stress and disease course. *American Psychologist, 49,* 389–404.

Carver, C. S., Pozo, C., Harris, S. D., Noriega, B., Scheier, M. F., Robinson, D. S., Ketcham, A. S., Moffat, F. L., Jr., & Clark, K. C. (1993). How coping mediates the effect of optimism on distress: A study of women with early stage breast cancer. *Journal of Personality and Social Psychology, 65,* 375–390.

Cassileth, B. R., Lusk, E. J., Miller, D. S., Brown, L. L., & Miller, C. (1985). Psychosocial correlates of survival in advanced malignant disease? *New England Journal of Medicine, 312,* 1551–1555.

Colon, E. A., Callies, A. L., Popkin, M. K., & McGlave, P. B. (1991). Depressed mood and other variables related to bone marrow transplantation survival in acute leukemia. *Psychosomatics, 32,* 420–425.

Derogatis, L. R., Abeloff, M. D., & Melisaratos, N. (1979). Psychological coping mechanisms and survival time in metastatic breast cancer. *Journal of the American Medical Association, 242,* 1504–1508.

Fox, B. H. (1978). Premorbid psychological factors as related to cancer incidence. *Journal of Behavioral Medicine, 1,* 45–133.

Fox, B. H., Temoshok, L., & Dreher, H. (1988). Mind–body and behavior in cancer incidence. *Advances, 5,* 41–56.

Given, C. W., Given, B. A., & Stommel, M. (1994). The impact of age, treatment, and symptoms on the physical and mental health of cancer patients: A longitudinal perspective. *Cancer Supplement, 74,* 2128–2138.

Greer, S. (1991). Psychological response to cancer and survival. *Psychological Medicine, 21,* 43–49.

Greer, S., Morris, T., & Pettingale, K. W. (1979). Psychological response to breast cancer: Effect on outcome. *Lancet, 2,* 785–787.

Heckhausen, J., & Schulz, R. (1995). A life-course theory of control. *Psychological Review, 102,* 284–304.

Hislop, G. T., Waxler, N. E., Coldman, A. J., Elwood, J. M., & Kan, L. (1987). The prognostic significance of psychosocial factors in women with breast cancer. *Journal of Chronic Diseases, 40,* 729–735.

Jamison, R. N., Burish, T. G., & Wallston, K. A. (1987). Psychogenic factors in predicting survival of breast cancer patients. *Journal of Clinical Oncology, 5,* 768–772.

Jensen, A. B. (1991). Psychosocial factors in breast cancer and their possible impact upon prognosis. *Cancer Treatment Reviews, 18,* 191–210.

Levenson, J. L., & Bemis, C. (1991). The role of psychological factors in cancer onset and progression. *Psychosomatics, 32,* 124–132.

Morgenstern, H., Gellert, G. A., Walter, S. D., Ostfeld, A. M., & Siegel, B. S. (1984). The impact of a psychosocial support program on survival with breast cancer: The importance of selection bias in program evaluation. *Journal of Chronic Diseases, 37,* 273–282.

Mroczek, D. K., Spiro, A., III, Aldwin, C. M., Ozer, D. J., & Bosse, R. (1993). Construct validation of optimism and pessimism in older men: Findings from the Normative Aging Study. *Health Psychology, 12,* 406–409.

Norem, J. K., & Cantor, N. (1986). Anticipatory and post hoc cushioning strategies: Optimism and defensive pessimism in "risky" situations. *Cognitive Therapy and Research, 10,* 347–362.

Norem, J. K., & Illingworth, K. S. (1993). Strategy dependent effects of reflecting on self and tasks: Some implications of optimism and defensive pessimism. *Journal of Personality and Social Psychology, 65,* 822–835.

Phillips, D. P., & Smith, D. G. (1990). Postponement of death until symbolically meaningful occasions. *Journal of the American Medical Association, 263,* 1947–1951.

Phillips, D. P., Todd, E. R., & Wagner, L. M. (1993). Psychology and survival. *Lancet, 342,* 1142–1145.

Radloff, L. S. (1977). The CES–D scale: A self-report depression scale for research in the general population. *Applied Psychological Measurement, 1,* 385–401.

Redd, W. H., Silberfarb, P. M., Andersen, B. L., Andrykowski, M. A., Bouberg, D. H., Burish, T. G., Carpenter, P. J., Cleeland, C., Dolgin, M., & Levy, S. M. (1991). Physiologic and psychobehavioral research in oncology. *Cancer, 67,* 813–822.

Ryff, C. D. (1991). Possible selves in adulthood and old age: A tale of shifting horizons. *Psychology & Aging, 6,* 286–295.

Scheier, M. F., & Bridges, M. W. (1995). Person variables and health: Personality predispositions and acute psychological states as shared determinants for disease. *Psychosomatic Medicine, 57,* 255–268.

Scheier, M. F., & Carver, C. S. (1985). Optimism, coping, and health: Assessment and implications of generalized outcome expectancies. *Health Psychology, 4,* 219–247.

Scheier, M. F., Carver, C. S., & Bridges, M. W. (1994). Distinguishing optimism from neuroticism (and trait anxiety, self-mastery, and self-esteem): A re-evaluation of the Life Orientation Test. *Journal of Personality and Social Psychology, 67,* 1063–1078,

Schulz, R., & Heckhausen, J. (in press). A life-span model of successful aging. *American Psychologist.*

Schulz, R., Heckhausen, J., & Locher, J. L. (1991). Adult development, control and adaptive functioning. *Journal of Social Issues, 47,* 177–196.

Silberfarb, P. M., Anderson, K. M., Rundle, A. C., Holland, J. C. B., Cooper, M. R., & McIntyre, O. R. (1991). Mood and clinical status in patients with multiple myeloma. *Journal of Clinical Oncology, 9,* 2219–2224.

Spiegel, D., Bloom, J. R., Kraemer, H. C., & Gottheil, E. (1989). Effect of psychosocial treatment on survival of patients with metastatic breast cancer. *Lancet, 338,* 888–891.

Temoshok, L. (1991). Malignant melanoma, AIDS, and complex search for psychosocial mechanisms. *Advances, 7,* 20–28.

Temoshok, L., & Dreher, H. (1992). *The Type C connection: The mind–body link to cancer and your health.* New York: Penguin.

Zonderman, A. B., Costa, P. T., & McCrae, R. R. (1989). Depression as a risk for cancer morbidity and mortality in a nationally representative sample. *Journal of the American Medical Association, 262,* 1191–1195.

AFTERWORD

COPING WITH CANCER:
A Personal Odyssey

Henry P. David

1. Introduction

This article builds on my experience as a cancer patient and my reading about psycho-oncology. I will discuss the psychological impact cancer can make on patients, factors facilitating adaptation, prevalence of distress, barriers to psychological care and counseling, and mind–body linkages.

In mid-August 1995, while traveling abroad, my wife noticed what looked like an ingrown hair on my cheek just below the right eye. I thought little of it until the growth hardened. By great good fortune, I already had an early September appointment with my dermatologist for an entirely different reason. When I showed him the growth he took a biopsy. A week later he telephoned, asking me to come to his office that afternoon to have the growth removed. After the surgery he informed me that the biopsy indicated the presence of a malignant Merkel cell carcinoma, a very rare and aggressive skin cancer [Haag et al., 1995]. Indeed, in 40 years of clinical practice my dermatologist had seen only three such cases. I was the fourth. Subsequent examination of the specimen reconfirmed the diagnosis. My dermatologist recommended a 6-month waiting period after which he would examine me again.

Following a few days of shock I asked a physician friend at the (US) National Institutes of Health to arrange access to the limited medical literature on Merkel cell carcinoma. As a psychologist experienced in research, I endeavored to learn all I could about this life-threatening disease and then consider available treatment options. I found that the prognosis was not good for delaying further intervention. With the help of my internist, an appointment was arranged with the head of a major oncology group practice. In this practice with over 6,000 cancer cases in the files, I was only the second Merkel patient. To be certain, the diagnosis was confirmed by still a third pathologist. My reading of the medical literature helped me to understand

Reprinted from *Patient Education and Counseling, 37*, 293–297. (1999). Copyright © 1999 by the Elsevier Science Ireland Ltd. Used with permission of the author.

Adapted from a presentation made at the Congress of the World Federation for Mental Health, July 6–11, 1997 in Lahti, Finland.

The author is pleased to acknowledge the insights of Dr. Jimmie C. Holland to his understanding of psycho-oncology and the excellent clinical contributions of Drs. Crawford S. Brown, James Brown, Petr Hausner, and Irving Mizus to the treatment of Merkel cell carcinoma.

the risks and alternatives regarding the optimal therapy for Merkel cell carcinoma. Although a variety of tests and scans suggested that the cancer had not spread, my oncologist recommended, and I quickly agreed to an aggressive course of treatment: radiation with adjuvant chemotherapy, beginning immediately. Treatments were completed in late January 1996. Thus far, regular follow up examinations have not shown any evidence of recurrence. My dermatologist also continues to examine me periodically.

Patient participation in the treatment decision process is somewhat unusual in oncology practices. Many, if not most patients are so devastated by the diagnosis that they prefer to leave all decisions to their physicians. In part this may be because the centuries old belief that cancer equals death is still widespread. It was so strong that many physicians followed the dictum that patients should not be told of their diagnosis. This practice changed only gradually after survival rates improved in the late 1960s. Indeed, the European trained physician at the National Institutes of Health who had been so helpful in identifying the latest medical literature at first refused to give me the reprints, offering instead to forward them to my oncologist. Only after my vigorous protest did he relent and made copies for me as well. And so it was that in my initial meeting with my oncologist I gave him the reprints. He commented that it was the first time in his practice that a patient had done so. Reading about the limited clinical experience with Merkel cell carcinoma and the diverse prognoses (nearly all bad) with different treatment modalities in small groups of patients enhanced my understanding of this unusually aggressive cancer and allowed me to participate in the decision to initiate aggressive treatment. It gave me the feeling that I had not abrogated all responsibility but had retained some control over my destiny and had joined the battle against the cancer. My psychological well-being and that of my wife were enhanced by the sensitivity of my oncologist who explained to us what to expect. To help me cope, I started a diary and charted the results of the repeated laboratory tests. I was determined to survive now, as I had as a teenager fleeing Nazi Germany, as an American soldier in World War II, and following two heart attacks in the late 1980s.

2. Psycho-Oncology

As I read about the psychological impact of cancer, I became increasingly aware of the pioneering contributions of Jimmie C. Holland, M. D. Psycho-oncology emerged over the past 2 decades as a subspecialty of oncology with its own body of information, training, and research [Holland, 1993; Holland & Rowland, 1989]. Psycho-oncologists are trained in psychiatry and psychology with additional training in a cancer center to learn the particular problems faced by cancer patients and their families. Known as psychosocial oncology in Europe, psycho-oncology focuses on two major issues: (a) the psychological impact of cancer on the patient, the family, and caregivers and (b) the influence of cultural, psychological, and behavioral factors on cancer risk and survival. The main techniques are counseling and education. While there is more factual knowledge and more open discussion about cancer, the old fears still linger in popular culture.

2.1. Phases

Learning that one has cancer can be a catastrophic event. Receiving this often dev-astating information, despite apparent good health at the time, creates a personal crisis. Dr. Holland has identified three phases. Phase I is usually marked by disbelief, denial, or despair, generally lasting about a week or so. In the subsequent Phase II, reality is slowly recognized. Some patients may become anxious and depressed, show poor concentration and appetite, and experience difficulty in sleeping and maintaining a daily routine.

Fortunately, I did not experience Phase II. Perhaps I rationalized by accepting reality and seeking anxiety-reduction by reading available medical literature. My wife was encouraging, my work absorbed my time, and my appetite remained good. Phase II usually lasts 1–2 weeks and may include seeking a second opinion. In my case, with the clock ticking and the scarcity of medical experience with Merkel cell car-cinoma, my oncologist and I decided to initiate aggressive treatment immediately. This therapeutic alliance with the oncologist strengthened my feelings of optimism, of beating the cancer. The battle had begun.

Phase III generally represents a longer term adaptation, lasting weeks to months. The patient adjusts to the diagnosis and treatment and relies on successful past ways of coping with life crises. The quality of that adaptation largely depends on the prior level of adjustment and emotional maturity. Individuals have their own coping styles and respect for different personal approaches is important. In my case I rose at the regular time each morning, dressed, and went to work in my home office, continuing to write and edit a book. Somehow, I did not consider myself incapacitated by a major illness and tried to cope with problems much as I had always done. While there was anxiety at times, I was never clinically depressed. Instead I cursed a lot, made up a derogatory song about 'Merkelman,' and insisted that this beast was not going to get me. These mechanisms worked until the discomforts of extensive ra-diation and the fatigue induced by chemotherapy forced adjustments in my daily routine, reducing my capacity for productive work and requiring more frequent brief naps on my office couch.

2.2. Adaptation Factors

For many patients the response to catastrophic news is often similar at the time of diagnosis. Emotions may range from feelings of vulnerability, sadness, and fears related to self and family to problems reflecting discrete psychiatric disorders. The factors which contribute most to adaptation are derived from three areas: societal attitudes towards cancer, personal attributes the patient brings to illness, and the clinical reality of cancer to which the patient must adapt.

The society-derived factors are dynamic, changing as people change their per-ceptions of medicine, illness and cancer. While cancer is no longer a taboo topic, it is still greatly feared by large segments of the population. Society's demands for informed consent and better knowledge of treatment options and prognoses have not reduced uncertainty about treatment outcome.

Patient-derived factors depend largely on maturity at the time of illness and past experience in coping with stress. Cancer-derived factors constitute the clinical realities: disease stage of time of diagnosis, cancer site, symptoms, prognosis, types of treatment required and their impact on function, altered body structure and image (such as mastectomy and temporary loss of hair), and the psychological sensitivity of the treatment team.

In my experience, maintaining a positive attitude, self-esteem, and close relations with family members helped to ward off depression. The strong belief that I would overcome this cancer was important in maintaining a sense of control and in dealing with treatment side effects. Severe nausea was experienced only once during one session of chemotherapy and treated promptly.

An example of coping was dealing with the loss of body hair. Being totally bald for a time did not stop my social life or activities in public places. When hair returned to my head, my beard regrew only on my left cheek. My physicians had warned me that the radiation of my right cheek (the site of the original excision) would probably prevent future hair growth in that area. For several months I had only a one-sided beard. People either did not notice or were reluctant to ask. In the meantime I grew a mustache. Then gradually fuzz began to grow on the right side. My barber trimmed the left side to achieve some balance with the right. I was jubilant. I had beaten the odds and the predictions of the physicians. My beard was back, a visible symbol of victory over Merkel.

Psychologically healthy individuals generally emerge from cancer treatment without serious psychological sequelae or disorder. However, some psychological counseling may well be indicated to help patients cope with subtle psychological distress, such as lower self-esteem, sexual performance problems, and altered career goals.

3. Prevalence of Distress

When patients cope with serious illness, responses of fear, worry and sadness are expected and normal. Usually they are transient and dissipate as a crisis passes, as was true in my case. However, these normal emotions can become so persistent, pervasive, and distressing, that they deter treatment. At that point, worry and sadness exceeding clinically normal expectations become identifiable as anxiety and depression. Such 'symptoms' should be evaluated and, if significant, treated clinically. Sensitivity to this dimension of care requires ability to evaluate a psychological symptom, recognize the clusters of symptoms which represent a psychiatric disorder, and identify treatment options and resources.

The most common form of distress in patients with cancer is anxiety. The next most common is depression. They are often seen together. Anxiety is best considered as a symptom which exists on a continuum ranging from normal fears to situational anxiety and, finally, to a disabling anxiety disorder. Depression is on a continuum from sadness to reactive depression and, finally, to its most severe form, major depression. Prior vulnerability to depressions generally predicts recurrence during physical illness.

In my case, whether it was denial or a well established daily life routine, I did not experience incapacitating depression. I did not allow myself to feel 'sick,' to stay in bed, or not to work. That and the strong support of my wife helped me to endure.

4. Barriers to Psychological Counseling

Barriers to dealing with patients' psychological distress come from patients themselves, physicians, and institutions. Some patients are reluctant to draw attention to psychological problems because they fear stigma and embarrassment. Physicians seldom ask about distress because of fear of opening a Pandora's box or reluctance to invest extra time. Institutions usually place a low priority on expensive psychological services. Too often psychological distress is ignored, unrecognized, and untreated in the management of patients who are especially vulnerable, such as individuals without life companions.

5. Mind–Body Linkages

There has been a growing interest in the medical community and the public in the mind's effect on health. Intriguing findings have been reported linking various psychological states to changes in the endocrine and immune systems [Benson with Stark, 1996]. In Dr. Holland's view, the psychological and the spiritual come together when people are very ill. At her Memorial Sloan Kettering counseling center, patients create art—much of which adorns the center's walls—describing their spiritual triumphs in battling cancer [Ryan, 1998]. Similarly, the concept of psycho-immunology has gained increasing credibility with popular articles and books exhorting patients to 'think positively' and to 'fight' the illness. While there is no firm scientific evidence of the extent to which such advice can affect cancer, I am convinced that it helped me. I personalized 'Mr. Merkel' and was determined to fight this 19th century German anatomist for whom the facial cancer had been named. As a survivor of Hitler Germany, my recurrent dreams of being pursued by Nazis reflected this inner struggle. Perhaps my assertive style of decision making and/or the protective karma that had shielded me in previous life crises came to my rescue once again. I stopped to rest only when assaulted by intermittent bouts of fatigue which increased as the treatments progressed. I was determined to beat 'Mr. Merkel' and to continue my scientific work.

6. General Conclusion

While the literature does not suggest that any single style of coping with cancer is better than another, and that much depends on the stage and type of cancer, the power of belief appears to be a natural source of bodily health and psychological strength. Cancer patients can participate more assertively in their treatment and, in the process, alleviate the terrifying sense of helplessness that can accompany diagnosis with a deadly disease. I am certain that my positive attitude contributed to my recovery and to the smiles it brought to my treatment team. While no one knows whether Merkel will return some day, I am vigilant of its potential threat but enjoy life to the fullest. It would be very welcome to hear about the experience of others.

References

Benson H, with Stark M. The power and biology of belief. New York: Scribner, 1996.

Haag ML, Glass LF, Fenske NA. Merkel cell carcinoma: diagnosis and treatment. Dermatol Surg 1995;21:669–83.

Holland JC. Principles of psycho-oncology. In: Holland JF et al., editor. Cancer medicine, 3rd edition, Philadelphia: Lea and Febinger, 1993, pp. 1017–33.

Holland JC, Rowland JH, editors, Handbook of psycho-oncology. Oxford: Oxford University Press, 1989.

Ryan M., They help patients cope with fear. Parade, 1998, 20 September, 8–9.